Carpal Ligament Surgery

Emmanuel Camus • Luc Van Overstraeten
Editors

Carpal Ligament Surgery

Before Arthritis

Springer

Editors
Emmanuel Camus
Hand Surgery Unit
SELARL Chirurgie de la Main
Polyclinique du Val de Sambre
Maubeuge
France

Luc Van Overstraeten
Hand Surgery Unit
HFSU
Tournai
Belgium

Additional material to this book can be downloaded from http://extras.springer.com

ISBN 978-2-8178-0550-4 ISBN 978-2-8178-0379-1 (eBook)
DOI 10.1007/978-2-8178-0379-1
Springer Paris Heidelberg New York Dordrecht London

Printed on acid-free paper

Springer is part of Springer Science+Business Media (www.springer.com)

Video Contents

Tournai Belgium 2009
Carpal Instability

Recorded at the
Franco Belgian Congress: Carpal Ligament Surgery
With French and Belgian Hand Groups
Tournai – Belgium 2009 April 17th–18th

English Audio Translation

Extra Materials on http://extras.springer.com

Communications of the Techniques Session

1. Ligament Debridement – Pinning	L. Van Overstraeten. Tournai – Belgium
2. Technique of Repair of Scapholunate Ligament by Arthrotomy (Taleisnik's Technique)	C. Rizzo. Lyon – France
3. Discussion about Debridement and Taleisnik's Procedure	
4. Treatment of Chronic Scapholunate Lesions. Arthroscopic Dorsal Capsulodesis	Ch. Mathoulin. Paris – France
5. Treatment of Scapholunate Instabilities by Blatt's Capsulodesis	L. Van Overstraeten. Tournai – Belgium
6. Berger's Capsulodesis with Dorsal Intercarpal Ligament in Chronic Scapholunate Instability	N. Dréant. Nice – France
7. Viegas' Dorsal Carpal Capsulodesis	E. Camus. Maubeuge – France
8. Capsulofibrodesis, a New Procedure in the Treatment of Scapholunate Dissociation	O. Delattre. Fort de France – France
9. Discussion about Treatement of Chronic Scapholunate Lesions – Arthroscopic Dorsal Capsulodesis – Blatt – Berger – Viegas – Capsulofibrodesis	
10. Brunelli's Tenodesis	F. Schuind. Bruxelles – Belgium
11. My Preference for the Treatment of Chronic Reducible Scapholunate Dissociation	J.K. Stanley. London – Great Britain
12. Tenodesis 3LT	L. De Smet. Leuven – Belgium
13. Treatment of Chronic Scapholunate Lesions. ECRB Ligamentplasty	Ch. Mathoulin. Paris – France
14. Scapholunate Ligament Reconstruction Using a Bone–Tissue–Bone Graft	J. Goubau. Brugge – Belgium
15. Reduction and Association of the Scaphoid and Lunate (RASL)	J. Goubau. Brugge – Belgium
16. Chronic Luno Triquetral Ligament Injuries. Arthrodesis vs. Capsulodesis	L. De Smet. Leuven – Belgium
17. Scaphocapitate Arthrodesis	F. Deletang. Orléans – France

Cadaver Workshops

Foreword

Ligamentous Surgery of the Wrist by Emmanuel Camus and Luc Van Overstraeten is an ambitious undertaking. It begins with a detailed discussion of the ligamentous anatomy, followed by chapters on wrist biomechanics and pathomechanics. Two chapters on wrist imaging thoroughly cover the standard imaging modalities including x-ray/CT/arthrography and ultrasound followed by an eloquent chapter devoted to MRI of normal and pathological wrist ligament anatomy. The methodology of a standard diagnostic arthroscopy is well covered by a master in the field, followed by two more in-depth chapters on its applications in the arthroscopic diagnosis and treatment of scapholunate instability. This includes a detailed description of a novel arthroscopic capsulodesis procedure. Open treatment methods of acute and chronic tears are well covered and include chapters on open repair, two methods of dorsal capsulodesis, tendon graft reconstruction including the Brunelli capsulodesis and tri-ligament tenodesis, bone ligament bone reconstruction, the RASL procedure as well as a new concept of capsulofibrodesis. Treatment of lunotriquetral ligament injuries through arthrodesis or capsulodesis is also covered in addition to additional chapters on midcarpal instability, axial dislocations and the emerging approach of arthroscopic treatment of perilunate dislocations. The book is replete with clinical examples of wrist ligament injuries and treatment. Few books have covered all aspects of wrist instability in such a comprehensive manner. The authors should be congratulated for their organized and in-depth approach to an often confusing subject. For students of the wrist and its disorders, this book is a must have.

David J. Slutsky, M.D., F.R.C.S (C)

Preface

It is today admitted that a traumatic carpal ligamentary lesion may lead to an instability and then to a carpal degenerative arthritis. However, the variety of anatomopathological classifications and the multiplicity of surgical repair techniques reflect the difficulty to conceive this ligamentary pathology. Truly, the clinical analysis and traditional techniques of investigation face to the complexity of the wrist and to the small size of its components, especially the carpal bones.

The mechanical complexity of the wrist is due to the number of synchronized bones in every movement of the hand, since the forearm to the palm there is not less than 15 in a few volume.

Clinical analysis is in this wrist joint insufficient to measure exactly the mobility, normal or pathologic, of these carpal bones. Paraclinical examinations have a particular place. From x-ray to arthroscopy, including arthro-CT scan and soon MRI, the tools are today available.

Talking about the repairing techniques, their diversity must not hide that a biomechanical and physiological principle is looming and must be sought.

This book is the result of a reflection of an expert group of wrist pathology. It attempts to analyze, to understand, to explain and to make logical, if not obvious, the reflection which must accompany each practitioner in diagnosis and treatment of the carpal ligamentary lesions. This book has voluntarily left aside the degenerative carpal pathology, which usually benefits more visibility in various scientific works.

We hope that with this work the reader may apprehend more globally quite dispersed knowledge and find in this beginning of synthesis the matter to rethink a difficult and sometimes thankless surgery to make a surgical adventure of the twenty-first century.

Emmanuel Camus
Luc Van Overstraeten

Preface (French Edition 2009)

Carpal ligament wrist surgery before arthritis. From trauma to instability.

It is just about time that someone has thought of writing the account of more than 30 years of anatomical, biomechanical studies and experiments and setting them out against results of clinical practice. One must commend the courage of Emmanuel Camus (a French Hand surgeon) and that of Luc van Overstraeten (a Belgian Hand surgeon), both fascinated by the wrist, for undertaking such a vast and complex subject.

Can we, in 2009, sift through all these works?

Can we propose a classification that enables us to propose a treatment with a reasonable benefit/risk ratio to symptomatic patients?

What is the available validated data to choose one technique over another?

These questions and many others have engaged the authors to search for answers.

The most difficult task is to present hand surgeons with an algorithm for early lesions whose evolution pattern is unknown. What are the factors predicting unfavourable evolution, i.e. what are the criteria of instability of these lesions?

Due to the great importance of these works that will be immediately useful to all hand surgeons, it was in order that the Société Française de Chirurgie de la Main and the Belgian Hand Group both sponsor this initiative.

Christian Dumontier, M.D.
General Secrétary of the GEM-SFCM

Acknowledgements

Editors particularly want to thank:

- J. Goubau for the audio translation of the DVDs
- H. Khalifa (Surgitranslation) for the English relecture. Chapters 3, 4, 6, 7, 9, 15, 16, 22, 24, 29, 30 and 31.
- Sauramps Medical – Montpellier, Paris – France. Publisher of the French version 2009.

Contents

Contributors

C. Alexieva Hand Surgery Unit, CHU et SOS mains de Fort-de-France, Fort-de-France, Martinique

B. Allemon Department of Medical Imaging, Universitair Ziekenhuis Brussel, Brussels, Belgium

B. Berghs Hand and Upper Limb Unit, Department of Orthopaedics and Trauma, AZ St Jan AV Brugge – Oostende, Bruges, Belgium

E. Camus Hand Surgery Unit, SELARL Chirurgie de la Main, Polyclinique du Val de Sambre, Maubeuge, France

P. Ceuterick Department of Orthopaedics and Hand Surgery, Cliniques de l'Europe, Brussels, Belgium

G. Dautel Service de Chirurgie Plastique et Reconstructrice de l'Appareil Locomoteur, Centre Chirurgical Emile Gallé, Nancy, France

M. De Maeseneer Department of Medical Imaging, Universitair Ziekenhuis Brussel, Brussels, Belgium

L. De Smet Department of Orthopedic Surgery, U.Z. Pellenberg, Lubbeek (Pellenberg), Belgium

O. Delattre Hand Surgery Unit, CHU et SOS mains de Fort-de-France, Fort-de-France Martinique, Martinique

F. Delétang SOS Mains Orléans Val de Loire, Polyclinique des Longues Allées, Saint-Jean-de-Braye, France

J.-C. Dosch Hand Surgery Unit, Service de Radiologie et de la Main Illkirch, CHU Strasbourg, Hôpital de Hautepierre, Stransbourg, Cedex, France

Centre de Chirurgie Orthopédique, Strasbourg, Cedex, France

N. Dréant Pole Urgence Main Nice, Nice, France

F. Duroux Hand Surgery Unit, CHU et SOS mains de Fort-de-France, Fort-de-France, Martinique

W. El Kazzi Department of Orthopaedics and Traumatology, Erasme University Hospital, Brussels, Belgium

V. Feipel Laboratoire d'Anatomie Fonctionnelle, Institut des Sciences de la Motricité, Université Libre de Bruxelles, Brussels, Belgium

J. Garret Hand and Upper Extremity Unit, Clinique du Parc, Lyon, France

A. Gazarian Hand and Upper Extremity Unit, Clinique du Parc, Lyon, France

S. Goeminne Hand Surgery Unit, Department of Orthopedic Surgery, U.Z. Pellenberg, Lubbeek (Pellenberg), Belgium

J. Goubau Hand and Upper Limb Unit, Department of Orthopaedics and Trauma, AZ St Jan AV Brugge – Oostende, Bruges, Belgium

Department of Orthopaedics and Traumatology, University Hospital Brussels, Brussels, Belgium

V. Guigal Hand and Upper Extremity Unit, Clinique du Parc, Lyon, France

I. Janssens Department of Orthopedic Surgery, U.Z. Pellenberg, Lubbeek (Pellenberg), Belgium

S. Joulie Hand Surgery Unit, CHU et SOS mains de Fort-de-France, Fort-de-France Martinique, Martinique

D. Kerckhove Hand and Upper Limb Unit, Department of Orthopaedics and Trauma, AZ St Jan AV Brugge – Oostende, Bruges, Belgium

Ch. Mathoulin Hand Surgery Unit, Institut de la main, Clinique Jouvenet, Paris, France

T. Moser Département de Radiologie, CHUM, Hôpital St Luc, Montréal, QC, Canada

A. Pagliei Hand Surgery Unit, Institut de la main, Clinique Jouvenet, Paris, France

E. Papadogeorgou Hand Surgery Unit, Institut de la main, Clinique Jouvenet, Paris, France

N. Pouliart Department of Medical Imaging, Universitair Ziekenhuis Brussel, Brussels, Belgium

S. Provyn Department of Experimental Anatomy, Vrije Universiteit Brussel, Brussels, Belgium

C. Rizzo Hand and Upper Extremity Unit, Clinique du Parc, Lyon, France

J.-L. Roux Hand Surgery Unit, Institut Montpelliérain de la Main, Montpellier, France

F. Schuind Department of Orthopaedics and Traumatology, Erasme University Hospital, Brussels, Belgium

M. Shahabpour Department of Medical Imaging, Universitair Ziekenhuis Brussel, Brussels, Belgium

L. Stratan Hand Surgery Unit, CHU et SOS mains de Fort-de-France, Fort-de-France, Martinique

A.-P. Uzel MCU-PH Chirurgie, Orthopédique, CHU, Guadeloupe, France

P. Van Hoonacker Hand and Upper Limb Unit, Department of Orthopaedics and Trauma, AZ St Jan AV Brugge – Oostende, Bruges, Belgium

L. Van Overstraeten Hand and Foot Surgery Unit SPRL, Tournai, Belgium

W. Van De Sande Department of Orthopedic Surgery, U.Z. Pellenberg, Lubbeek (Pellenberg), Belgium

J. Vogels Hand Surgery Unit, CHU et SOS mains de Fort-de-France, Fort-de-France Martinique, Martinique

Part I
Fundamentals

Anatomy of the Carpal Ligaments

V. Feipel

Variable descriptions and nomenclatures of the ligaments of the wrist have been presented. Classical anatomical textbooks describe more than 30 different ligaments related to the carpus. Differences of description, classification, and nomenclature increase the complexity of understanding this region [7, 24, 36, 51, 55, 89]. More recently, researchers proposed a simplified description of the carpal ligaments using various classifications [7, 22, 36, 51, 55, 78, 88]. Several authors also mention a variability of carpal ligament anatomy [20, 22, 36, 50, 59, 85], which could contribute to explain the differences found in the literature. Sennwald and Segmüller [78] presented a classification of the wrist ligaments in five groups. More recently, Sennwald et al. [79] redescribed the palmar scaphotriquetral ligament that had fallen into oblivion for 90 years.

This lack of unanimity concerning carpal ligament anatomy could have effects on the diagnosis and the treatment of the ligamentous lesions of the wrist. The existence of various classifications of carpal instability reinforces this assumption [31, 32, 52, 54, 89].

Morphometric studies about the carpal ligaments are rare. The majority of them relate to the measurement of ligament cross-sectional areas of the with an aim of determining their mechanical properties [47, 56, 63, 72, 74]. Few studies concerned the evaluation of ligament dimensions in situ and their variations [14, 21, 45, 74, 85, 86]. This kind of information could nevertheless improve our knowledge in the field of carpal anatomy and pathology, refine the therapeutic choices, and provide a partial explanation to the individual variations of carpal kinematics highlighted by several studies [17, 19, 23, 72, 74], since the capsular ligaments are probably the principal structures which limit and control carpal motions.

V. Feipel
Laboratoire d'Anatomie Fonctionnelle,
Faculté des Sciences de la Motricité, Université Libre de Bruxelles,
808 route de Lennik, CP 619, B-1070 Brussels, Belgium
e-mail: vfeipel@ulb.ac.be

E. Camus, L. Van Overstraeten (eds.), *Carpal Ligament Surgery*,
DOI 10.1007/978-2-8178-0379-1_1, © Springer-Verlag France 2013

In this chapter, we will attempt to summarize the principal lessons that can be drawn from the literature concerning the functional anatomy of the carpal ligaments. We will use, for this description, the classification suggested by Sennwald and Segmüller [78] as a basis while taking into account structures which are not included in this classification.

1 Flexor and Extensor Retinacula

Sennwald and Segmüller [78] describe these structures as an extra-capsular group of ligaments. In our view, the retinacula belong to the muscular apparatus. We thus will not extend on the description of these structures. Nevertheless, their role, and especially that of the flexor retinaculum, in the stability of the wrist remains discussed.

Table 1 presents the various functions of the flexor retinaculum as well as the effects of its section [26, 28, 29, 37, 46, 65, 70, 80].

2 Proximal and Distal Interosseous Ligaments

Figure 1 schematizes the anatomy of the interosseous ligaments. The functions of this group are maintaining transverse cohesion, and thus stability, as well as limiting and/or guiding of the segmental movements. The stiffness of the interosseous ligaments is lower than that of the extrinsic ligaments, because of a more important type III collagen content, which allows interosseous ligaments to lengthen more compared to extrinsic ligaments. Their failure load is regarded as higher than that of the extrinsic ligaments [3–5, 11, 18, 24, 27, 30, 34, 35, 38, 43, 44, 49, 55, 56, 58, 63, 69, 71, 73, 77, 78, 81–83, 87, 92, 95].

The distal interosseous ligaments are shorter and more resistant than the proximal ones, offering thus less freedom of movement to the bones of the distal carpus. The distal ligaments present a dorsal part, connecting the dorsal faces of the adjacent bones and a deep portion, located palmarly and connecting the interosseous faces of

Table 1 Roles of the flexor retinaculum and effects of its section [26, 28, 29, 37, 46, 65, 70, 80, 97]

Roles	Section
Anchoring of thenar and hypothenar muscles	⬂ of carpal tunnel pressure
Transverse carpal stability	⬂ of intrinsic and extrinsic muscle force
Pulley for the flexor tendons	⬀ of carpal tunnel width and volume
	⬂ of gliding resistance between nerve, tendons and synovial sheath
	Δ of scaphoid kinematics

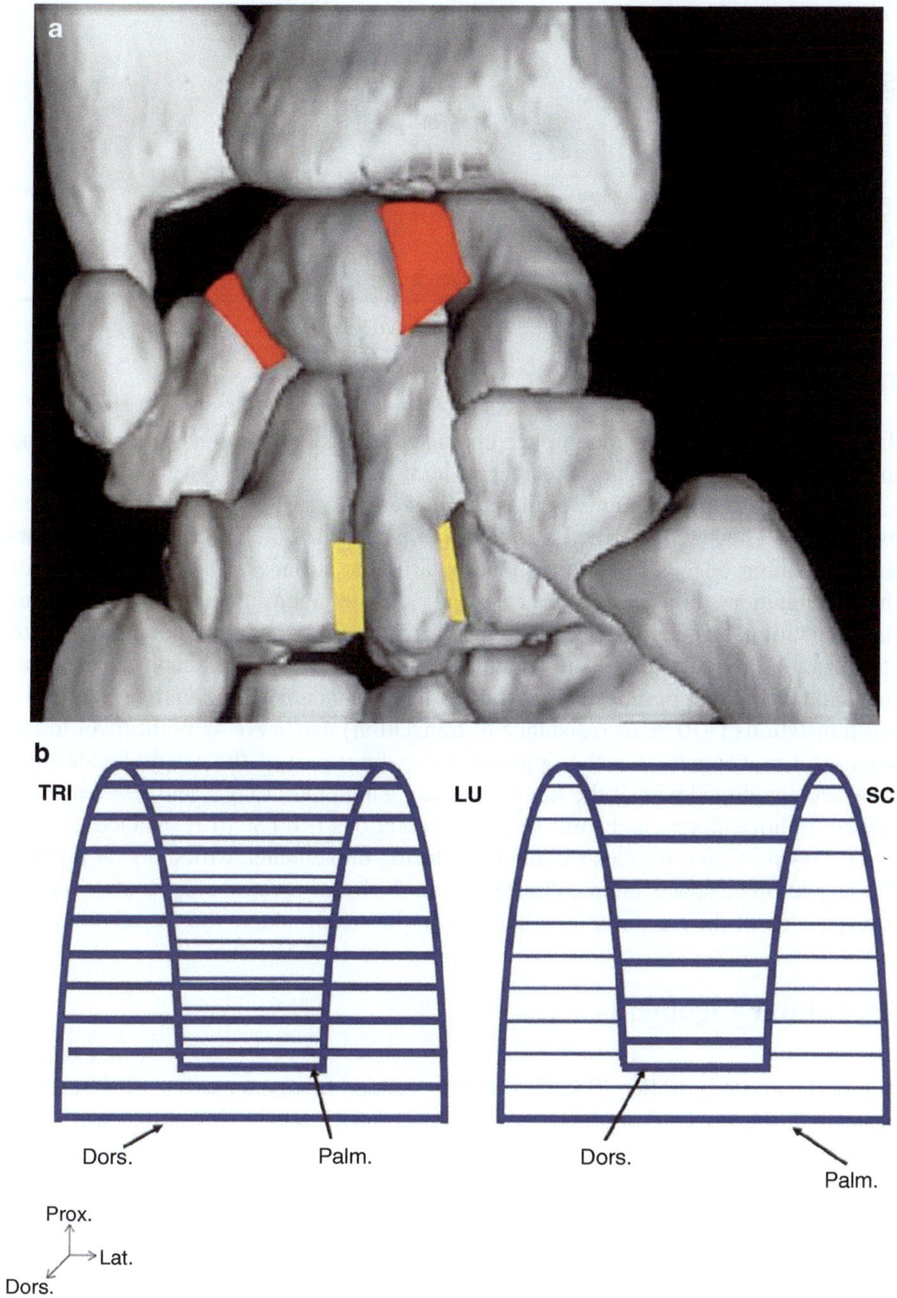

Fig. 1 Interosseous ligaments. (**a**) Palmar view of a 3D model showing the location of the proximal (*red*) and distal (*yellow*) interosseous ligaments. (**b**) Schematic representation of the proximal interosseous ligaments according to [3, 42–44, 71]. (**c**) Failure load of the proximal interosseous ligaments according to [63, 69, 73, 87, 94]. Abbreviations: TRI: triquetrum, LU: lunate, SC: scaphoid, SL: scapholunate interosseous ligament, LT: lunotriquetral interosseous ligament

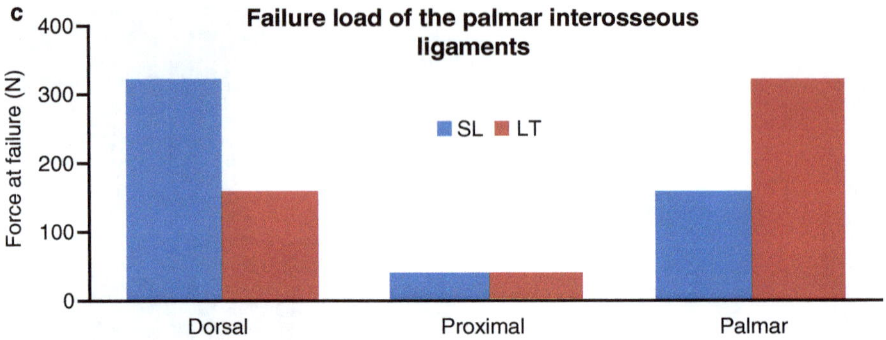

Fig. 1 (continued)

the adjacent bones. Their incomplete character allows communication between the midcarpal space and the carpometacarpal joint spaces.

The interosseous ligaments of the proximal carpus (Fig. 1b, c) have been studied extensively. They are described as a crown or a cap, surrounding the proximal, dorsal, and palmar edges of the corresponding articular surfaces. The proximal part of the two ligaments consists of fibrocartilage, with collagen fibers without preferential orientation. This part carries the radiocarpal cartilage but does not contribute to stabilization or limitation of movements. The dorsal part of the scapholunate ligament and the palmar part of the lunotriquetral ligament are short and resistant, limiting translations (~70 % of resistance to translation) and serve as point pivot to the segmental movements. On the opposite, the palmar part of the scapholunate ligament and the dorsal part of the lunotriquetral ligament are longer and less resistant, present oblique fibers, and limit segmental rotations (~60 % of resistance to rotation). This provision implies a cam effect during movements, with a dorsal pivot in the scapholunate space and a palmar pivot on the lunotriquetral side. It also implies a suspension of the lunate in torsion between the scaphoid and the triquetrum.

3 Palmar Ligaments

Sennwald and Segmüller [78] present the palmar ligaments as two "V"-shaped structures, the proximal palmar "V" and the distal palmar "V" (Fig. 2a). These structures include part of the radiocarpal (except the short radiolunate ligament) and ulnocarpal (except the ulnocapitate and ulnotriquetral ligaments) ligaments from the classical descriptions (Fig. 2c). The dimensions of the main palmar ligaments are presented in Table 2 [2, 3, 6, 8, 11, 14, 16, 21, 25, 39, 51, 55, 57, 60, 61, 63, 69, 71, 73, 75, 78, 84, 93, 94, 96].

Fig. 2 Palmar ligaments. (**a**) Palmar view of a 3D model showing the palmar "Vs" (*red lines*) according to Sennwald and Segmüller [78]. (**b**) Palmar view of a 3D model showing the ligaments of the scaphotrapezio-trapezoidal joint (scaphotrapezial in *yellow*, scaphocapitate in *orange*, and capitotrapezial in *green*). (**c**) Palmar radio- and ulnocarpal ligaments. (**d**) Distal view of the inferior epiphysis of the radius showing the attachment zones of the palmar radiocarpal ligaments. Attachment sites of short radiolunate ligament in *yellow*, long radiolunate ligament in *red* and radiocapitate ligament in *blue*

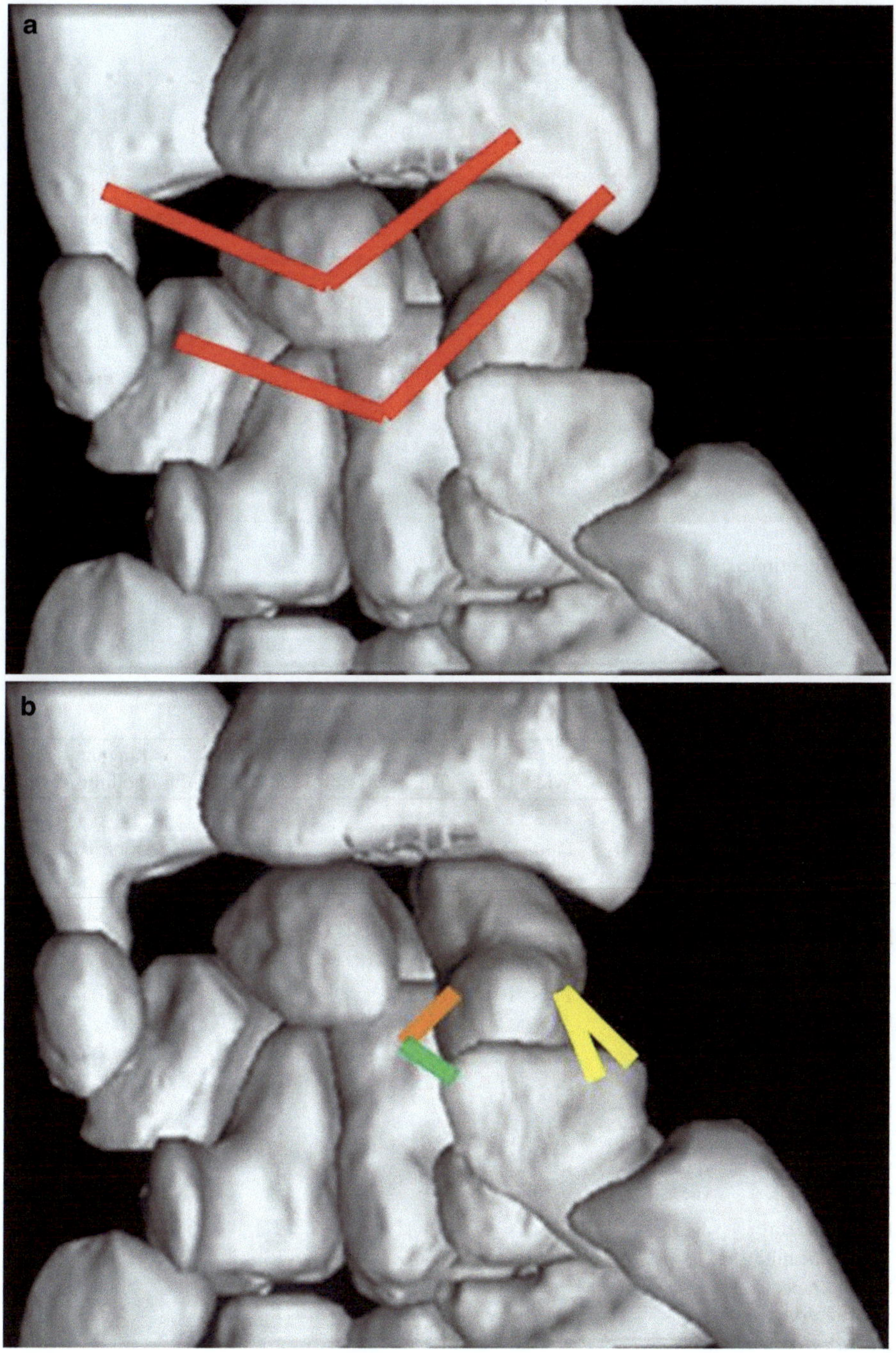
a
b

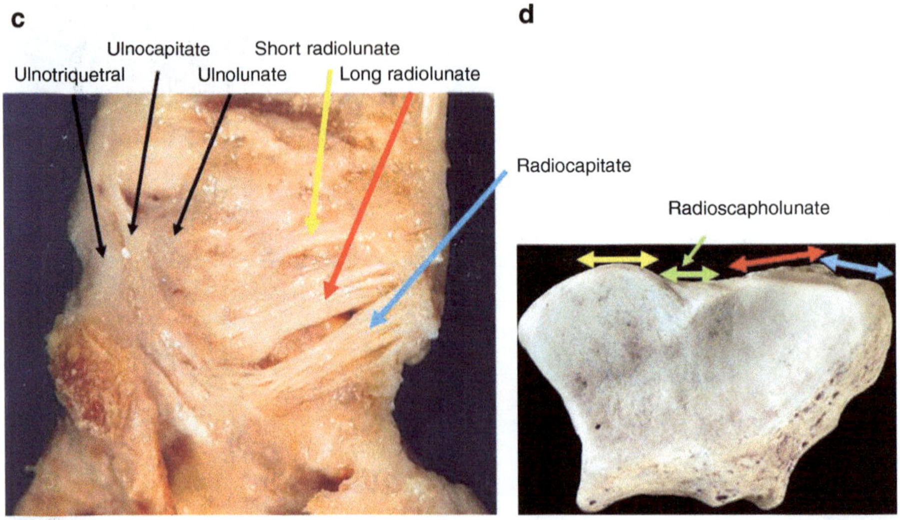

Fig. 2 (continued)

Table 2 Dimensions and mechanical properties of the carpal ligaments according to [14, 18, 21, 38, 62, 69, 73, 75, 94]

	Length (mm)	Width (mm)	Thickness (mm)	Coronal inclination (°)	Tangent modulus (MPa)
Interosseous					
Scapholunate	Palm: 2–4	Palm: 6	Palm: 1		Dors: 100–300
	Dors: 5–6	Dors: 6	Dors: 2–3		
	Prox: 4	Prox: 11	Prox: 1		
Lunotriquetral	Palm: 3–5	Palm: 6	Palm: 2		
	Dors: 3	Dors: 6	Dors: 1		
	Prox: 2	Prox: 10	Prox: 1		
Distal interosseous					>300
Palmar					
Ulnolunate	12–23	2–5	1	151	<100
Ulnotriquetral	18	5			<100
Ulnocapitate	29	3			<100
Radiolunate	11–17	8	1–2	34	<100
Radiocapitate	25–29	8	1–2	44	<100
Lunotriquetral	8–11	5–7	1	27	
Triquetrocapitate	11–13	4–7	2–4	139	<100
Scaphotrapezio-trapezoidal					>300
Dorsal					
Radiocarpal	18–22	8–13	1	28	<100
Intercarpal	33–41	6–7	1–2	167	<100

Besides their attachment at the palmar surface of the capitate, the ulnocapitate and radiocapitate ligaments merge through interwoven fibers in front of the lunocapitate joint line (Fig. 2c).

The radioscapholunate ligament is a loose and little organized connective tissue, constituting the vascular sheath of the proximal arteries for the scaphoid and lunate. Its mechanical resistance is low compared to the other palmar ligaments (failure load of 40 N and elongation to failure of 174 % versus 150 N and 125 % for the radiocapitate ligament, for instance).

The main roles of the palmar ligaments are the limitation of radial (ulnocarpal ligaments) and ulnar deviation (radiocarpal ligaments), as well as of dorsal flexion. They also prevent ulnar, anterior, and posterior translations. They have an important role in carpal stability and are supposed to contribute to the determination of movements. Moreover, the radiocarpal ligaments limit intracarpal pronation and maintain the scaphoid.

Berger and Amadio [6] and Siegel and Gelberman [84] showed that the knowledge of ligamentous insertions on the distal radius (Fig. 2d) could contribute to the evaluation of functional implications of distal radius fractures or styloidectomy.

Also, most studies describe the radiocarpal ligaments as displaying a relatively constant morphology, in contrast with the ulnocarpal ligaments. The latter vary significantly, concerning their general morphology as well as their dimensions. However, the presence of two radiolunate ligaments (long and short), described in many studies, was not observed in 40 % of the cases in our work [22].

The palmar scaphotriquetral ligament was not described by most authors. Sennwald et al. [79] showed its situation deep to the palmar ligaments, crossing the palmar surface of the head of the capitate and connecting the waist of the scaphoid to the palmar surface of the triquetrum.

The support of the distal pole of the scaphoid is ensured by the scaphotrapezial, scaphocapitate, and capitotrapezial ligaments (Fig. 2b).

4 Dorsal Ligaments

At the dorsal aspect of the carpus, the dorsal radiocarpal or dorsal radiotriquetral ligament and the dorsal intercarpal or dorsal scaphotriquetral ligament form a "V"-shaped structure with its apex at the level of the ligamentous crest of the triquetrum (Fig. 3). This structure constitutes the dorsal "V" of Sennwald and Segmüller [78].

The morphological variability of the dorsal ligaments is much larger than that of the palmar ligaments, as shown by many studies [11, 14, 16, 21, 22, 33, 49, 53, 55, 59, 69, 71, 73, 77, 78, 91, 94, 96]. The dimensions of the dorsal ligaments are presented in Table 2.

The dorsal radiotriquetral ligament limits intracarpal supination, radial deviation, palmar flexion, and ulnar translation of the carpus. As a whole, the "V" dorsal limits palmar flexion. These ligaments contribute also significantly to carpal

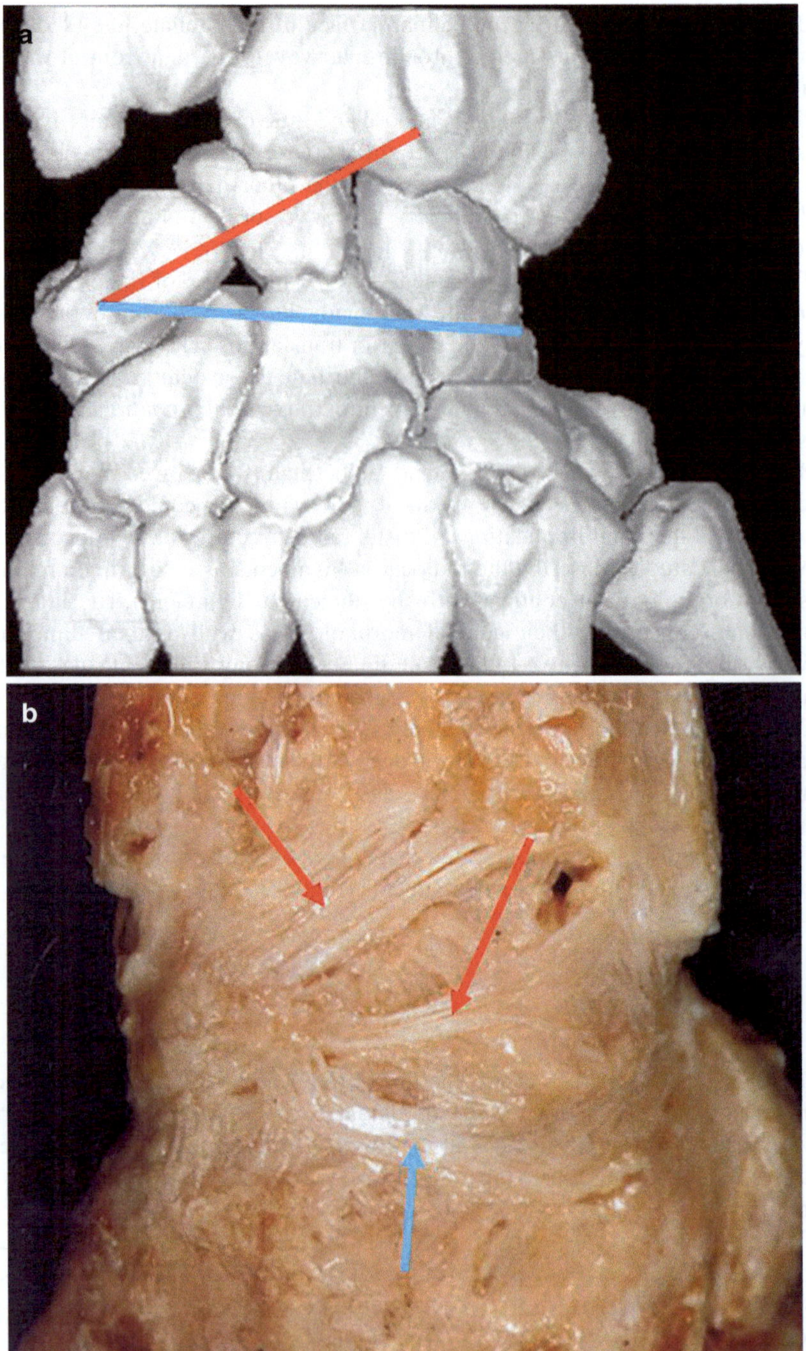

Fig. 3 Dorsal ligaments. (**a**) Dorsal view of a 3D model showing the dorsal "V," dorsal radiocarpal ligament in *red*, dorsal intercarpal ligament in *blue*. (**b**) Anatomical specimen presenting one of the variations of the dorsal "V," double radiotriquetral ligament (*red arrows*) (type II of Viegas et al. [94]). Dorsal intercarpal ligament (*blue arrow*)

stability by the support offered to the lunate and their role in longitudinal and transverse wrist cohesion. The dorsal radiocarpal ligament is a relatively strong structure, displaying a failure load of approximately 150 NR and a tangential modulus of 30 MPa, in spite of a low thickness (1 mm). The dorsal intercarpal ligament is characterized by a failure load of approximately 80 NR and a tangential modulus of 45 MPa.

Finally, the dorsal ligaments are very rich in nervous endings compared to the palmar ligaments. Approximately 80 % of these terminations are observed near ligament insertions and 80 % in the epi-ligamentous sheath.

5 Triangular Fibrocartilage Complex

Regarded as the pulley of the extensor carpi ulnaris, the triangular fibrocartilage complex (Fig. 4) consists of several poorly dissociated elements. The triangular fibrocartilage itself is supplemented by several associated structures, the palmar and dorsal radioulnar ligaments, the palmar ulnolunate ligament, the ulnotriquetral ligament, the ulnocapitate ligament, the ulnocarpal meniscus, the prestyloid recess, the ulnar collateral ligament, and the sheath of the extensor carpi ulnaris. The dimensions of the components of this complex are presented in Tables 2 and 3 [1, 15, 16, 64, 66–68, 75, 76, 78, 90].

The triangular fibrocartilage is attached to the distal margin of ulnar notch of the radius. Its ulnar attachments are located at the level of the lateral surface of the ulnar styloid process, the fovea of the ulnar head and the deep surface of the articular capsule or the ulnar collateral ligament. It is broader laterally and thicker medially. Its central part is avascular. The distal part of its fibers originating from the radius extends distally to attach on the medial surface of the triquetrum and hamate; this constitutes the ulnocarpal meniscus. The access to the prestyloid recess is located between the fibrocartilage itself and the meniscus. The palmar and dorsal radioulnar ligaments reinforce the edges of the triangular fibrocartilage. The ulnocarpal ligaments are also attached at the palmar margin of the fibrocartilage. The sheath of the extensor carpi ulnaris is closely blended with the posterior part of the complex.

The ulnar complex, as it is frequently named, plays a central role in the stability of the distal radioulnar joint and the ulnar carpus. In addition, it participates in the transmission of constraints between the hand and the forearm. In this context, it is frequently described as a cushion interposed between the carpus and the ulna.

During axial loading experiments, Adams et al. [1] showed that an average force of 440 N caused avulsion of the fibrocartilage at the level of its ulnar attachments, without macroscopic lesions of fibrocartilage substance. The average elongation was 17 %, more important in the radial portion (28 %).

Let us finally note that nervous endings (free endings and proprioceptors) are mainly found in the ulnar portion of the complex, which explains the absence of instability in case of lesion of the radial part of the fibrocartilage.

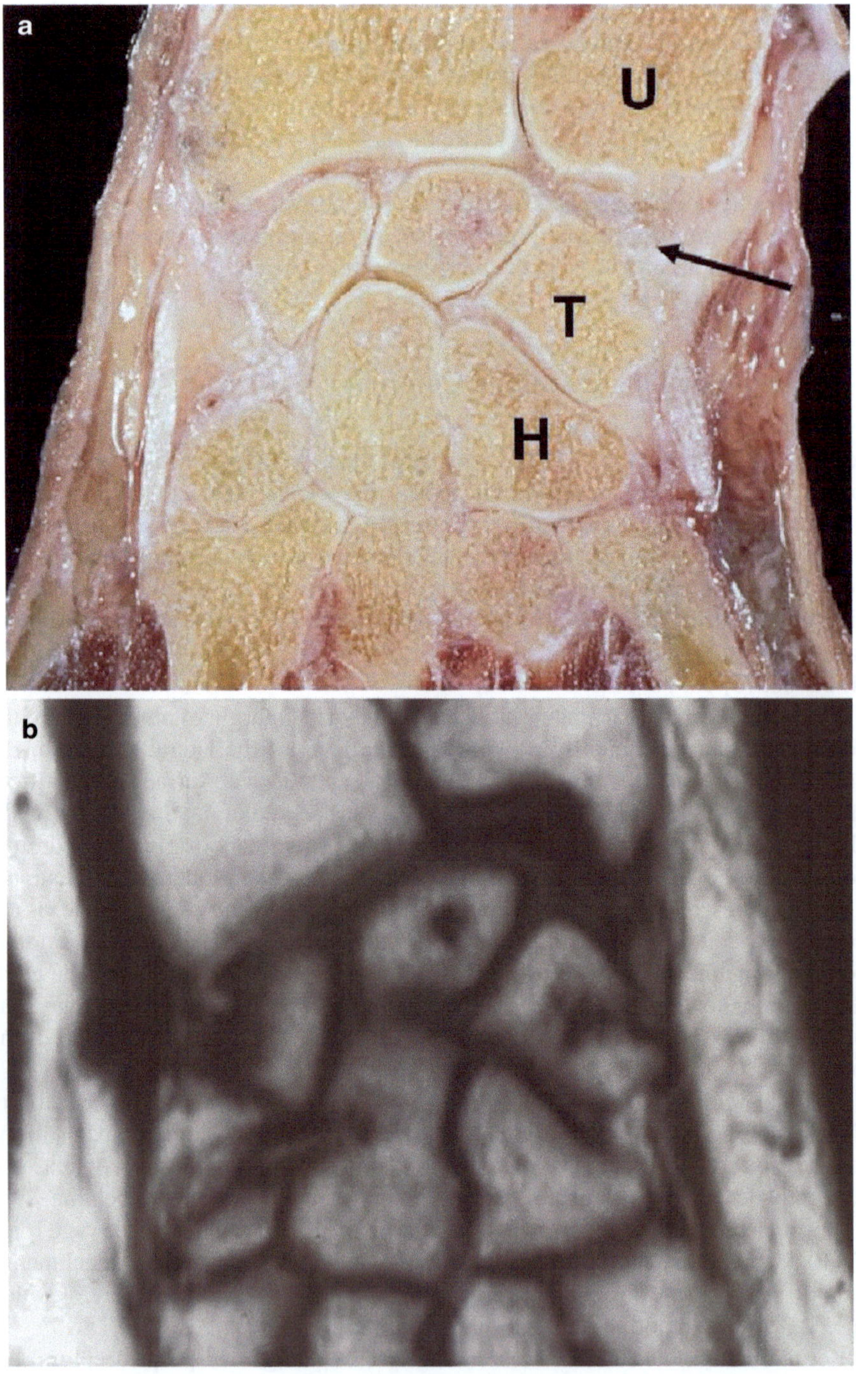

Fig. 4 Triangular fibrocartilage complex. (**a**) Frontal section of an anatomical specimen. (**b**) Frontal section (MRI T1). *U* ulna, *T* triquetrum, *H* hamate, *arrow* triangular fibrocartilage complex

Table 3 Dimensions of the main components of the triangular fibrocartilage complex according to [75]

	Length (mm)	Width (mm)	Thickness (mm)
Proximal part (*FCT*)			
Palmar	12.5 (2.4)		1.7 (0.5)
Central	11.4 (2.1)		1.0 (0.5)
Dorsal	11.8 (2.5)		1.4 (0.4)
Radial		14.3 (2.0)	1.7 (0.5)
Ulnar		4.0 (1.2)	2.0 (0.5)
Distal part (*meniscus*)	8.5 (1.6)	13.2 (1.2)	2.1 (0.5)

6 Collateral Ligaments

The collateral ligaments have not been included in the classification of Sennwald and Segmüller [78]. Several authors indicate that these ligaments are loaded during opposed deviation, serve as support to the scaphoid and constitute the anchoring point of rotation axes.

On the other hand, the majority of the authors consider that such ligaments do not exist or are not contributive because they would prevent lateral deviations. Other studies showed a variable morphology of the collateral ligaments, incompatible with a stabilizing function of the carpus. Dynamic collateral stabilization is ensured by the muscular apparatus: abductor pollicis longus and extensor pollicis brevis on the radial side and extensor carpi ulnaris on the ulnar side [9–13, 16, 21, 22, 24, 25, 30, 36, 40, 41, 44, 48, 50, 59, 88, 95].

7 Conclusion

The anatomy of the carpal ligaments is complex. This chapter tried to provide insight on current knowledge in the field of functional anatomy of the carpal ligaments. We will have noticed that certain data remain little explored. The capsular ligaments of the wrist present morphological and morphometric variations. These relate to mainly the ulnar and dorsal ligaments. They could explain the biomechanical variations reported in the literature and the diversity of classifications and treatment methods suggested for carpal instability, although further studies are necessary to confirm this assumption.

References

1. Adams BD, Samani JE, Holley KA (1996) Triangular fibrocartilage injury: a laboratory model. J Hand Surg Am 21A:189–193
2. Berger RA, Blair WF (1984) The radioscapholunate ligament: a gross and histologic description. Anat Rec 210:393–405

3. Berger RA (1996) The gross and histologic anatomy of the scapholunate interosseous ligament. J Hand Surg Am 21A:170–178
4. Berger RA, Imeada T, Berglund L, An KN (1999) Constraint and material properties of the subregions of the scapholunate interosseous ligament. J Hand Surg Am 24A:953–962
5. Berger RA (2001) The anatomy of the ligaments of the wrist and distal radioulnar joints. Clin Orthop 383:32–40
6. Berger RA, Amadio PC (1994) Predicting palmar radiocarpal ligament disruption in fractures of the distal articular surface of the radius involving the palmar cortex. J Hand Surg Br 19B:108–113
7. Berger RA, Landsmeer JMF (1990) The palmar radiocarpal ligaments: a study of adult and fetal human wrist joints. J Hand Surg Am 15A:847–854
8. Bettinger PC, Linscheid RL, Berger RA, Cooney WP, An KN (1999) An anatomic study of the stabilizing ligaments of the trapezium and trapeziometacarpal joint. J Hand Surg Am 24A:786–798
9. Boabighi A, Kuhlmann JN, Kenesi C, Guerin-Surville H (1989) Etude élastométrique du complexe ligamentaire scaphoïdien distal et du ligament scapho-lunaire. Bull Assoc Anat 73:5–10
10. Boabighi A, Kuhlmann JN, Kenesi C (1993) The distal ligamentous complex of the scaphoid and scapho-lunate ligament. An anatomical, histological and biomechanical study. J Hand Surg Br 18B:65–69
11. Bonjean P, Honton L, LInarte R, Vignes J (1981) Anatomical bases for the dynamic exploration of the wrist joint. Anat Clin 3:73–85
12. Braus H (1929) Anatomie des Menschen. Springer, Berlin
13. Brunelli GA, Brunelli GR (1995) Une nouvelle intervention pour la dissociation scapho-lunaire. Ann Chir Main 14:207–213
14. Canovas E, Ledoux D, Bonnel E (1998) Biometry of the capsular ligaments of the wrist. Ann Chir Main 17(3):207–214
15. Cavalcante ML, Rodriguez CJ, Mattar R (2004) Mechanoreceptors and nerve endings of the triangular fibrocartilage in the human wrist. J Hand Surg Am 29A:432–435
16. Connell D, Page P, Wright W, Hoy G (2001) Magnetic resonance imaging of the wrist ligaments. Australas Radiol 45:411–422
17. Craighen MAC, Stanley JK (1995) Wrist kinematics: row, column or both? J Hand Surg Br 20B:165–170
18. Cuénod P, Charrière E, Papaloizos MY (2002) A mechanical comparison of bone-ligament-bone autografts from the wrist for replacement of the scapholunate ligament. J Hand Surg Am 27A:985–990
19. De Lange A, Huiskes R, Kauer JMG (1990) Wrist-joint ligament length changes in flexion and deviation of the hand: an experimental study. J Orthop Res 8:722–730
20. Efremov S, Oberlin C (1996) The pisiformtriquetral complex: an anatomical study. J Hand Surg Br 21B:20
21. Feipel V, Rooze M (1999) The capsular ligaments of the wrist: morphology, morphometry and clinical applications. Surg Radiol Anat 21:175–180
22. Feipel V, Rooze M (1997) The capsular ligaments of the wrist. Eur J Morphol 35:87–94
23. Feipel V, Rooze M, Louryan S, Lemort M (1994) Functional anatomy of the carpus in radioulnar deviation and in flexion and extension: a bi- and three-dimensional CT study. In: Schuind F, An KN, Cooney WP, Garcia-Elias M (eds) Advances in the biomechanics of the hand and wrist. Plenum Press, New York, pp 255–270
24. Fick R (1904) Handbuch der Anatomie und Mechanik der Gelenke. Fischer-Verlag, Jena
25. Fisk GR (1984) The wrist. J Bone Joint Surg Br 66B:396–407
26. Fuss FK, Wagner TF (1996) Biomechanical alterations in the carpal arch and hand muscles after carpal tunnel release. Clin Anat 9:100–108
27. Garcia-Elias M (2003) Lésions du complexe lunotriquetral: principes thérapeutiques. Chir Main 22:57–64

28. Garcia-Elias M, AN KN, Cooney WP, Linscheid RL, Chao EY (1989) Stability of the transverse carpal arch: an experimental study. J Hand Surg Am 14A:277–282
29. Garcia-Elias M, Sanchez-Freijo JM, Salo JM, Lluch AL (1992) Dynamic changes of the transverse carpal arch during flexion-extension of the wrist: effects of sectioning the transverse carpal ligament. J Hand Surg Am 17A:1017–1019
30. Garcia-Elias M, Smith DK, Ruby LK, Horii E, An KN, Linscheid RL, Chao EYS, Cooney WP (1994) Normal and abnormal carpal kinematics. In: Schuind F, An KN, Cooney WP, Garcia-Elias M (eds) Advances in the biomechanics of the hand and wrist. Plenum Press, New York, pp 247–254
31. Gilula LA, Weeks PM (1978) Post-traumatic ligamentous instabilities of the wrist. Radiology 129:641–651
32. Green DP, O'Brien ET (1980) Classification and management of carpal dislocations. Clin Orthop 149:55–72
33. Hagert E, Garcia-Elias M, Forsgren S, Ljung BO (2007) Immunohistochemical analysis of wrist ligament innervation in relation to their structural composition. J Hand Surg Am 32:30–36
34. Harvey EJ, Hanel D, Knight JB, Tencer AF (1999) Autograft replacements for the scapholunate ligament: a biomechanical comparison of hand-based autografts. J Hand Surg Am 24A:963–967
35. Hofstede DJ, Ritt MJ, Bos KE (1999) Tarsal autografts for reconstruction of the scapholunate interosseous ligament: a biomechanical study. J Hand Surg Br 24A:968–976
36. Hogikyan JV, Louis DS (1992) Embryologic development and variations in the anatomy of the ulnocarpal ligamentous complex. J Hand Surg Am 17A:719–723
37. Ishiko T, Puttlitz CM, Lotz JC, Diao E (2003) Scaphoid kinematics after division of the transverse carpal ligament. J Hand Surg Am 28A:267–271
38. Johnston RB, Seller JG, Miller EJ, Drvaric DM (1995) The intrinsic and extrinsic ligaments of the wrist. A correlation of collagen typing and histologic appearance. J Hand Surg Br 20B:750–754
39. Katz DA, Green JK, Werner FW, Loftus JB (2003) Capsulo-ligamentous restraints to dorsal and palmar carpal translation. J Hand Surg Am 28A:610–613
40. Kauer JM (1975) The articular disc of the hand. Acta Anat 93:590–605
41. Kauer JMG (1979) The collateral ligament function in the wrist joint. Acta Morphol Neerl Scand 17:252–253
42. Kauer JM (1980) Functional anatomy of the wrist. Clin Orthop 149:9–20
43. Kauer JM, de Lange A (1987) The carpal joint: anatomy and function. Hand Clin 3:23–29
44. Kauer JMG, Savelberg HHCM, Huiskes R, Kooloos JGM (1994) Role of the wrist ligaments with respect to carpal kinematics and carpal mechanism. In: Schuind F, An KN, Cooney WP, Garcia-Elias M (eds) Advances in the biomechanics of the hand and wrist, vol A 256, NATO ASI series. Plenum Press, New York, pp 271–280
45. Kim HK, Ryu J, Han JS, Yang SB, Kish V (1994) A new cross-sectional area measurement technique for intrinsic and extrinsic human wrist ligaments: in-situ MRI study. In: Proceedings of the SIROT inter-meeting, Boston, 1994
46. Kiritsis PG, Kline SC (1995) Biomechanical changes after carpal tunnel release: a cadaveric model for comparing open, endoscopic, and step-cut lengthening techniques. J Hand Surg Am 20A:173–180
47. Kooloos JGM, Savelberg HHCM (1992) Measurements of cross-sectional areas in selected human wrist-joint ligaments. Acta Anat 144:325–328
48. Kuhlmann JN (1979) Les mécanismes de l'articulation du poignet. Ann Chir 33:711–719
49. Kuhlmann JN, Landet C, Luboinski A, Boabighi A, Landjerit B, Guerin-Surville H, Baux S (1988) Les structures fibreuses du poignet. II – Etude biomécanique. Bull Assoc Anat 72:31–35
50. Lewis OJ, Hamshere RJ, Bucknill TM (1970) The anatomy of the wrist joint. J Anat 106:539–552

51. Linscheid RL (1986) Kinematic considerations of the wrist. Clin Orthop 202:27–39
52. Linscheid RL, Dobyns JH, Beabout JW, Bryan RS (1972) Traumatic instability of the wrist: diagnosis, classification and pathomechanics. J Bone Joint Surg Br 54A:1612–1632
53. Mayfield JK (1980) Mechanism of carpal injuries. Clin Orthop 149:45–54
54. Mayfield JK (1984) Patterns of injury to carpal ligaments. Clin Orthop 187:36–42
55. Mayfield JK, Johnson RP, Kilcoyne RF (1976) The ligaments of the wrist and their functional significance. Anat Rec 186:417–428
56. Mayfield JK, Williams WJ, Erdman AG, Dahlof WJ, Wallrich MA, Kleinhenz WA, Moody NR (1979) Biomechanical properties of human carpal ligaments. Orthop Trans 3:143–144
57. Meade TD, Schneider LH, Cherry K (1990) Radiographic analysis of selective ligament sectioning at the carpal scaphoid: a cadaver study. J Hand Surg Am 15A:855–862
58. Mitsuyasu H, Patterson RM, Shah MA, Buford WL, Iwamoto Y, Viegas SF (2004) The role of the dorsal intercarpal ligament in dynamic and static scapholunate instability. J Hand Surg Am 29A:279–288
59. Mizuseki T, Ikuta Y (1989) The dorsal carpal ligaments: their anatomy and function. J Hand Surg Br 14B:91–98
60. Moritomo H, Viegas SF, Nakamura K, DaSilva MF, Patterson RM (2000) The scaphotrapezio-trapezoidal joint. Part 1: an anatomic and radiographic study. J Hand Surg Am 25A:899–910
61. Moritomo H, Murase T, Arimitsu S, Oka K, Yoshikawa H, Sugamoto K (2008) Change in the length of the ulnocarpal ligaments during radiocarpal motion: possible impact on triangular fibrocartilage complex foveal tears. J Hand Surg Am 33A:1278–1286
62. Nagao S, Patterson RM, Buford WL, Andersen CR, Shah MA, Viegas SF (2005) Three-dimensional description of ligamentous attachments around the lunate. J Hand Surg Am 30A:685–692
63. Nowak MD, Logan SE (1991) Distinguishing biomechanical properties of intrinsic and extrinsic human wrist ligaments. J Biomech Eng 113:85–93
64. Ohmori M, Azuma H (1998) Morphology and distribution of nerve endings in the human triangular fibrocartilage complex. J Hand Surg Br 23B:522–525
65. Okutsu I, Ninomiya S, Hamanaka I, Kuroshima N, Inanmani H (1989) Measurement of pressure in the carpal canal before and after endoscopic management of carpal tunnel syndrome. J Bone Joint Surg Am 71A:679–683
66. Palmer AK (1989) Triangular fibrocartilage complex lesions: a classification. J Hand Surg Am 14A:594–606
67. Palmer AK (1990) Triangular fibrocartilage disorders: injury patterns and treatment. Arthroscopy 6:125–132
68. Palmer AK, Werner FW (1981) The triangular fibrocartilage complex of the wrist-anatomy and function. J Hand Surg Am 6:153–162
69. Patterson MR, Moritomo H, Yamaguchi S, Mitsuyasu H, Shah M, Buford WL, Viegas SF (2003) Scaphoid anatomy and mechanics: update and review. Oper Tech Orthop 13:2–10
70. Richman JA, Gelberman RH, Rydevik BL, Hajek PC, Braun RM, Gylys-Morin VM, Berthoty D (1989) Carpal tunnel syndrome: morphologic changes after release of the transverse carpal ligament. J Hand Surg Am 14A:852–857
71. Ritt MJPF, Bishop AT, Berger RA, Linscheid RL, Berglund LJ, An KN (1998) Lunotriquetral ligament properties: a comparison of three anatomic subregions. J Hand Surg Am 23A:425–431
72. Salvia P, Klein P, David JH, Rooze M (1994) The envelope of active wrist circumduction: an in vivo electrogoniometric study. In: Schuind F, An KN, Cooney WP, Garcia-Elias M (eds) Advances in the biomechanics of the hand and wrist, vol 256, NATO ASI series. Plenum Press, New York, pp 313–328
73. Savelberg HHCM, Kooloos JGM, Huiskes R, Kauer JMG (1992) Stiffness of the ligaments of the human wrist joint. J Biomech 25:369–376

74. Savelberg HHCM, Otten JDM, Kooloos JGM, Huiskes R, Kaner JMG (1993) Carpal bone kinematics and ligament lengthening for the full range of joint movement. J Biomech 26:1389–1404
75. Schmidt HM (2004) Die Anatomie des ulnokarpalen Komplexes. Orthopade 33:628–637
76. Schuind F, An KN, Berglund L et al (1991) The distal radioulnar ligaments. A biomechanical study. J Hand Surg Am 16A:1106–1114
77. Sennwald G (1987) L'entité radius-carpe. Springer, Berlin
78. Sennwald G, Segmüller G (1986) Base anatomique d'un nouveau concept de stabilité du carpe. Int Orthop 10:25–30
79. Sennwald G, Zdravkovic V, Oberlin C (1994) The anatomy of the palmar scaphotriquetral ligament. J Bone Joint Surg Br 76B:147–149
80. Seradge H, Seradge E (1989) Piso-triquetral pain syndrome after carpal tunnel release. J Hand Surg Am 14A:858–862
81. Shin AY, Bishop AT (1998) Treatment options for lunotriquetral dissociation. Tech Hand Up Extrem Surg 2:2–17
82. Short WH, Werner FW, Green JK, Masaoka S (2002) Biomechanical evaluation of ligamentous stabilizers of the scaphoid and lunate. J Hand Surg Am 27A:991–1002
83. Short WH, Werner FW, Green JK, Masaoka S (2005) Biomechanical evaluation of the ligamentous stabilizers of the scaphoid and lunate: part II. J Hand Surg Am 30A:24–34
84. Siegel DB, Gelberman RH (1991) Radial styloidectomy: an anatomical study with special reference to radiocarpal intracapsular ligamentous morphology. J Hand Surg Am 16A:40–44
85. Smith DK (1993) Dorsal carpal ligaments of the wrist: normal appearance on multiplanar reconstructions of three-dimensional Fourier transform MR imaging. Am J Roentgenol 161:119–125
86. Smith DK (1993) Volar carpal ligaments of the wrist: normal appearance on multiplanar reconstructions of three-dimensional Fourier transform MR imaging. Am J Roentgenol 161:353–357
87. Sokolow C, Saffar P (2001) Anatomy and histology of the scapholunate ligament. Hand Clin 17:77–81
88. Taleisnik J (1976) The ligaments of the wrist. J Hand Surg Am 1:110–118
89. Taleisnik J (1980) Post-traumatic carpal instability. Clin Orthop 149:73–82
90. Tang JB, Ryu J, Kish V (1998) The triangular fibrocartilage complex: an important component of the pulley for the ulnar wrist extensor. J Hand Surg Am 23A:986–991
91. Tomita K, Berger EJ, Berger RA, Kraisarin J, An KN (2007) Distribution of nerve endings in the human dorsal radiocarpal ligament. J Hand Surg Am 32A:450–458
92. Upal MA, Crisco JJ, Moore DC, Sonenblum SE, Wolfe SW (2006) In vivo elongation of the palmar and dorsal scapholunate interosseous ligament. J Hand Surg Am 31:1326–1332
93. Viegas SF, Patterson RM, Ward K (1995) Extrinsic wrist ligaments in the pathomechanics of ulnar translation instability. J Hand Surg Am 20A:312–318
94. Viegas SF, Yamaguchi S, Boyd NL, Patterson RM (1999) The dorsal ligaments of the wrist: anatomy, mechanical properties, and function. J Hand Surg Am 24A:456–468
95. Virchow H (1902) Die Weiterdrehung des Naviculare carpi bei Dorsalflexion, und die Bezeichnungen der Handbänder. Anat Anz 21:111
96. Xu J, Tang JB (2009) In vivo length changes of selected carpal ligaments during wrist radioulnar deviation. J Hand Surg Am 34A:401–408
97. Yoshii Y, Zhao C, Henderson J, Zhao KD, Zobitz ME, An KN, Amadio PC (2008) Effects of carpal tunnel release on the relative motion of tendon, nerve, and subsynovial connective tissue in a human cadaver model. Clin Biomech 23:1121–1127

Carpal Biomechanics: Application to Ligamentous Injuries

E. Camus

1 Introduction

Since Destot in 1905, the study of intracarpal injuries has interested many authors who were faced with wrist traumatisms [1–7]. Therefore, the analysis of the sole traumas is not enough to understand carpal biomechanics. Studies have thus been led in different directions to solve injuries' mechanism.

Imaging studies dealt with the radiography of healthy subjects [8–17], with the in vitro measure of intracarpal movements [18–27] and then in vivo by CT scan [28–40]. The radiographic studies of healthy subjects enabled to measure the shift of the bones that could be seen on front and profile views. But the bone superposition and the out-of-the-radiographic-plane position of some bones do not allow to measure all the displacements. Cadaveric studies allowed researchers to fix markers on carpal bones to differentiate them better and measure their movements. The authors of these studies mostly resorted to metallic markers, which shifting was recorded by stereoradiography. Yet, the necessary surgical approach to introduce the markers and their presence inside the wrist involve a doubt on the similarity in between in vivo results [23, 28, 29]. Recent CT scan studies measured in vivo the in-plane and out-of-plane movements of the bones [28, 29, 36, 38–40]. These studies enabled to draw an accurate view of carpal biomechanics.

In vitro studies on carpal ligament sections were useful to start some ligamentous traumatic sequences. Several carpal restraints are thus described [7, 41–50].

Works on forces transmission enabled to explain the different strains applied to the moving wrist [51–58].

As the study and the diagnosis of carpal ligamentous injuries are difficult, it seems necessary to present a biomechanical synthesis of the available data on the topic.

E. Camus
Hand Surgery Unit, SELARL Chirurgie de la Main,
Polyclinique du Val de Sambre,
162, route de Mons, 59600 Maubeuge, France
e-mail: ejcamus@wanadoo.fr, emmanuel.camus@wanadoo.fr

E. Camus, L. Van Overstraeten (eds.), *Carpal Ligament Surgery*,
DOI 10.1007/978-2-8178-0379-1_2, © Springer-Verlag France 2013

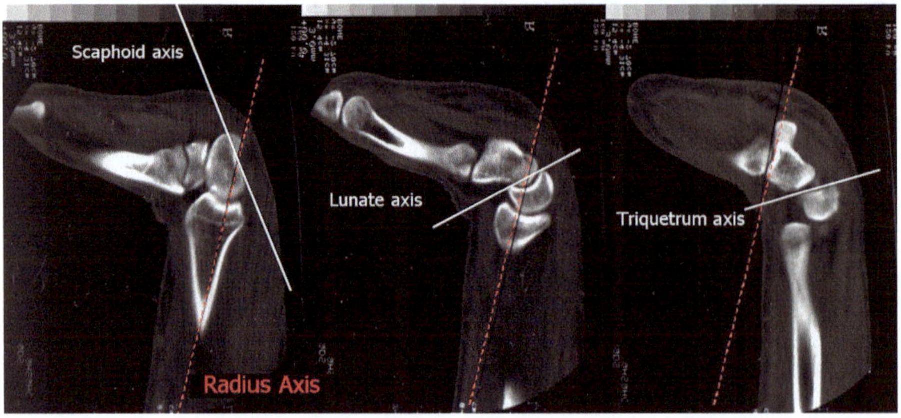

Fig. 1 Sagittal section of the extended wrist column by column. *Red* radius axis, *Black* wrist bone axis

2 Kinematics of the Wrist

2.1 Flexion and Extension of the Wrist

Under the action of carpal flexor or extensor tendons, both carpal rows flex or extend jointly, with varied ranges of motion [29, 40]. As the movements of both rows have the same direction in the sagittal plane, the ranges of motions add up. The tilting movements in the frontal plane are not important [29, 40]. Usually, it is said the radiocarpal space is mainly mobilized during flexion and the mediocarpal space during extension [59]. In fact, thorough CT scan studies prove this is oversimplified [40, 60] (Fig. 1). Flexion is predominant in STT, radiolunar and ulnotriquetral spaces (Fig. 2). Extension is predominant in radioscaphoid, lunocapital and triquetrohamate spaces (Fig. 3).

The main flexion and extension lines of the wrist are thus described. These lines represent the space which is the most mobile in each motion. The scapholunate ligament is where those lines cross and reverse (Fig. 4).

2.2 Radial and Ulnar Deviation of the Wrist

Both carpal rows deviate in the same direction in the frontal plane. The radial or ulnar deviation of both rows adds up [17]. But in the sagittal plane, different movements coexist.

During radial deviation, the proximal row (R1) flexes, and the distal row (R2) extends. With such inverse movements, one neutralizes each other and this allows to

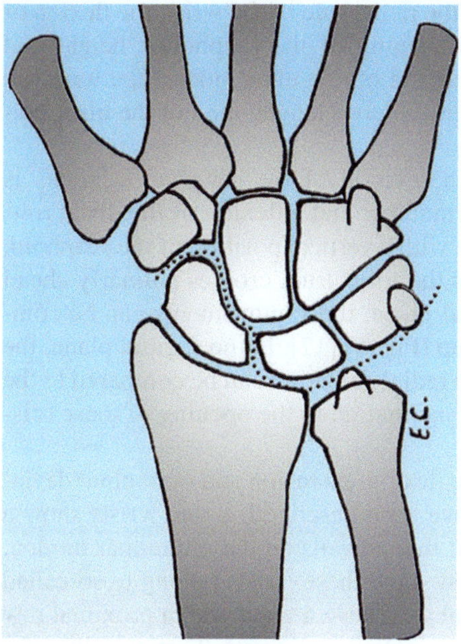

Fig. 2 Wrist main flexion line

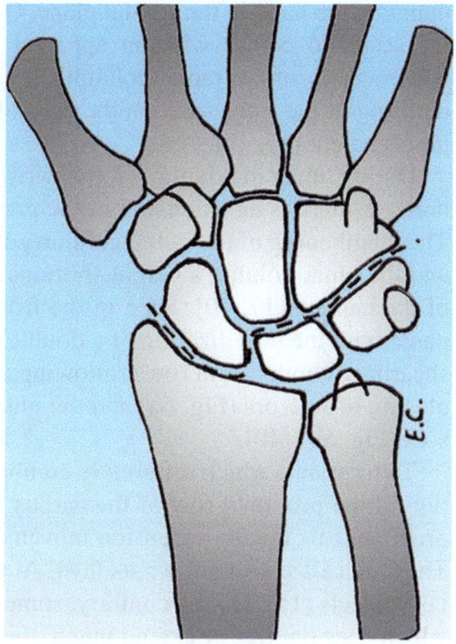

Fig. 3 Wrist main extension line

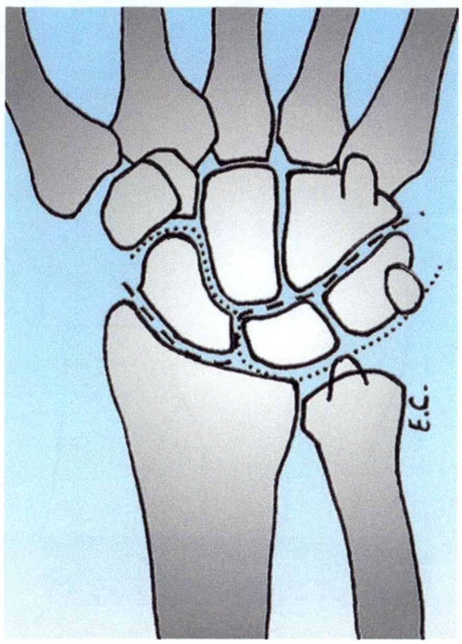

Fig. 4 Junction of the of flexion and extension main lines within the scapholunate ligament

maintain the hand in the frontal plane. On the radial side of the wrist, the flexion of the scaphoid comes with an apparent shortening of the scaphoid's height and consequently of the radial column's height, and on the ulnar side of the wrist, an uplifting of the triquetrum on the hamate engenders a lengthening of the ulnar column's height [17, 40].

During ulnar deviation of the wrist, a reversal of the rows' movements is noticed; there is an extension of the proximal row and a flexion of the distal row. The lengthening of the radial column goes with a vertical position of the scaphoid, and the ulnar column's height shortens as the triquetrum crosses palmarly ahead of the hamate [17, 40]. Seen in the frontal plane, those movements can be compared with the mobilization of a double cup (Fig. 5) [17]. In the sagittal plane, the shearing of both carpal rows following the radial deviation can be compared to the closing of scissors (Fig. 6a) and the ulnar inclination to the opening of these scissors (Fig. 6b) [40].

Two variants which differently combine flexion-extension and radioulnar deviation of the proximal row of the carpus have been described. Some wrists show a proximal row flexion-extension movement that prevails on the radioulnar motion. They are called column wrists [14]. At first sight, these wrists belong to so-called lax subjects [15]. On the contrary, some subjects have a wrist with a proximal row which does not flex or extend much; they are called row wrists. They usually refer to rigid wrists. The influence of gender on both these biomechanical variants is still under consideration [14, 16].

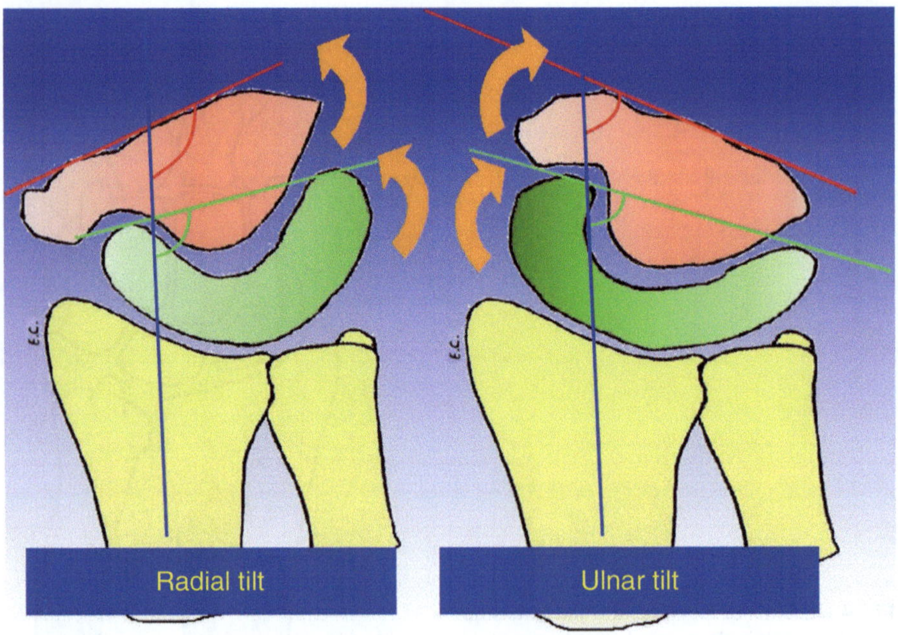

Fig. 5 Pattern of both carpal rows mobility following the double-cup description. *Blue* radius axis, *red* distal row transverse axis, *green* proximal row transverse axis

3 Actions of the Ligaments and Peripheral Tendons

3.1 Ligaments

Ligaments are passive brakes which authorize movements inside and between the rows and maintain the spacial coherence of the carpus [61]. They allow intra-row movements, which are adaptative for congruence movements, and inter-row movements which are efficient movements to mobilize the hand [17]. The limit of range depends on their length. For didactic reasons, intrinsic and deep extrinsic ligaments (Fig. 7) and extrinsic superficial ligaments will be separately represented (Fig. 8).

The scapholunate ligament links both bones (Fig. 7-1). The fibres which constitute the ligament are not symmetrically distributed. The dorsal part of the ligament is the most fibrous and thickest and also the most resistant [62]. It is considered as the main stabilizer of the scapholunar couple. It is always injured in scapholunar instability [63–65]. This ligamentous injury involves an increase flexion of the scaphoid from 3° to 6° [47–50, 62, 66], an extension of the lunate of 5° [50] and a dorsal translation of the scaphoid's proximal pole more than 2 mm [62]. Tang also noticed a possible displacement of the rotation centre of the wrist [67].

The radioscapholunate ligament (Fig. 7-2) is thin; it is a neurovascular pedicle [62, 68] and not a real ligament.

The lunotriquetral ligament (Fig. 7-3). Its fibres are asymmetric too. On the palmar part, these fibres are thicker and resist to traction. They lock up the palmar translation of the lunate. Dorsal fibres are the most torsion resistant. They lock up both the lunate's dorsal translation and the torsion by differential flexion-extension between the two bones [41]. When the ligament is injured, it engenders

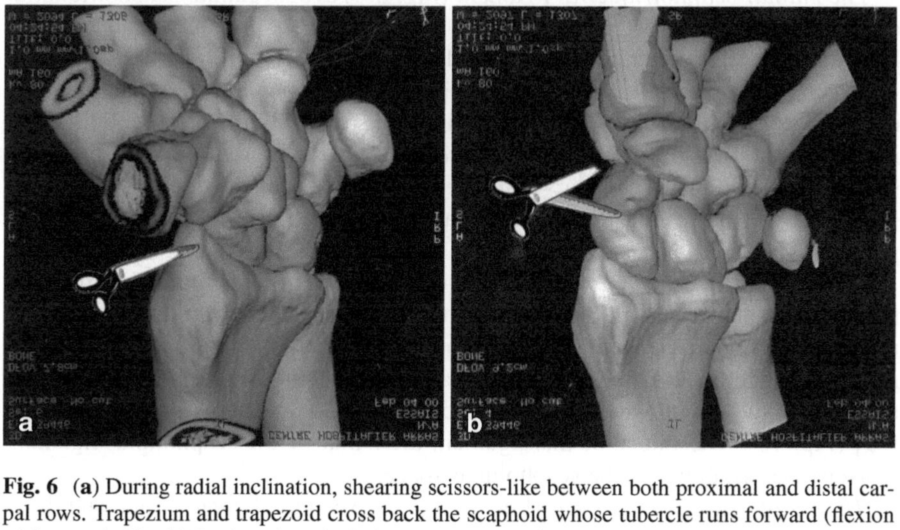

Fig. 6 (**a**) During radial inclination, shearing scissors-like between both proximal and distal carpal rows. Trapezium and trapezoid cross back the scaphoid whose tubercle runs forward (flexion of the scaphoid). (**b**) During ulnar deviation, trapezium and trapezoid run distally to the scaphoid. The distal row flexes when the proximal row extends

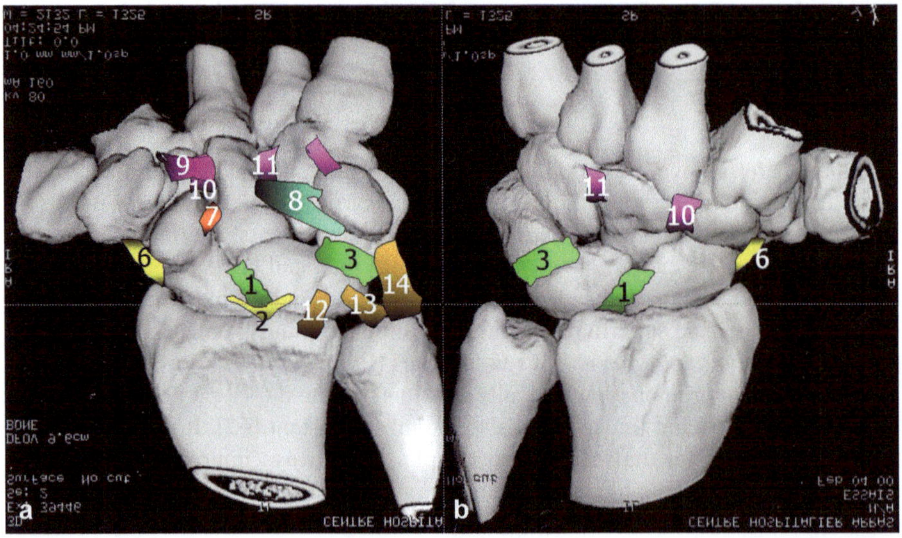

Fig. 7 Intrinsic and deep extrinsic ligaments. (**a**) Palmar view. (**b**) Dorsal view. *1* Scapholunate ligament, *2* Radioscapholunate ligament, *3* Lunotriquetral ligament, *6* Scaphotrapezial ligament, *7* Scaphocapitate ligament, *8* Triquetrohamatocapitate ligament, *9* Capitotrapezial ligament, *10* Capitotrapezoidal ligament, *11* Capitohamate ligament, *12* Short radioulnar ligament, *13* Ulnolunar ligament, *14* Ulnotriquetral ligament

a lunotriquetral instability with VISI and sometimes a gap with supination of the triquetrum [42].

The palmar scaphotriquetral ligament (Fig. 8-4) avoids palmar scaphotriquetral dissociation and indirectly scapholunate dissociation. It probably maintains the head of the capitate when the wrist extends [66].

The radioscaphocapitate ligament (Fig. 8-5) is a powerful palmar ligament ensuring carpal cohesion. It is tensed against the scaphoid tubercle which lifts it in radial inclination of the wrist (Fig. 9). It avoids the dorsal translation of the proximal scaphoid pole and is a secondary stabilizer of the scapholunate couple [63]. If it is injured, it can be responsible for the scaphoid's instabilities with DISI and scapholunar gap [64].

The scaphotrapezial ligament (Fig. 7-6) is V. pattern ligament attached to the radial side of the scaphoid, the proximal point and at distal joint on the palmar and radial sides of the trapezium [68]. It is another secondary stabilizer of the scapholunar couple together with the radioscaphocapitate ligament. For Moritomo et al., it is also one of the points where the scaphoid's flexion-extension axis passes through [69] (Fig. 10). The injury of this ligament after that of the scapholunar ligament worsens the instability of the scapholunar space.

The scaphocapitate ligament (Fig. 7-7) is the second element which stabilizes the scaphoid with the distal carpal row [68]. It also plays a part in the materialization of the scaphoid's flexion-extension axis (Fig. 10).

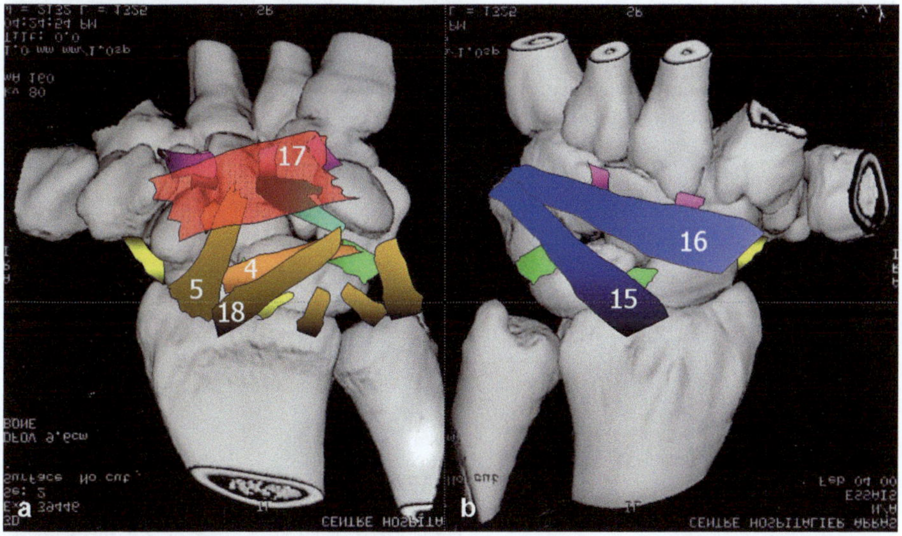

Fig. 8 Extrinsic ligaments. (**a**) Palmar view. (**b**) Dorsal view. *4* Scaphotriquetral ligament, *5* Radioscaphocapitate ligament, *15* Dorsal radiocarpal ligament, *16* Dorsal intercarpal ligament, *17* Carpal anterior annular ligament, *18* Radiolunotriquetral ligament

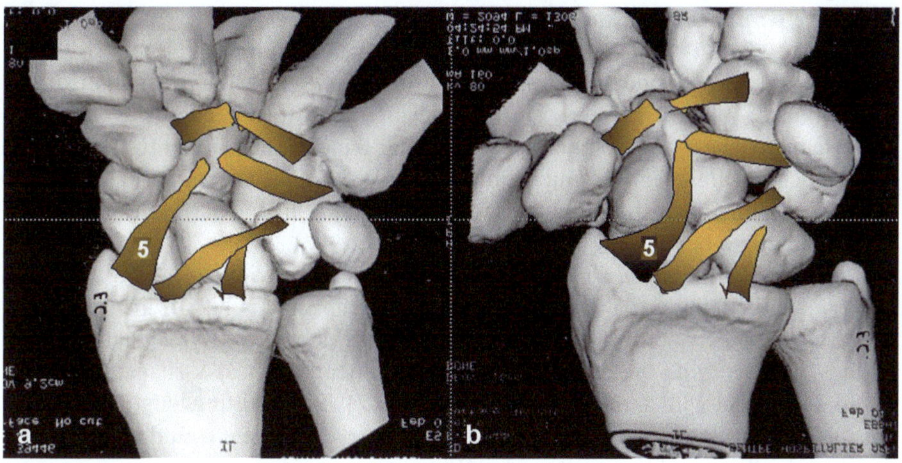

Fig. 9 Lifting of the radioscaphocapitate ligament by the scaphoid tubercle during radial inclination. (**a**) Ulnar inclination. (**b**) Radial inclination. *5* Radioscaphocapitate ligament

The triquetocapitate ligament (Fig. 7-8) is tensed from the radial angle distal from the triquetrum to the ulnar part of the capitate's body [68]. It takes attachment from the hamate bone, and its fibres go to the ulnotriquetral ligament to describe the ulnocapitate ligament. It is the ulnopalmar stabilizer of the mediocarpal space.

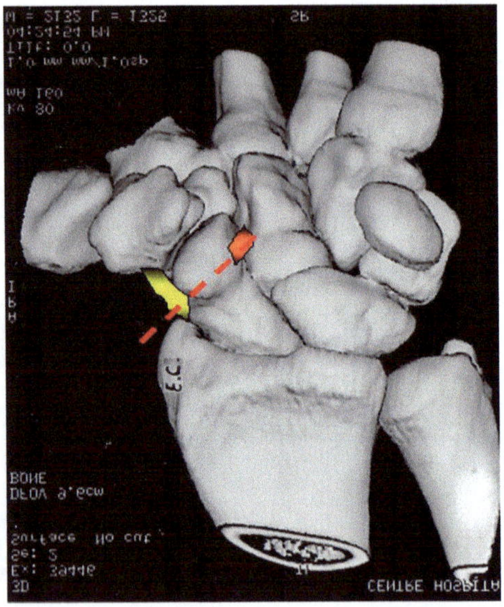

Fig. 10 Materialization of the axis of flexion-extension of the scaphoid. *Orange* scaphocapitate ligament, *yellow* scaphotrapezium ligament, *dotted line* scaphoid's flexion/extension axis according to Moritomo

The long radiolunotriquetral ligament (Fig. 8-18) is the palmar part of Kuhlmann's triquetral sling [8, 61]. It prevents the ulnar translation of the carpal bones. When this ligament is injured, the perilunar region becomes deeply unstable and thus promotes the perilunar dislocation of the carpal bones [7].

The dorsal radiocarpal ligament (Fig. 8-15) is radiolunotriquetral. It is the dorsal part of Kuhlmann's triquetral sling [8, 11, 61]. It is a secondary stabilizer of the carpal bones. When it is injured, it is as destabilizing for the carpus as when the radioscaphocapitate and scaphotrapezial palmar bundles are injured [65]. The dorsal radiocarpal ligament is injured in more than 50 % of the carpal instabilities, often in association with the interosseous scapholunar ligament, but it may be the only ligament to be injured [70].

The dorsal intercarpal ligament (Fig. 8-16) links the triquetrum and the distal scaphoid and continues on the trapezium and the trapezoid in half of the cases. It is the last secondary stabilizer of the carpal bones [65]. For Viegas, this ligament constitutes, together with the dorsal radiocarpal ligament, a dorsal V-shaped radioscaphoidal ligament with a transversal orientation [47]. The resulting length varies, but the ligament is always tensed. A direct radioscaphoid ligament would be either lax, to allow the flexion of the wrist, and inefficient or tensed in a neutral position, preventing flexion and giving stiffness. This transversal V-shaped ligament remains tensed whatever the position of flexion or extension of the wrist thanks to the movement of the branches of the V which modify the angle (Fig. 11) and whatever the radioulnar inclination of the wrist as it goes together with the linked movements of flexion/extension of the scaphoid.

The transverse anterior annular ligament of the carpal bones (Fig. 8-17) completes the system. If it were sectioned, there would be an extension of the scaphoid

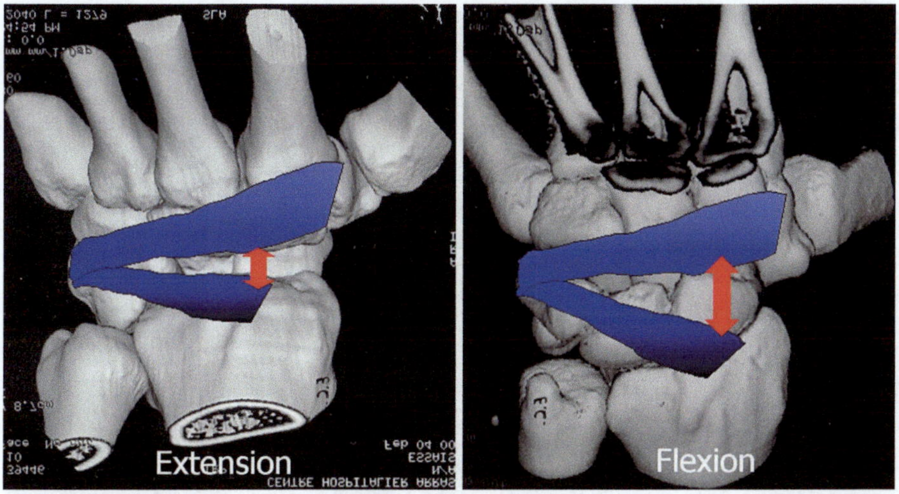

Fig. 11 Opening variation of the angle of the dorsal ligamentous V

of 58 % during the carpal ulnar drift and probably an increase of the restraints on the other ligaments [48].

To sum up, the scapholunar instability is often the result of an interosseous injury. The problem increases if other ligaments, mainly the palmar secondary stabilizers (radioscaphocapitate ligament or scaphotrapezial ligament) or the dorsal secondary stabilizers (dorsal radiocarpal or dorsal intercarpal), are affected [63–65, 71].

If the ligamentous injury starts at the distal pole of the scaphoid and affects the STT ligamentous system, there is also a destabilizing of the scaphoid, what can lead to STT arthritis if no surgical repair is made [72]. This situation of distal scaphoidal ligamentous injury can be compared to the partial osseous resections which are used in scaphotrapezial arthritis [73]. The distal scaphoidal resection separates the scaphoid from the trapezium and the trapezoid. It engenders a DISI in half of the cases [74], but the isolated trapeziectomy does not destabilize the wrist. The injury of the scaphotrapezial ligament only seems to have no impact on the scaphoid's stability. It must be linked with a scaphotrapezoidal ligamentous injury or maybe a scaphocapitate ligamentous injury to produce a scaphoidal destabilization by its distal pole.

The lunotriquetral instability is linked to an injury of the lunotriquetral ligament, the palmar radiolunotriquetral ligament and the dorsal radiocarpal ligament [7, 42]. It is often associated to an ulnocarpal hyper pressure or to an injury of the TFCC. There may be a responsibility of the injured triquetrocapitate and palmar scaphotriquetral ligaments, but this has not been studied yet.

A ligamentous injury is not necessarily unstable at once. If one of the restraints of the different compartments is affected, there is often merely an occult ligamentous laxity, which can only be seen by arthroscopy. However, the repetition of movements in a wrist where there is such a laxity can engender a real instability by

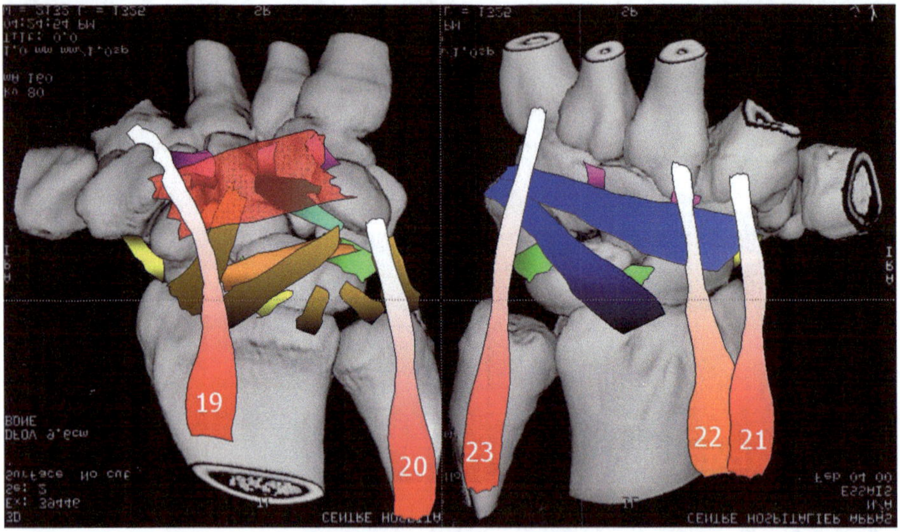

Fig. 12 Motor tendons of the carpus. *19* Flexor carpi radialis, *20* Flexor carpi ulnaris, *21* Extensor carpi radialis longus, *22* Extensor carpi radialis brevis, *23* Extensor carpi ulnaris

the fatigability of previously sane restraints. Berger asserted that carpal destabilization is linked to the number of cycles of movements imposed to the wrist. This assertion is checked for the scapholunar compartment [63–65] and for the lunotriquetral compartment [42].

3.2 *Tendons*

The peripheral tendons come stabilizing the wrist with the carpal ligaments. The carpal motors muscles and tendons are the flexor carpi radialis and the flexor carpi ulnaris, the extensor carpi radialis brevis and longus and the extensor carpi ulnaris. Their direction is mostly axial (Fig. 12). This layout makes them play a role in the cohesion of the carpal bones. Intracarpal pressures are mainly due to the traction impressed on the hand by the motor tendons. The traction strengths stiffen the tendons which become like the bars of a cage around the carpal bones [51].

Schematically, there are four muscular groups, often contracting two by two, surrounding the wrist [75]. The action of the palmaris longus is insignificant. The radial and ulnar flexors and extensors act two by two and simultaneously, in the elementary movements of the carpus. For instance, the neutral extension of the wrist is the result of the simultaneous contraction of the radial and ulnar carpal extensors (Table 1). The dart thrower's motion (DTM) is produced by the alternative contraction of flexor carpi ulnaris and the extensor carpi radialis longus and brevis [76].

Table 1 Combined action of the carpal motor muscular groups

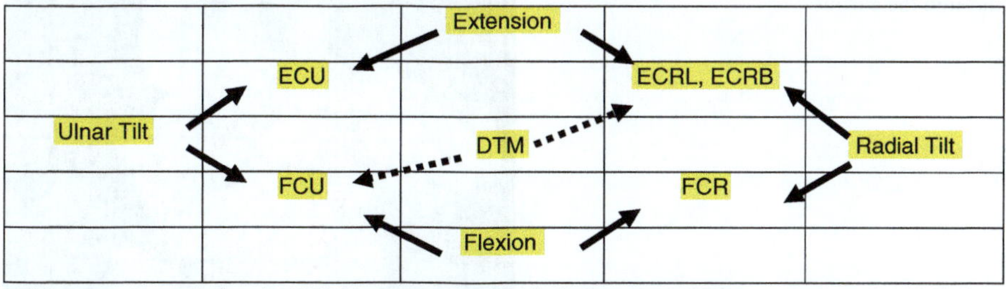

ECU extensor carpi ulnaris, *ECRL* extensor carpi radialis longus, *ECRB* extensor carpi radialis brevis, *FCU* flexor carpi ulnaris, *FCR* flexor carpi radialis, *DTM* dart thrower's motion. In this motion, the ECR and FCU tendons do not have a combined but an alternative action (*dotted arrow*)

This tension applied to the tendons makes them become rigid. They are variable brakes of carpal dislocation according to their tension degree. The motors of the fingers have a distinguished action from the motors of the wrist. The extension of the carpus increases the efficiency of the fingers flexors [59]. When the wrist moves, the agonist groups are tense and the antagonist groups are lax. This imbalance of tension of the different groups produces the hand mobilization. On the contrary, in the powerful grasp, the osseous cohesion is possible thanks to the tension of the finger flexors and the wrist extensors. This leads to the tendinous caging of the carpal bones in association with the ligaments to maintain carpal coherence [51].

The flexor carpi radialis stabilizes the scaphoid distal pole. The fibres of its sheath are closely combined to those of the scaphotrapezial capsule [77]. Its role is important since 40–70 % of the tension created by this tendon enables the stabilization of the scaphoid and prevents its collapse by flexion [52]. At the back of the wrist, the extensors carpi radialis longus and brevis stabilize the proximal pole [52, 67]. When the scapholunar ligament is injured, the course of these three tendons, which are necessary to move the hand, is lengthened and requires to develop more strength [67]. Chronicle STT instability can rupture the flexor carpi radialis [78, 79].

4 Absorption and Transmission of Axial Pressures

The pressures going through the carpus originate in the muscular contraction and in the tendinous tension of the motors of the hand. This results in an axial compression which tends to dislocate the carpus. The tenoligamentous system creates cohesion which limits collapse. Axial pressures are normally transmitted to the forearm without carpal exhaustion that give the motor muscles a stable support to move the hand. These pressures are not spread at random. In the neutral position of the wrist, pressure in the radioscaphoid fossa is superior to pressure recorded at the radiolunate or ulnotriquetral spaces [53]. Radioscaphoid pressure represents 45–55 % of total pressure, radiolunar pressure from 30 to 40 % and pressure under TFCC from 9.7 to 22 %. The radius thus receives from 80 to 90.3 % of the total pressure distributed through the carpus [52, 54–57].

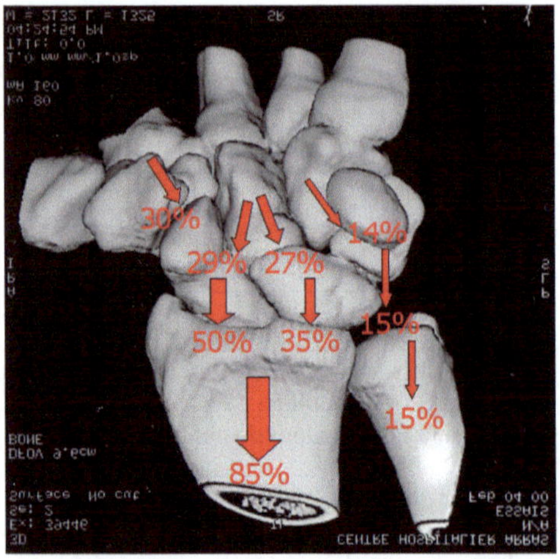

Fig. 13 Distribution of the pressures through the carpus

In the mediocarpal space, the scaphoid receives from 28 to 30.7 % of the total pressure through STT and from 26 to 32 % through the scaphocapitate space. The lunate receives from 26 to 29 % of the pressure through the capitate, and the triquetrum receives from 10.5 to 17 % of the total pressure which is transmitted by the hamate [56, 57] (Fig. 13). According to Schuind, intracarpal pressure is concentrated towards the scaphoid when it is transmitted from the mediocarpal to the radiocarpal spaces [56]. During the contraction of the motors of the hand, tendinous tension and consequently carpal caging increase as laxity decreases. The carpus is in a maximal position of interlocking [51]. Pressure in the different columns of the carpus may vary during motion. It is redistributed towards the scaphoid in radial tilt of the wrist but towards the lunate in ulnar tilt or during a grasp movement [50, 55, 57]. These physiological variations of pressure in the carpus can undergo a post-traumatic evolution. After a scapholunar dissociation, there is a decrease of pressure in the scaphoid fossa of the radius and an increase of pressure in the radiolunar and lunocapital joints [50, 58]. Consequently, the lunate becomes overworked. The scaphoid does not take its responsibility as it is unbolt and escapes from pressure by flexion instead of transmitting it. But when flexion is too important, its proximal pole bumps into the dorsal margin of the radius and engenders a dorsal radioscaphoid hyperpressure. The apparition of carpal arthritis comes as a consequence of this phenomenon [58].

5 Balance of the Carpal Proximal Row

The movements of the proximal row, which automatically associate flexion and radial tilt and extension and ulnar tilt, prove the carpal proximal row is in constant balance. The compaction strengths on the radial column of the carpus flex the scaphoid that drives the proximal row to follow scaphoid in flexion. The compaction

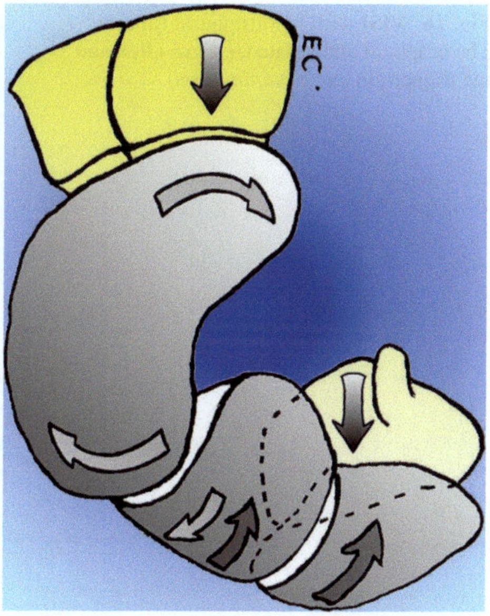

Fig. 14 Carpal proximal row in equilibrium. Scaphoid flexion counterbalances triquetrum extension

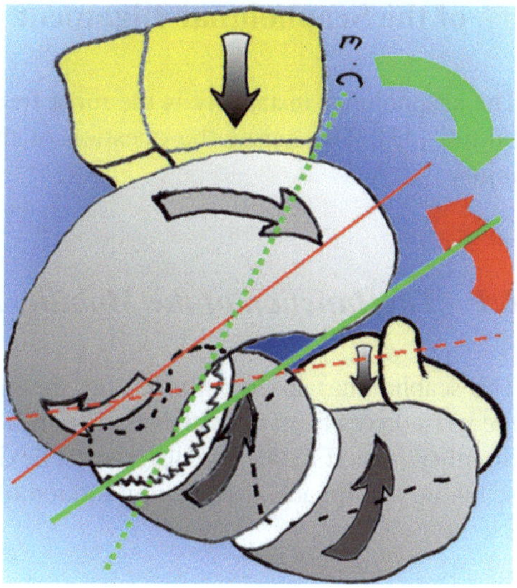

Fig. 15 DISI with scapholunar ligament rupture. The scaphoid flexes (*green axis*) and the lunate (*red axis*) and triquetrum extend

strengths on the ulnar column of the wrist extend the triquetrum which drives the proximal row in the same direction [40].

During the grasp, the compaction strengths of the carpus are global. The radial strengths which flex the proximal row are counterbalanced by the ulnar strengths which extend the proximal row. The carpal proximal row is thus in a state of balance under pressure (Fig. 14). At that stage, the injury of one of the intrinsic ligaments can make the lunate go out from its axis, with DISI (Fig. 15) or VISI (Fig. 16).

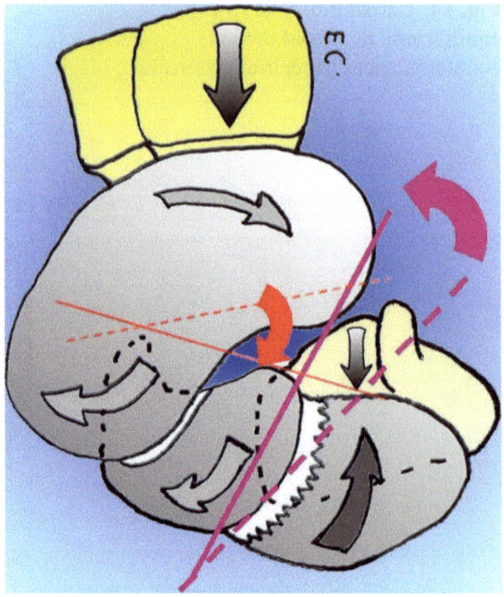

Fig. 16 VISI with lunotriquetral rupture. The scaphoid and lunate (*red axis*) flex and the triquetrum extends (*pink axis*)

6 Particular Factors of Vulnerability of the Scapholunar Ligament

The scapholunar instability is the most frequent of the post-traumatic carpal instabilities [43]. This raises the question of the factors which facilitate this frequent injury.

6.1 The Junction of the Mobility Main Lines

The scapholunar space is the seat of the maximal constraints of movements when the wrist drives from flexion to extension. This is where the main lines of intracarpal mobility cross (Fig. 4). The differential flexion/extension value is about 30° between scaphoid and lunate, absorbed by torsion of the ligament [40].

6.2 The Capitate's Transmitted Pressure

The head of the capitate is just facing the scapholunar ligament in the neutral position and in the ulnar tilt of the carpus. In case of axial load, the head tends to dissociate the scapholunar space as a quoin [80]. This becomes obvious in case of scapholunate collapse with the shortening of the carpal height. The head of the capitate is usually locked in the scapholunar space.

6.3 Concentration and Reverse Absorption of Pressures

The lunate is in equilibrium when it is under pressure (*see above*: *balance of the proximal row*). It remains in a neutral position as it absorbs the flexion constraints transmitted by the scaphoid and the extension constraints transmitted by the triquetrum. Since most of the axial loads are directed towards the radius via the scaphoid, the loads which flex the scaphoid are stronger than the loads of the ulnar column which extend the triquetrum. This should result in an imbalance in flexion of the whole carpal proximal row. But the lunate often has a dorsal horn which is thinner than the palmar horn [81]. The axial pressure transmitted by the capitate thus helps the triquetrum to extend the lunate. The triquetrolunate ligament is not the only piece that maintains the lunate in equilibrium. This ligament is thus less affected than the scapholunar ligament in overload injuries.

7 Conclusion

Because the scapholunar ligament is exposed to axial constraints of mobility and loads, it represents a weak point of the proximal row. But it is protected by quite a complete system of extrinsic ligaments which contribute to unify the wrist. There are a palmar ligamentous plane, a dorsal ligamentous plane and a distal scaphoidal ligamentous complex. The different tendons around the wrist can also have a cohesion effect of the carpus. A ligamentous injury is less likely to happen if the scapholunar ligament is unaffected. In that case, the lunotriquetral ligament is most likely injured. Seldom the extrinsic ligaments can be the only one to be affected, astride on the radiocarpal or the mediocarpal spaces. Once all the biomechanical aspects are put together, it is possible to understand the different mechanisms of the carpal collapse, which result from the application of the mechanical loads to the carpus, badly absorbed or badly redirected, by bones badly locked when they should sustain load. The different ligament injuries explain the varieties of carpal instabilities. Consequently, clinical, paraclinical and arthroscopic exams have to explore those different ligamentous restraints for the best. This aims to enable a ligamentous repair as physiological as possible.

References

1. Destot E (1905) Lésions du poignet et accidents du travail. Vigot, Paris
2. Wagner CJ (1956) Perilunar dislocations. J Bone Joint Surg 38 A:1198–1207
3. Linscheid R, Dobyns JH, Beabout JW, Bryan RS (1972) Traumatic instability of the wrist. J Bone Joint Surg 54-A:1612–1632
4. Meyrueis JP, Cameli M, Pan P (1978) Instabilité du carpe. Diagnostic et formes cliniques. Ann Chir 32:555–560

5. Allieu Y et al (1984) Table ronde sur l'instabilité du carpe. Ann Chir Main 3:277–367
6. Gilula LA, Destouet JM, Weeks PM, Young LV, Wray RC (1984) Roentgenographic diagnosis of the painful wrist. Clin Orthop Relat Res 187:52–64
7. Mayfield JK (1984) Patterns of injury to carpal ligaments. Clin Orthop Relat Res 187:36–42
8. Kuhlmann N (1979) Les mécanismes de l'articulation du poignet. Ann Chir 33:711–719
9. Lanoy JF, Mazas Y, Mazas F, Rengeval JP (1982) Etude radiologique des centres de rotation du poignet. Ann Chir Main 1:227–232
10. Schernberg F, Gérard Y (1983) L'exploration radiologique du poignet. Rev Chir Orthop 69:521–531
11. Kapandji A (1987) Biomécanique du carpe et du poignet. Ann Chir Main 6:147–169
12. Schernberg F (1990) Roentgenographic examination of the wrist. J Hand Surg 15B:210–228
13. Sennwald GR, Zdravkovic V, Kern HP, Jacob H (1993) Kinematics of the wrist and its ligaments. J Hand Surg 18A:805–814
14. Craigen MA, Stanley JK (1995) Wrist kinematics. Row, column or both? J Hand Surg 20B:165–170
15. Garcia-Elias M, Ribe M, Rodriguez J, Cots M, Casas J (1995) Influence of joint laxity on scaphoid kinematics. J Hand Surg 20B:379–382
16. Nuttall D, Trail IA, Stanley JK (1998) Movement of the scaphoid in the normal wrist. J Hand Surg Br 23:762–764
17. Camus EJ, Millot F, Larivière J, Rtaimate M, Raoult S (2008) The double-cup carpus: a demonstration of the variable geometry of the carpus. Chir Main 27(1):12–19
18. Youm Y, Mcmurtry RY, Flatt A, Gillespie TE (1978) Kinematics of the wrist. J Bone Joint Surg 60 A:423–431
19. Kuhlmann N, Gallaire M, Pineau H (1978) Déplacements du scaphoïde et du semi-lunaire au cours des mouvements du poignet. Ann Chir 32:543–553
20. De Lange A, Kauer JM, Huiskes R (1985) Kinematic behaviour of the human wrist joint: a roentgen-stereophotogrammetric analysis. J Orthop Res 3:56–64
21. Ruby LK, Cooney WP, An KN, Linscheid RL, Chao EY (1988) Relative motion of selected carpal bones: a kinematic analysis of the normal wrist. J Hand Surg 13A:1–10
22. Savelberg HH, Koolos JG, De Lange A, Huiskes R, Kauer JM (1991) Human carpal recruitment and three-dimensional carpal motion. Orthop Res 9:693–704
23. Kobayashi M, Berger RA, Nagy L, Linscheid RL, Ushiyama S, Ritt M, An KN (1997) Normal kinematics of carpal bones: a three dimensional analysis of carpal bone motion relative to the radius. J Biomech 30:787–793
24. Berger RA, Crowninshield RD, Flatt AE (1982) The three-dimensional rotational behaviors of the carpal bones. Clin Orthop 167:303–310
25. Berger RA, Blair WF, Crowninshield RD, Flatt AE (1982) The scapholunate ligament. J Hand Surg 7A:87–91
26. Werner FW, Short WH, Fortino MD, Palmer AK (1997) The relative contribution of selected carpal bones to global wrist motion during simulated planar and out-of-plane wrist motion. J Hand Surg 22A:708–713
27. Ishikawa JI, Cooney WP, Niebur G, An KN, Minami A, Kaneda K (1999) The effects of wrist distraction on carpal kinematics. J Hand Surg 24A:113–120
28. Crisco JJ, Mcgovern RD, Wolfe SW (1999) Noninvasive technique for measuring in vivo three-dimensional carpal bone kinematics. J Orthop Res 17:96–100
29. Moojen TM, Snel JG, Ritt MJ, Kauer JM, Venema HW, Bos KE (2002) Three-dimensional carpal kinematics in vivo. Clin Biomech 17:506–514
30. Moutet F, Chapel A, Cinquin PH, Rosepitet L (1990) Imagerie du carpe en trois dimensions. Ann Chir Main Mbre Sup 9:32–37
31. Patterson RM, Nicodemus CL, Viegas SF, Elder KW, Rosenblatt J (1998) High-speed, three-dimensional kinematic analysis of the normal wrist. J Hand Surg 23A:446–453
32. Moritomo H, Viegas SF, Elder K, Nakamura K, Dasilva MF, Patterson RM (2000) The scapho-trapezio-trapezoidal joint. Part 2: a kinematic study. J Hand Surg 25A:911–920

33. Wolfe SW, Crisco JJ, Katz LD (1997) A non-invasive method for studying in vivo carpal kinematics. J Hand Surg 22B:147–152
34. Sun JS, Shih TTF, Ko CM, Chang CH, Hang YS, Hou SM (2000) In vivo kinematic study of normal wrist motion: an ultrafast computed tomographic study. Clin Biomech 15:212–216
35. Patterson RM, Elder KW, Viegas SF, Buford WL (1995) Carpal bone anatomy measured by computer analysis of three-dimensional reconstructions of computed tomography images. J Hand Surg 20A:923–929
36. Feipel V, Rooze M (1999) Three-dimensional motion patterns of the carpal bones: an in-vivo study using three-dimensional computed tomography and clinical applications. Surg Radiol Anat 21:125–131
37. Wolfe SW, Neu C, Crisco JJ (2000) In vivo scaphoid, lunate and capitate kinematics in flexion and in extension. J Hand Surg 25A:860–869
38. Moojen TM, Snel JG, Ritt MJ, Venema HW, Kauer JM, Bos KE (2002) Scaphoid kinematics in vivo. J Hand Surg 27A:1003–1010
39. Moojen TM, Snel JG, Ritt MJ, Venema HW, Kauer JM, Bos KE (2003) In vivo analysis of carpal kinematics and comparative review of the literature. J Hand Surg 28A:81–87
40. Camus EJ, Millot F, Larivière J, Rtaimate M, Raoult S (2004) Kinematics of the wrist using 2D and 3D analysis. Biomechanical and clinical deductions. Surg Radiol Anat 26:399–410
41. Ritt MJ, Bishop AT, Berger RA, Linscheid RL, Berglund LJ, An KN (1998) Lunotriquetral ligament properties: a comparison of three anatomic subregions. J Hand Surg Am 23:425–431
42. Ritt MJ, Linscheid RL, 3rd Cooney WP, Berger RA, An KN (1998) The lunotriquetral joint: kinematic effects of sequential ligament sectioning, ligament repair, and arthrodesis. J Hand Surg Am 23(3):432–445
43. Mitsuyasu H, Patterson RM, Shah MA, Buford WL, Iwamoto Y, Viegas SF (2004) The role of the dorsal intercarpal ligament in dynamic and static scapholunate instability. J Hand Surg Am 29(2):279–288
44. Short WH, Werner FW, Green JK, Weiner MM, Masaoka S (2002) The effect of sectioning the dorsal radiocarpal ligament and insertion of a pressure sensor into the radiocarpal joint on scaphoid and lunate kinematics. J Hand Surg Am 27(1):68–76
45. Larsen CF, Amadio PC, Gilula LA, Hodge JC (1995) Analysis of carpal instability: I. Description of the scheme. J Hand Surg Am 20(5):757–764
46. Hodge JC, Gilula LA, Larsen CF, Amadio PC (1995) Analysis of carpal instability: II. Clinical applications. J Hand Surg Am 20(5):765–776
47. Viegas SF, Yamaguchi S, Boyd NL, Patterson R (1999) The dorsal ligament of the wrist: anatomy, mechanical properties, and function. J Hand Surg 24A:456–468
48. Ishiko T, Puttlitz CM, Lotz JC, Diao E (2003) Scaphoid behavior after division of the transverse carpal ligament. J Hand Surg 28A:267–271
49. Mayfield JK, Johnson RP, Kilcoyne RK (1980) Carpal dislocations: pathomechanics and progressive perilunar instability. J Hand Surg 5A:226–241
50. Short WH, Werner FW, Fortino MD, Palmer AK, Mann KA (1995) A dynamic biomechanical study of scapholunate ligament sectioning. J Hand Surg 20A:986–999
51. Kapandji AI, Martin-Bouyer Y, Verdeille S (1991) Three-dimensional CT study of the carpus under pronation-supination constraints. Ann Chir Main 10:36–47 [French]
52. Linscheid RL, Dobyns JH (2002) Dynamic carpal stability. Keio J Med 51:140–147
53. Koebke J, Fehrmann P, Mockenhaupt J (1989) Stress on the normal and pathologic wrist joint. Handchir Mikrochir Plast Chir 21:127–133
54. Werner FW, Glisson RR, Murphy DJ, Palmer AK (1986) Force transmission trough the radioulnar carpal joint: effect of ulnar lengthening and shortening. Handchir Mikrochir Plast Chir 18:304–308
55. Hara T, Horii E, An KN, Cooney WP, Linscheid RL, Chao EY (1992) Force distribution across the wrist joint: application of pressure-sensitive conductive rubber. J Hand Surg 17A:339–347

56. Schuind F, Cooney WP, Linscheid RL, An KN, Chao EYS (1995) Force and pressure transmission trough the normal wrist. A theoretical two-dimensional study in the posteroanterior plane. J Biomech 28:587–601
57. Genda E, Horii E (2000) Theoretical stress analysis in wrist joint – neutral position and functional position. J Hand Surg 25B:292–295
58. Sato S (1995) Load transmission trough the wrist joint: a biomechanical study comparing the normal and pathological wrist (abstract, art in Japanese). Nippon Seikeigeka Gakkai Zasshi 69:470–483
59. Dufour M, Pillu M (2006) Biomécanique fonctionnelle. Issy-les-Moulineaux/Elsevier, Masson [French], pp 371
60. Kaufmann RA, Pfaeffle HJ, Blankenhorn BD, Stabile K, Robertson D, Goitz R (2006) Kinematics of the midcarpal and radiocarpal joint in flexion and extension: an in vitro study. J Hand Surg 31A:1142–1148
61. Kuhlmann JN (2002) La stabilité et les instabilités radio- et médio-carpiennes. Sauramps Médical, Montpellier
62. Berger RA, Imeada T, Berglund L, An KN (1999) Constraint and material properties of the subregions of the scapholunate interosseous ligament. J Hand Surg 24A:953–962
63. Short WH, Werner FW, Green JK, Masaoka S (2002) Biomechanical evaluation of ligamentous stabilizers of the scaphoid and lunate. J Hand Surg 27A:991–1002
64. Short WH, Werner FW, Green JK, Masaoka S (2005) Biomechanical evaluation of ligamentous stabilizers of the scaphoid and lunate: part II. J Hand Surg 30A:24–34
65. Short WH, Werner FW, Green JK, Masaoka S (2007) Biomechanical evaluation of ligamentous stabilizers of the scaphoid and lunate: part III. J Hand Surg 32A:297.e1–297.e18
66. Sennwald GR, Zdravkovic V, Oberlin C (1994) The anatomy of the palmar scaphotriquetral ligament. J Hand Surg 76B:147–149
67. Tang JB, Ryu J, Kish V (1997) Scapholunate interosseous ligament sectioning adversely affects excursions of radial wrist extensor and flexor tendons. J Hand Surg 22A:720–725
68. Berger RA (2001) The anatomy of the ligaments of the wrist and distal radioulnar joints. Clin Orthop Relat Res Feb (383):32–40
69. Moritomo H, Viegas SF, Elder K, Nakamura K, Dasilva MF, Patterson RM (2000) The scapho-trapezio-trapezoidal joint. Part 1: an anatomic and radiographic study. J Hand Surg 25A:899–910
70. Slutsky DJ (2008) The incidence of dorsal radiocarpal ligament tears in patients having diagnostic wrist arthroscopy for wrist pain. J Hand Surg 33A:332–334
71. Gayet LE, Texereau J, Condroyer A, Duport G, Clarac JP (2000) Modélisation cinématique du carpe et instabilité. Rev Chir Orthop 86(suppl II):87 [French]
72. Sicre G, Laulan J, Rouleau B (1997) Scaphotrapeziotrapezoid osteoarthritis after scaphotrapezial ligament injury. J Hand Surg 22B:189–190
73. Herren DB, Lehmann O, Simmen BR (1998) Does trapeziectomy destabilize the carpus? J Hand Surg 23B:676–679
74. Garcia-Elias M, Lluch AL, Farreres A, Castillo F, Saffar P (1999) Resection of the distal scaphoid for scaphotrapeziotrapezoid osteoarthritis. J Hand Surg 24B:448–452
75. Saffar P, Semaan I (1994) The study of the biomechanics of wrist movements in an oblique plane. A preliminary report. In: Schuind F, An KN, Cooney WP III, Garcia-Elias M (eds) Advances in the biomechanics of the hand and wrist. Plenum Press, New York, NATO ASI Series A: life sciences. Vol. 256: pp 305–311
76. Moritomo H, Apergis EP, Herzberg G, Werner FW, Wolfe SW, Garcia-Elias M (2007) IFSSH committee report of wrist biomechanics committee: biomechanics of the so-called dart-throwing motion of the wrist. J Hand Surg 32A:1447–1453
77. Masquelet AC, Strube F, Nordin JY (1993) The isolated scapho-trapezio-trapezoid ligament injury. Diagnosis and surgical treatment in four cases. J Hand Surg 18B:730–735
78. Cowey AJ, Carmont MR, Tins B, Ford DJ (2007) Flexor carpi radialis rupture reined in! Inj Extra 38(3):90–93 (Elsevier Online)

79. Verkellen K, Dauwe D, Demuynck M, Kestelijn P, Vanden Berghe L (1992) Spontaneous ruptures of the flexor carpi radialis tendon secondary to STT osteoarthritis. Acta Orthop Belg 58:474–476
80. Oberlin C (1990) Carpal instability and desaxations. Anatomical bases. Clinical and Radiologic study. Elsevier – conférence d'enseignement de la SOFCOT. 38:235–50 [French]
81. Watson HK, Yasuda M, Guidera PM (1996) Lateral lunate morphology: an X-ray study. J Hand Surg 21A:759–763

Clinical Examination of Wrist Ligaments

C. Rizzo, J. Garret, V. Guigal, and A. Gazarian

1 Introduction

The wrist was considered to be a single bone up until 1860; over a century and a half with the progress of imaging techniques, it has currently become by far the most complex articulation of the human skeleton.

Imaging is necessary to establish the diagnosis of posttraumatic lesions as well as the choice of their treatment but needs to be guided by a meticulous clinical examination. This clinical examination dictates the choice of complementary investigations as well as which questions these investigations should answer.

2 Conditions of the Examination

Patient and examiner comfort are essential. They should be sitting facing each other separated by an examination table the height of a desk (about 1 m) and a width not exceeding 60 cm; if too wide, it would force the examiner to lean forwards; too narrow would be insufficient to allow the patient to extend the forearm while relaxing both the elbow and the hand simultaneously.

The patient should be sitting at the right height with both forearms bare till above the elbow to allow examination of the contralateral wrist (Fig. 1).

C. Rizzo (✉) • J. Garret • V. Guigal • A. Gazarian
Hand and Upper Extremity Unit,
Clinique du Parc,
Lyon 69006, France
e-mail: c.rizzo@cliniqueduparclyon.com; j.garret@cliniqueduparclyon.com

E. Camus, L. Van Overstraeten (eds.), *Carpal Ligament Surgery*,
DOI 10.1007/978-2-8178-0379-1_3, © Springer-Verlag France 2013

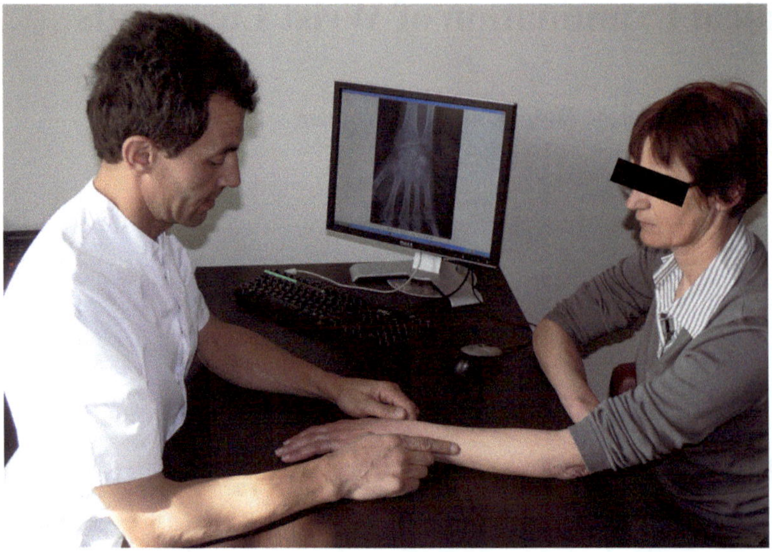

Fig. 1 Examination setup with the examiner and patient facing each other across a table of appropriate height and width

3 History Taking

This is the first part of the examination and is essential to orient the diagnosis. Age of the patient must be noted, the affected and dominant sides, his/her work and hobbies (sports, music, gardening, etc.). General history of the patient is first noted and then any symptoms present before the actual presenting symptoms (reason for consultation) followed by the date and circumstances of the trauma and the consequences. When the examination is conducted much later than the initial trauma, the examiner must strive to determine the main complaint of the patient.

3.1 General History

General history is taken including pathology that can affect treatment results, e.g. diabetes and tobacco.

3.2 Local History

Any ipsilateral upper limb pathology must be noted and considered; this can modify therapeutic indications.

3.3 Circumstances of the Injury

It is important to identify the circumstances of the trauma (fall from height while walking, skiing, car accident…) and specify if it is a low- or high-energy injury and if it is a domestic, sports or work accident and try to describe the mechanism of trauma as precisely as possible: direct or indirect, in forced extension or flexion, with impact on radial, ulnar or median nerves.

Hyperextension injuries, for example, orient towards a diagnosis of scapholunate lesion if the impact is to the thenar eminence and towards a TFCC lesion if it is directed to the hypothenar side, as do injuries in forced rotation 'reverse drill'.

The date of the accident sometimes becomes difficult to determine when it goes back weeks, months or even years before presentation but is directly relevant to the choice of treatment.

4 Pain

This is the most important symptom and several points are important to clarify during examination.

4.1 Site

It is crucial to get the patient to pinpoint the pain even if it is rarely excruciating in wrist ligament injuries.

The patient often just points to the whole wrist declaring 'my wrist is painful'.

The examiner should get the patient to specify whether pain is palmar or dorsal or in the inside of the wrist and then further localize it to the radial, ulnar or middle of the wrist.

It is useful to get the patient to use a finger to actually point out the point of maximal pain intensity. This simple gesture is very useful to guide the rest of the clinical examination.

4.2 Circumstances of Onset

Is the pain permanent, upon intense effort or on certain movements? It may be triggered by simple flexion/extension or by more complex movements such as extension with ulnar inclination or with certain actions such as pressure on the hand to lift oneself out of a chair, open a jar or hold a cooking pan. All these elements specified during the examination will help localize the site of pain and its repercussions on the use of the wrist.

4.3 Pain Intensity

This may be evaluated by the visual analogue scale that gives a numerical measurement reproducible for a series of examinations.

4.4 Functional Disability

It is important that the patient himself specifies the disabling effect of pain on the wrist, both on daily activities – such as opening a door, a jam jar or carrying a bottle of water – as well as professional ones. Validated and accepted questionnaires may be used. A comprehensive list of all the questionnaires is beyond the scope of this book, but the two most used globally are the DASH (disability of the arm, shoulder and hand) (Fig. 2) developed in 1994 by representatives of the Institute for Work and Health (IWH) and the American Academy of Orthopaedic Surgeons (AAOS) and translated from American to French by Dubert et al. [2] and the PRWE (patient-rated wrist evaluation) score developed by MacDermid in 1998 (Fig. 3) [3]. Besides being filled out by the patient far from surgeon' s influence, these are reproducible from one patient to another as well as for the same patient from one consultation to the next.

5 Sounds and Abnormal Phenomena

5.1 Benign Clicks

These are totally painless and fully reproducible at will without apprehension or discomfort. They are pneumatic such as generated upon forced flexion 'cracking' the metacarpophalangeal or proximal phalangeal joints.

5.2 Triggering

This is palpable, audible and sometimes visible. It can be benign in hyperlax wrists, but is most frequently pathological, with pain and sometimes apprehension. In this case it indicates scapholunate, lunotriquetral or midcarpal instability. The examination will attempt to then trace its origin.

5.3 Pathological Clicking

These are painful without obvious triggering and are provoked by specific movements. Ulnar clicking may denote underlying TFCC rupture.

Disabilities of the Arm, Shoulder and Hand

THE DASH

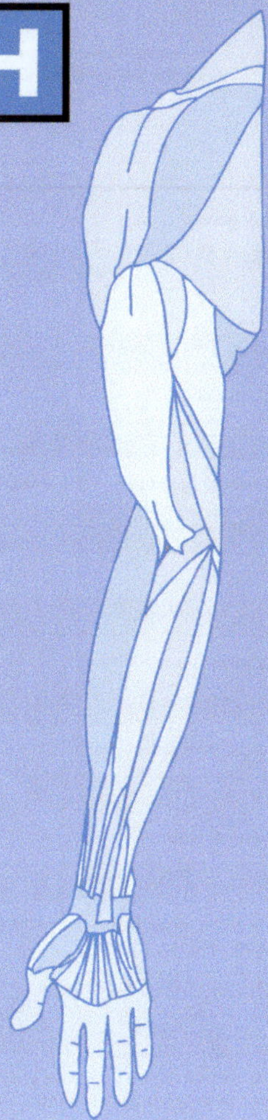

INSTRUCTIONS

This questionnaire asks about your symptoms as well as your ability to perform certain activities.

Please answer *every question*, based on your condition in the last week, by circling the appropriate number.

If you did not have the opportunity to perform an activity in the past week, please make your *best estimate* on which response would be the most accurate.

It doesn't matter which hand or arm you use to perform the activity; please answer based on your ability regardless of how you perform the task.

Fig. 2 DASH score (disability of arm, shoulder and hand) [2]

Disabilities of the Arm, Shoulder and Hand

Please rate your ability to do the following activities in the last week by circling the number below the appropriate response.

	NO DIFFICULTY	MILD DIFFICULTY	MODERATE DIFFICULTY	SEVERE DIFFICULTY	UNABLE
1. Open a tight or new jar.	1	2	3	4	5
2. Write.	1	2	3	4	5
3. Turn a key.	1	2	3	4	5
4. Prepare a meal.	1	2	3	4	5
5. Push open a heavy door.	1	2	3	4	5
6. Place an object on a shelf above your head.	1	2	3	4	5
7. Do heavy household chores (e.g., wash walls, wash floors).	1	2	3	4	5
8. Garden or do yard work.	1	2	3	4	5
9. Make a bed.	1	2	3	4	5
10. Carry a shopping bag or briefcase.	1	2	3	4	5
11. Carry a heavy object (over 10 lbs).	1	2	3	4	5
12. Change a lightbulb overhead.	1	2	3	4	5
13. Wash or blow dry your hair.	1	2	3	4	5
14. Wash your back.	1	2	3	4	5
15. Put on a pullover sweater.	1	2	3	4	5
16. Use a knife to cut food.	1	2	3	4	5
17. Recreational activities which require little effort (e.g., cardplaying, knitting, etc.).	1	2	3	4	5
18. Recreational activities in which you take some force or impact through your arm, shoulder or hand (e.g., golf, hammering, tennis, etc.).	1	2	3	4	5
19. Recreational activities in which you move your arm freely (e.g., playing frisbee, badminton, etc.).	1	2	3	4	5
20. Manage transportation needs (getting from one place to another).	1	2	3	4	5
21. Sexual activities.	1	2	3	4	5

Fig. 2 (continued)

DISABILITIES OF THE ARM, SHOULDER AND HAND

	NOT AT ALL	SLIGHTLY	MODERATELY	QUITE A BIT	EXTREMELY
22. During the past week, *to what extent* has your arm, shoulder or hand problem interfered with your normal social activities with family, friends, neighbours or groups? *(circle number)*	1	2	3	4	5

	NOT LIMITED AT ALL	SLIGHTLY LIMITED	MODERATELY LIMITED	VERY LIMITED	UNABLE
23. During the past week, were you limited in your work or other regular daily activities as a result of your arm, shoulder or hand problem? *(circle number)*	1	2	3	4	5

Please rate the severity of the following symptoms in the last week. *(circle number)*

	NONE	MILD	MODERATE	SEVERE	EXTREME
24. Arm, shoulder or hand pain.	1	2	3	4	5
25. Arm, shoulder or hand pain when you performed any specific activity.	1	2	3	4	5
26. Tingling (pins and needles) in your arm, shoulder or hand.	1	2	3	4	5
27. Weakness in your arm, shoulder or hand.	1	2	3	4	5
28. Stiffness in your arm, shoulder or hand.	1	2	3	4	5

	NO DIFFICULTY	MILD DIFFICULTY	MODERATE DIFFICULTY	SEVERE DIFFICULTY	SO MUCH DIFFICULTY THAT I CAN'T SLEEP
29. During the past week, how much difficulty have you had sleeping because of the pain in your arm, shoulder or hand? *(circle number)*	1	2	3	4	5

	STRONGLY DISAGREE	DISAGREE	NEITHER AGREE NOR DISAGREE	AGREE	STRONGLY AGREE
30. I feel less capable, less confident or less useful because of my arm, shoulder or hand problem. *(circle number)*	1	2	3	4	5

DASH DISABILITY/SYMPTOM SCORE = $\left[\left(\frac{\text{sum of n responses}}{n}\right) - 1\right] \times 25$, where n is equal to the number of completed responses.

A DASH score may <u>not</u> be calculated if there are greater than 3 missing items.

Fig. 2 (continued)

Disabilities of the Arm, Shoulder and Hand

WORK MODULE (OPTIONAL)

The following questions ask about the impact of your arm, shoulder or hand problem on your ability to work (including home-making if that is your main work role).

Please indicate what your job/work is:__________

❒ I do not work. (You may skip this section.)

Please circle the number that best describes your physical ability in the past week. Did you have any difficulty:

	NO DIFFICULTY	MILD DIFFICULTY	MODERATE DIFFICULTY	SEVERE DIFFICULTY	UNABLE
1. using your usual technique for your work?	1	2	3	4	5
2. doing your usual work because of arm, shoulder or hand pain?	1	2	3	4	5
3. doing your work as well as you would like?	1	2	3	4	5
4. spending your usual amount of time doing your work?	1	2	3	4	5

SPORTS/PERFORMING ARTS MODULE (OPTIONAL)

The following questions relate to the impact of your arm, shoulder or hand problem on playing *your musical instrument or sport or both*. If you play more than one sport or instrument (or play both), please answer with respect to that activity which is most important to you.

Please indicate the sport or instrument which is most important to you:__________

❒ I do not play a sport or an instrument. (You may skip this section.)

Please circle the number that best describes your physical ability in the past week. Did you have any difficulty:

	NO DIFFICULTY	MILD DIFFICULTY	MODERATE DIFFICULTY	SEVERE DIFFICULTY	UNABLE
1. using your usual technique for playing your instrument or sport?	1	2	3	4	5
2. playing your musical instrument or sport because of arm, shoulder or hand pain?	1	2	3	4	5
3. playing your musical instrument or sport as well as you would like?	1	2	3	4	5
4. spending your usual amount of time practising or playing your instrument or sport?	1	2	3	4	5

SCORING THE OPTIONAL MODULES: Add up assigned values for each response; divide by 4 (number of items); subtract 1; multiply by 25.
An optional module score may <u>not</u> be calculated if there are any missing items.

Institute for Work & Health | Research Excellence Advancing Employee Health

Fig. 2 (continued)

PATIENT-RATED WRIST EVALUATION

Name ______________________________ Date ______________________________

The questions below will help or understand how much difficulty you have had with your wrist in the past week. You will be describing your ***average*** *wrist symptoms* ***over the past week*** *on a scale of 0 to 10.* **Please provide an answer for ALL questions. If you did not perform an activity, please ESTIMATE the pain or difficulty you would expect.** If you have **never** performed an activity, you may leave it blank.

I. PAIN

Rate the average amount of pain in your wrist over the past week by circling the number that best describes your pain on a scale from 0 to 10, A zero (0) means that you did not have any pain and a ten (10) means that you had the worst pain you have ever experienced or that you could not do the activity because of pain.

Sample scale:	0 No pain	1	2	3	4	5	6	7	8	9	10 Worst ever
RATE YOUR PAIN:											
At rest	0	1	2	3	4	5	6	7	8	9	10
When doing a task with a repeated wrist movement	0	1	2	3	4	5	6	7	8	9	10
When lifting a heavy object	0	1	2	3	4	5	6	7	8	9	10
When it is at its worst	0	1	2	3	4	5	6	7	8	9	10
How often do you have pain?	0 Never	1	2	3	4	5	6	7	8	9	10 Always

2. FUNCTION

A. SPECIFIC ACTIVITIES

Rate the ***amount of difficulty*** *you experienced performing each of the items listed below, over the past week, by circling the number that describes your difficulty on a scale of 0 to 10. A zero (0) means you did not experience any difficulty and a ten (10) means it was so difficult you were unable to do it at all.*

Sample scale:	0 No difficulty	1	2	3	4	5	6	7	8	9	10 Unable to do
Turn a door knob using my affected hand	0	1	2	3	4	5	6	7	8	9	10
Cut meat using a knife with my affected hand	0	1	2	3	4	5	6	7	8	9	10
Fasten buttons on my shirt	0	1	2	3	4	5	6	7	8	9	10
Use my affected hand to push up from a chair	0	1	2	3	4	5	6	7	8	9	10
Carry a 10-pound object in my affected hand	0	1	2	3	4	5	6	7	8	9	10
Use bathroom tissue with my affected hand	0	1	2	3	4	5	6	7	8	9	10

B. USUAL ACTIVITIES

Rate the ***amount of difficulty*** *you experienced performing your usual activities on each of the areas listed below over the past week, by circling the number that best describes your difficulty on a scale of 0 to 10. By "usual activities," we mean the activities you performed before you started having a problem with your wrist. A zero (0) means that you did not experience any difficulty and a ten (10) means it was so difficult you were unable to do any of your usual activities.*

Personal care activities (dressing, washing)	0	1	2	3	4	5	6	7	8	9	10
Household work (cleaning, maintenance)	0	1	2	3	4	5	6	7	8	9	10
Work (your job or usual everyday work)	0	1	2	3	4	5	6	7	8	9	10
Recreational activities	0	1	2	3	4	5	6	7	8	9	10

Fig. 3 PRWE score (patient-rated wrist evaluation) developed by MacDermid et al. [3]

5.4 *Other Presentations*

These are usually associated with primary complaints discussed previously, and the examiner needs to help the patient accurately describe them. A frequent presentation is stiffness usually in flexion-extension or pronosupination and rarely in radial or ulnar inclination. Another is decreased force – usually secondary to pain.

5.5 Inspection

This is usually normal in chronic or subacute (more than 6 weeks) ligament injuries. A dorsal subluxation of the ulnar head may sometimes indicate distal radioulnar dislocation. In recent injuries, diffuse oedema is usual and adds little to the examination.

6 Clinical Measurements

6.1 Mobility

Active and passive mobility is compared to the contralateral side.

Flexion-extension:

The patient sits facing the examiner with the elbow on the table, the forearm vertical. The goniometer is placed on the dorsal aspect of the hand, wrist and forearm in flexion and palmarly in extension (Fig. 4). Normal values are approximately 80° and 70°, respectively [1].

6.2 Pronosupination

It is measured with elbow to trunk, flexed at 90°, and forearm horizontal. It is more difficult than flexion-extension and approximate measures should be avoided. A limb of the goniometer placed vertically in the axis of the arm and the other in the plane of the hand with the eye of the examiner at patient's hand level gives more precise readings (Fig. 5). Normal values of pronation and supination are 70–85° and 90°, respectively [1].

6.3 Radial and Ulnar Inclination

The hand is in supination with the goniometer placed on the dorsum of the forearm, wrist and hand, one limb along the third finger and the other in the axis of the mid-forearm (Fig. 6). Ulnar inclination is usually up to 40°, while radially it rarely exceeds 20°.

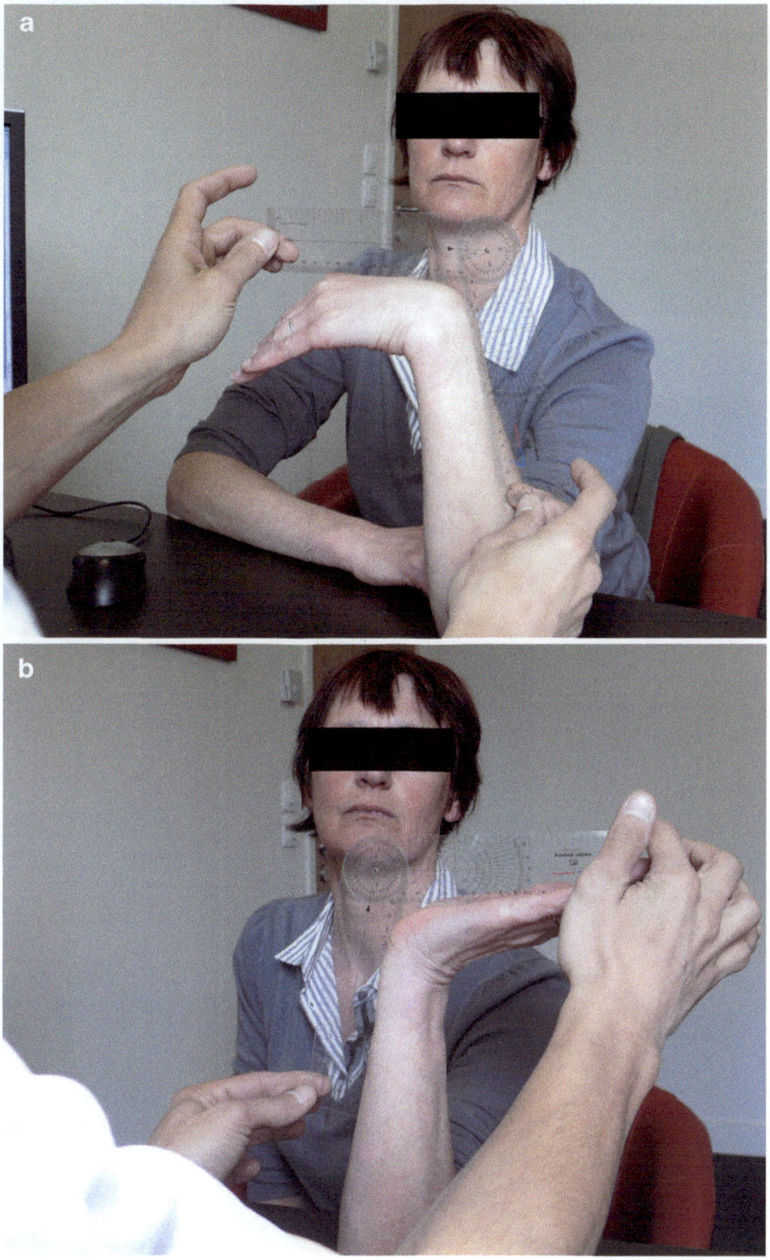

Fig. 4 Measurement of flexion (**a**) and extension (**b**) using the goniometer

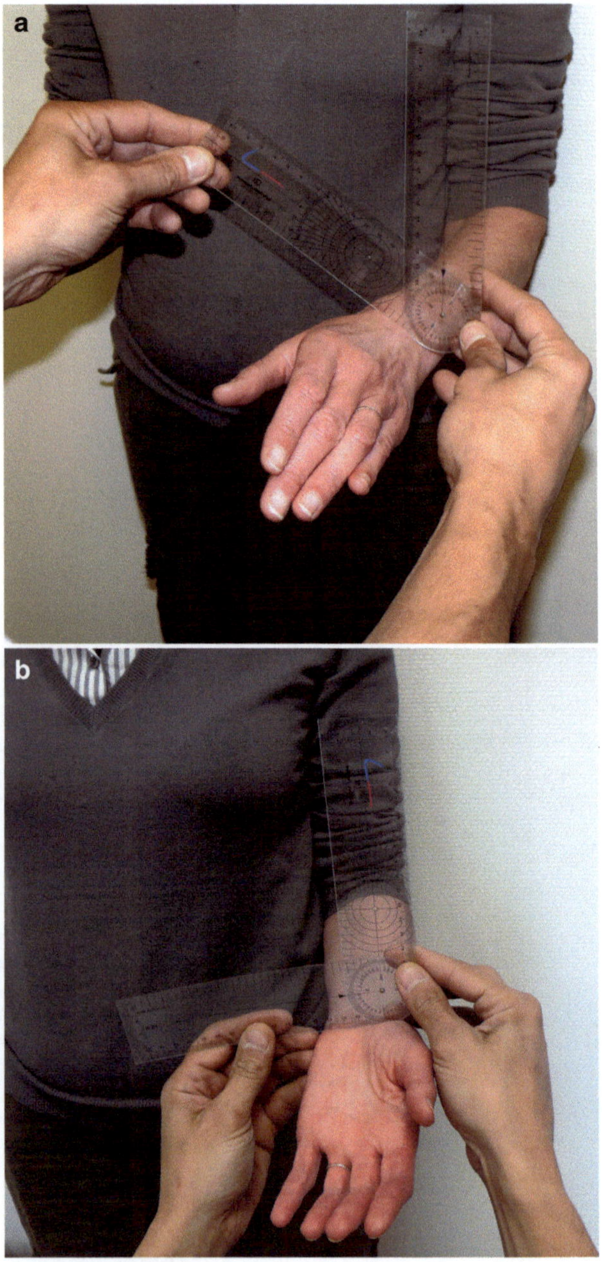

Fig. 5 Measurement of pronation (**a**) and supination (**b**) using the goniometer

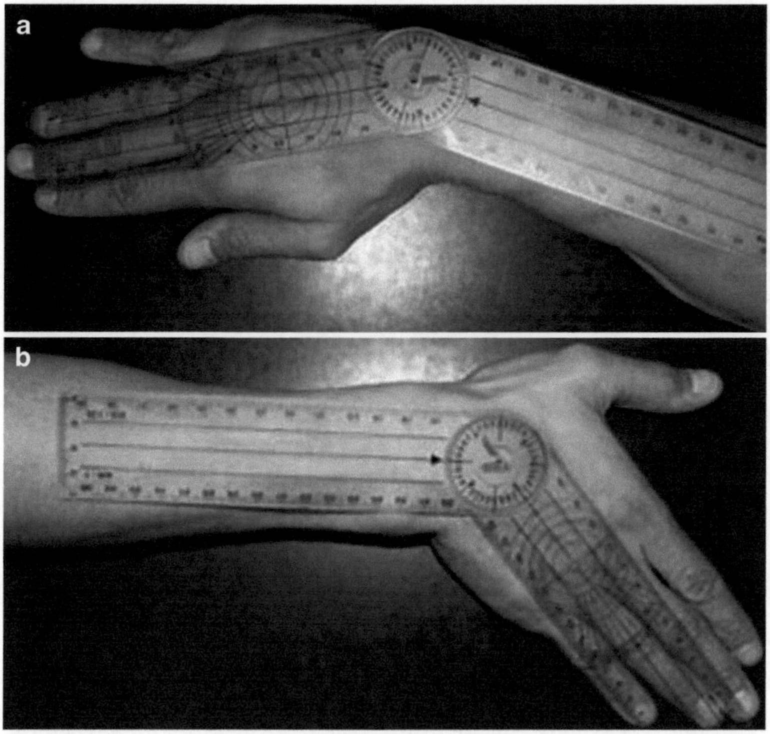

Fig. 6 Measurement of radial (**a**) and ulnar (**b**) inclination using the goniometer

7 Force

7.1 Grip Strength

Strength is measured using a dynamometer 'grip strength' (Fig. 7).

When a mechanical Jamar dynamometer is used, it should neither be too large nor too narrow and should be adjusted to the second spacing as shown by a study on 288 patients – 89 % of whom attained maximum force in this position [4]. The elbow is placed on the table, without resting the forearm, wrist or hand (Fig. 8).

Three measurements are taken for each side alternating rapidly between pathological and contralateral sides to detect potential malingerers. The patient is asked to grip strongly, maximally and briefly. This attitude seems the most logical and widely accepted; however, Haider et al. – in a study on 100 healthy volunteers – showed that the maximum values noted in a single measurement and the average of three measurements showed the same variation (about ±8 kg) and showed no

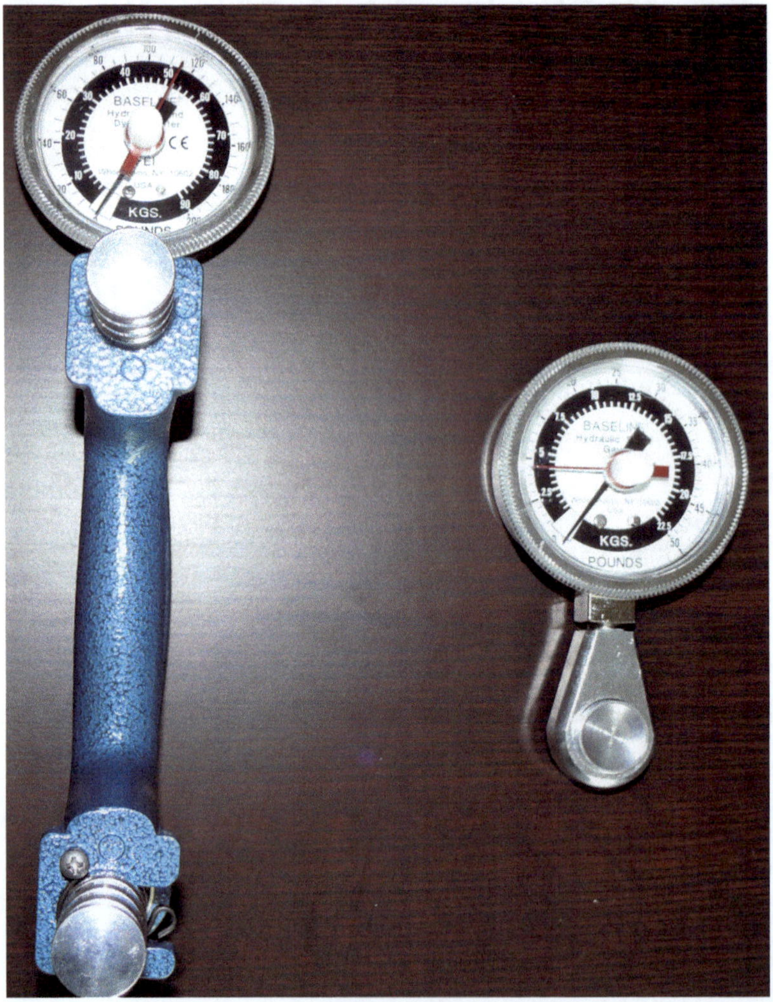

Fig. 7 Jamar dynamometer for grip strength measurement and pinch gauge dynamometer for pinch grip measurement

statistically significant difference [5]. In 2008, Gunther et al. studied 769 adult Caucasians (403 men and 366 women) aged 20–95 [6].

The normal values obtained are shown in Table 1. The authors noted a ratio of 95 % between right and left sides and that grip strength increases till the age of 35 when it slowly starts decreasing.

The force is directly correlated to several parameters such as the size of the hand or the girth of the forearm but is not significantly related to body mass index, work or dominant hand. Only one study, however, reports this conclusion, the others noting a correlation between dominance and grip strength [8–10].

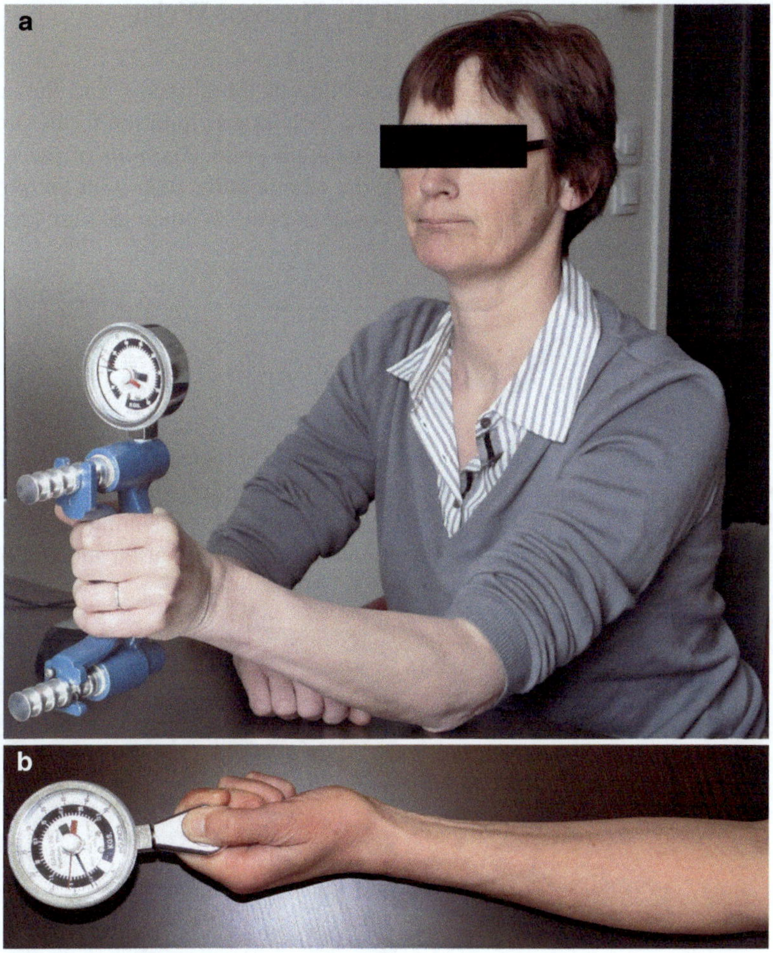

Fig. 8 Positioning for grip (**a**) and pinch (**b**) strength measurements

Table 1 Normal values of grip and pinch strength in kilograms according to Günther et al. [7, 10]

	Man ($n=403$)		Woman ($n=366$)	
Side	Right	Left	Right	Left
Grip strength (kg)	49	47	29	27
Pinch grip (kg)	10.4	9.7	6.6	6.1

7.2 Pinch Strength

The key pinch is measured using the pinch dynamometer held between thumb and index with the ulnar border of the hand, the wrist and forearm resting on the table (Fig. 5). The same recommendations for grip strength measurement apply (bilateral, rapid alternation, repetition). Normal values as reported by Günther et al. [10] are shown in Table 1.

8 The Anatomic Landmarks of the Normal Wrist

Wrist examination requires thorough knowledge of the anatomy and the surface landmarks. A systematic approach is advised without precipitation to the problem area so as not to miss another clinically significant point. The tour of the wrist is made ending at the starting point. Ideally the examination ends with the problem point designated by the patient. The bony dorsal and palmar landmarks are identified during this examination.

8.1 *The Dorsal Bony Landmarks (Fig. 9)*

From radial to palmar, the radial styloid can be easily palpated at the proximal wrist followed by the tubercle of Lister, the depression preceding the ulnar head corresponding to the distal radioulnar interval, the ulnar head (projecting in pronation, less obvious in supination) and the ulnar styloid (dorsal in pronation and ulnopalmar

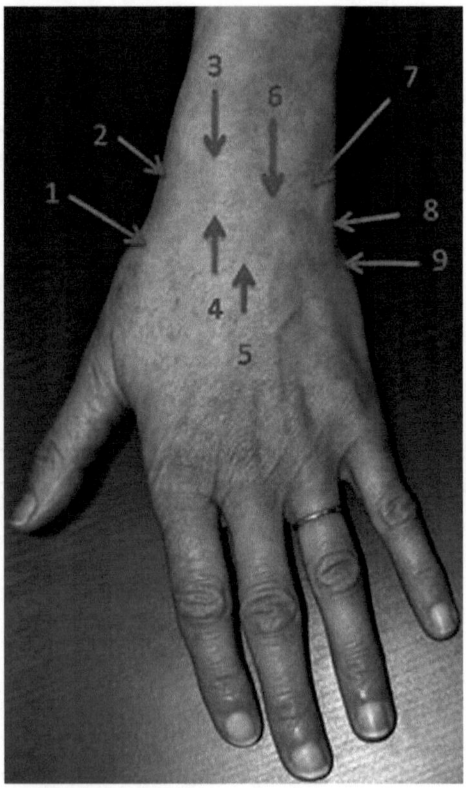

Fig. 9 Dorsal bony landmarks of the wrist: *1* snuff box and scaphoid, *2* radial styloid, *3* Lister's tubercle, *4* scapho-lunate space, *5* capitate's head, *6* distal radio-ulnar space, *7* ulnar head, *8* ulnar styloid, 9 ulnar snuff box and TFCC

in supination) [1]. Distally, the carpal bones can be palpated from radial to ulnar; the scaphoid body in the anatomical snuffbox while the proximal pole is made prominent by flexion and ulnar inclination of the wrist, about 2 cm distal to the tubercle of Lister. Immediately ulnar, still in flexion, is the scapholunate interval/ligament. The lunotriquetral interval is more readily palpable in flexion with radial deviation. Between these two points slightly distally is the depression dubbed the 'crucifixion fossa', which corresponds to the head of the capitate. Finally, the medial border of the wrist is the ulnar snuffbox between flexor carpi ulnaris and extensor carpi ulnaris denoting the TFCC.

8.2 *The Palmar Bony Landmarks (Fig. 10)*

It is important to carry out the examination in a circular and systematic manner [1] from the ulnar palmar border of the wrist. The ulnar head is palpated, then the pisiform distal to the flexion crease of the hypothenar eminence, and 1 cm distally and radially – the hamate and its hook. More radially, the anterior aspect of the radial styloid is palpated, more distally the tubercle of the scaphoid and the scaphotrapezial joint and finally the crest of trapezium at the base of the thenar eminence, and the base of the first metacarpal.

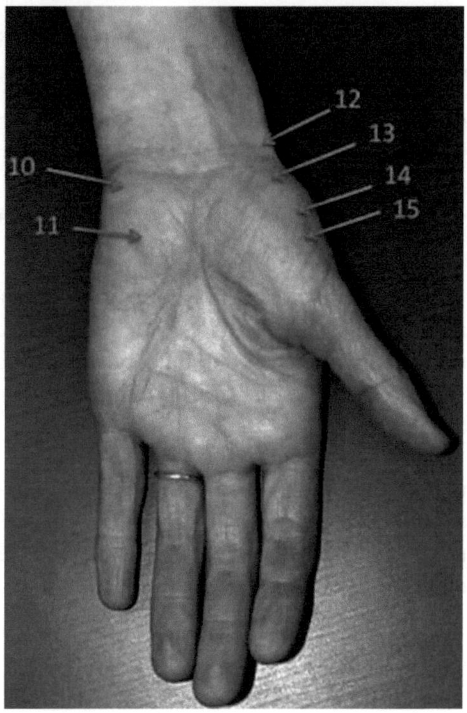

Fig. 10 Palmar bony landmarks of the wrist from ulnar to radial. *10* pisiform, *11* hook of hamate, *12* radial styloid, *13* scaphoid tubercle, *14* anterior crest of the trapezium and *15* first metacarpal

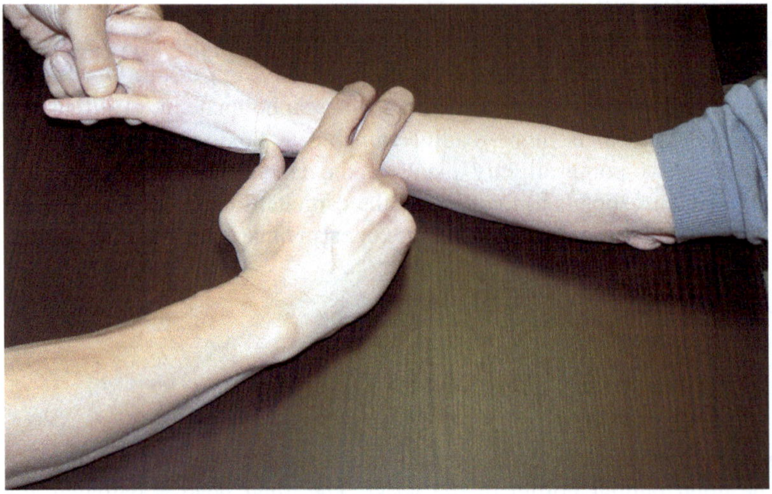

Fig. 11 Pressure on the ulnar styloid eliciting pain and denoting TFCC lesion

9 Palpation

According to Young et al. [11], there are three principles for palpation of the painful wrist:

- The exact point of pain is the site of pathology.
- If the exact point of pain is known, thus the anatomical structure is determined, then the diagnosis is made.
- The association of the positive and negative findings of the examination makes up the diagnosis.

As in the history, the examination, palpation, positional tests and dynamic tests allow precise localization of the pain. Correlated with the anatomy, a clinical diagnosis can be reached – to be confirmed by investigations.

The painful points in search of ligament pathology are on the dorsal and ulnar aspects.

The lunotriquetral interval – 2 cm distal to the tubercle of Lister in the radiocarpal depression – is difficult to palpate as it is situated at the ulnar border of the 4th extensor compartment (sometimes the 5th) and masked by the extensors. At the ulnar border of the wrist, pressure between the ulnar styloid and the triquetrum eliciting pain evokes a TFCC lesion [1, 11, 12] (Fig. 11).

10 Positional Tests

The examiner places the patient's wrist in the specific position triggering the pain and maintains it (pain, deformity).

Distal radioulnar instability can be evidenced by a pathognomonic dimple sign [1, 11, 12], where a depression immediately distal to the head of the ulna is observed on pressure by the examiner's thumb on the neck of the ulna (Fig. 12a) or spontaneously (Fig. 12b).

A TFCC lesion is suspected if pain is elicited by grinding this ligament between the carpal side of the ulnar head and the triquetrum. The examiner places the patient's wrist in pronation and slight extension and applies a forced ulnar inclination (Fig. 13). It is also possible to intensify the test by applying small pronation-supination movements in this position to elicit what Linscheid termed the 'grinding sign' [12].

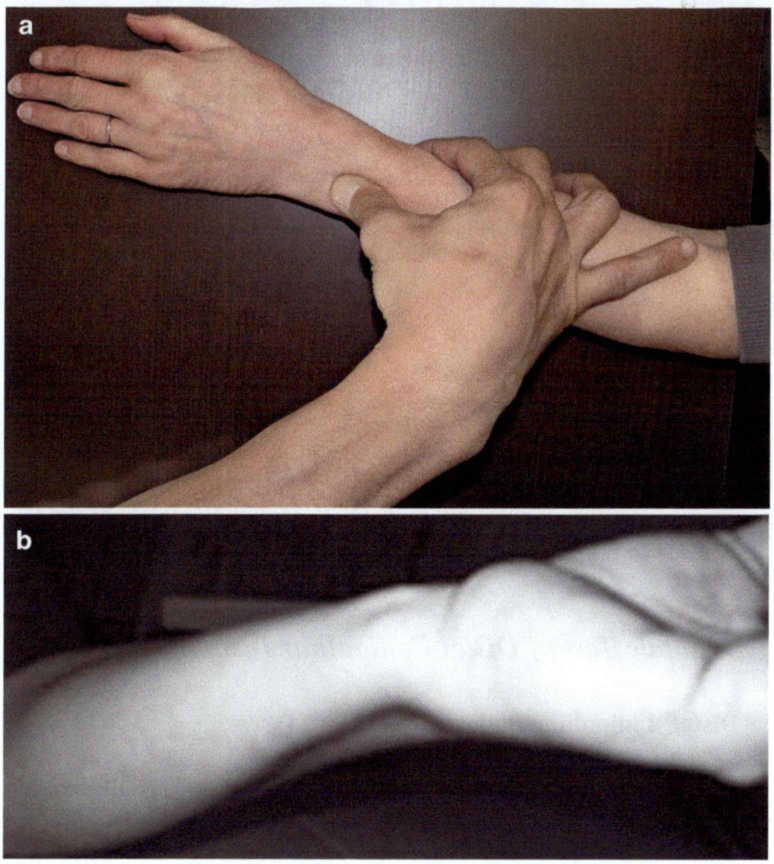

Fig. 12 The dimple sign is pathognomonic of distal radioulnar instability where the depression may be provoked by the examiner pressing on the ulnar neck (**a**) or spontaneously (**b**) (Photo by E. Camus)

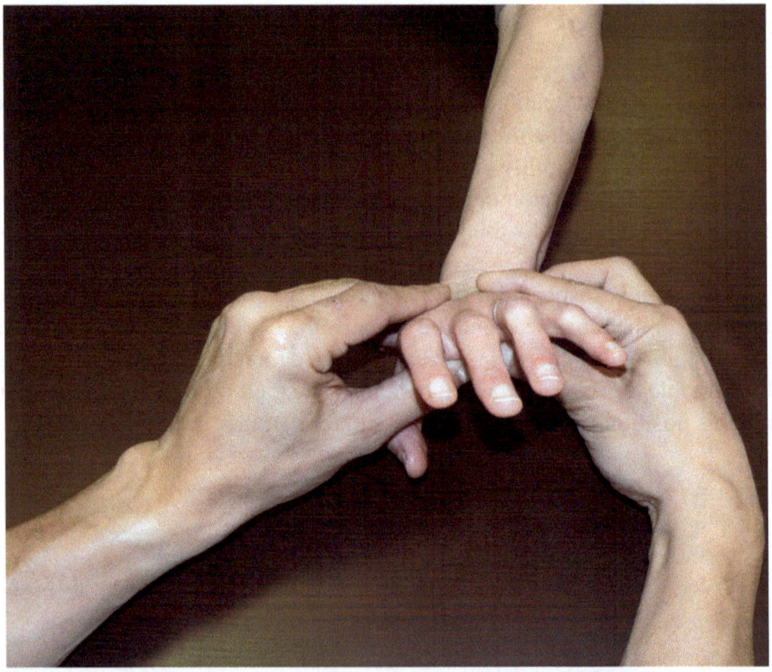

Fig. 13 A TFCC lesion is suspected if pain on the ulnar border of the wrist is elicited by grinding this ligament between the carpal side of the ulnar head and the triquetrum

11 Dynamic Tests

They differ from positional tests in that it is the movement from one position to another rather than maintaining a certain fixed position that triggers the pain thus giving a positive test. From proximal to distal, the following tests are used:

11.1 Dynamic Test of Distal Radioulnar Instability

11.1.1 Distal Radioulnar Ballottement (Fig. 14)

The forearm vertical as for scapholunate and lunotriquetral tests, the examiner stabilizes the radius between thumb and index and uses the other hand to move the ulnar head from palmar to dorsal direction in search of dorsal instability (more common) or from back to front for anterior instability (rarer).

A positive result denotes complete rupture of the stabilizing elements of the distal radioulnar joint especially the TFCC or the ECU sheath.

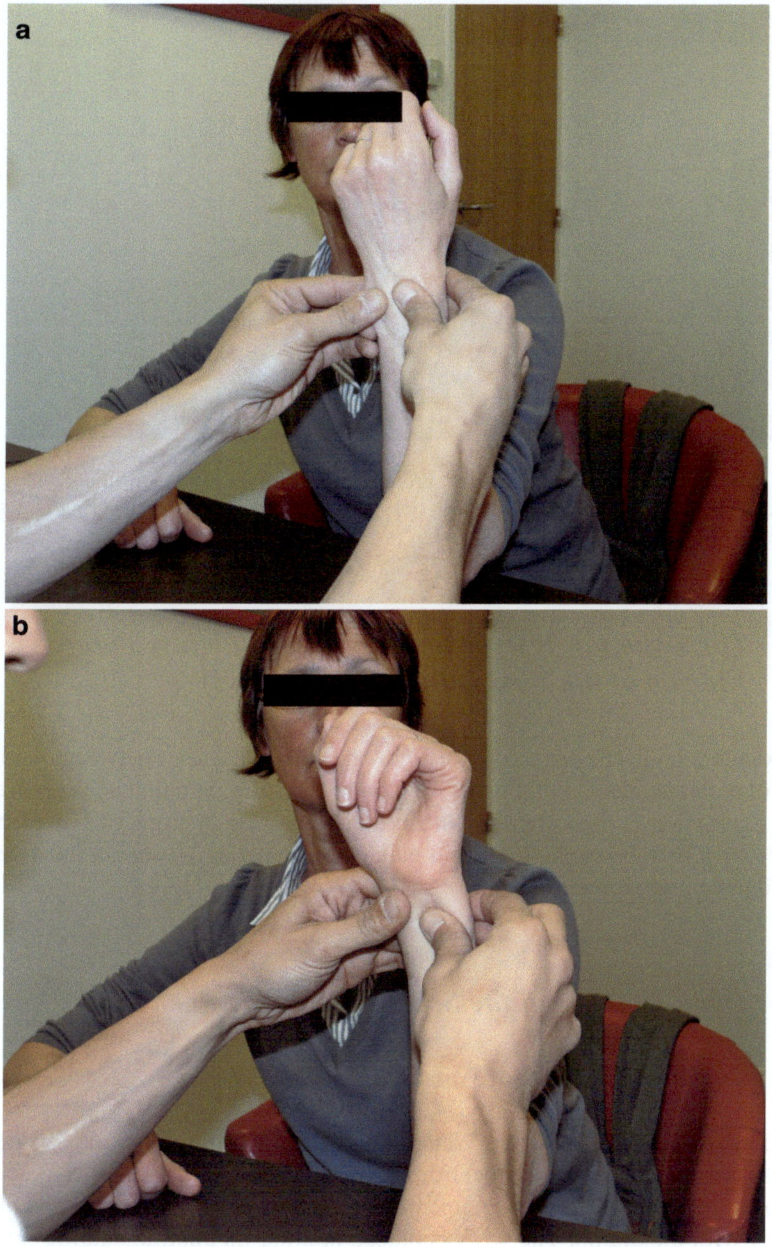

Fig. 14 Distal radioulnar ballottement detecting instability; it should be done in supination (**a**) and in pronation (**b**)

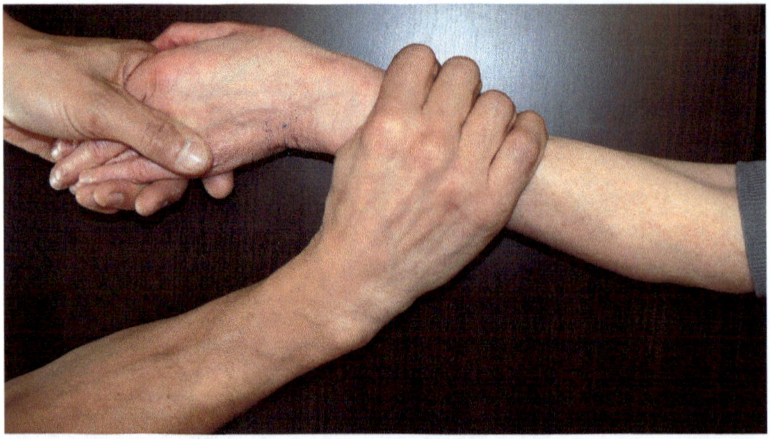

Fig. 15 The test for radiocarpal instability. From ulnar inclination, the examiner combines movement towards radial inclination and a posterior drawer – a painful click/triggering is a sign of instability

11.2 The Dynamic Test of Radiocarpal Instability: Forced Flexion of the First Carpal Row (Fig. 15)

The examiner holds the distal forearm with one hand and carpus between thumb and index of the other hand applying 10° of ulnar inclination. Simultaneous progressive radial inclination is then applied with posterior drawer. A triggering is then produced which may be physiologic and painless in hyperlax wrists but must be considered pathologic if painful [1].

11.3 Dynamic Tests of the Scapholunate Ligament SLL

11.3.1 **Scaphoid Shift Test of Watson** (Fig. 16)

Described in the mid-1980s by Watson et al. [13, 14], the scaphoid shift test is done by provoking dorsal dislocation of the scaphoid. The examiner places the thumb on the tubercle of the scaphoid and index on its posterior aspect and presses forcibly with the thumb. The wrist is placed in ulnar inclination and the scaphoid is thus maintained vertical (in extension). Bringing the wrist gently to radial inclination, the pressure exerted on the scaphoid prevents it from flexing and puts tension on the SLL. If the SLL is ruptured (even without visible radiological diastasis on static or dynamic views), this manoeuvre triggers acutely painful clicking. It is worthy of note that a non-pathological click may exist in young or hyperlax wrists.

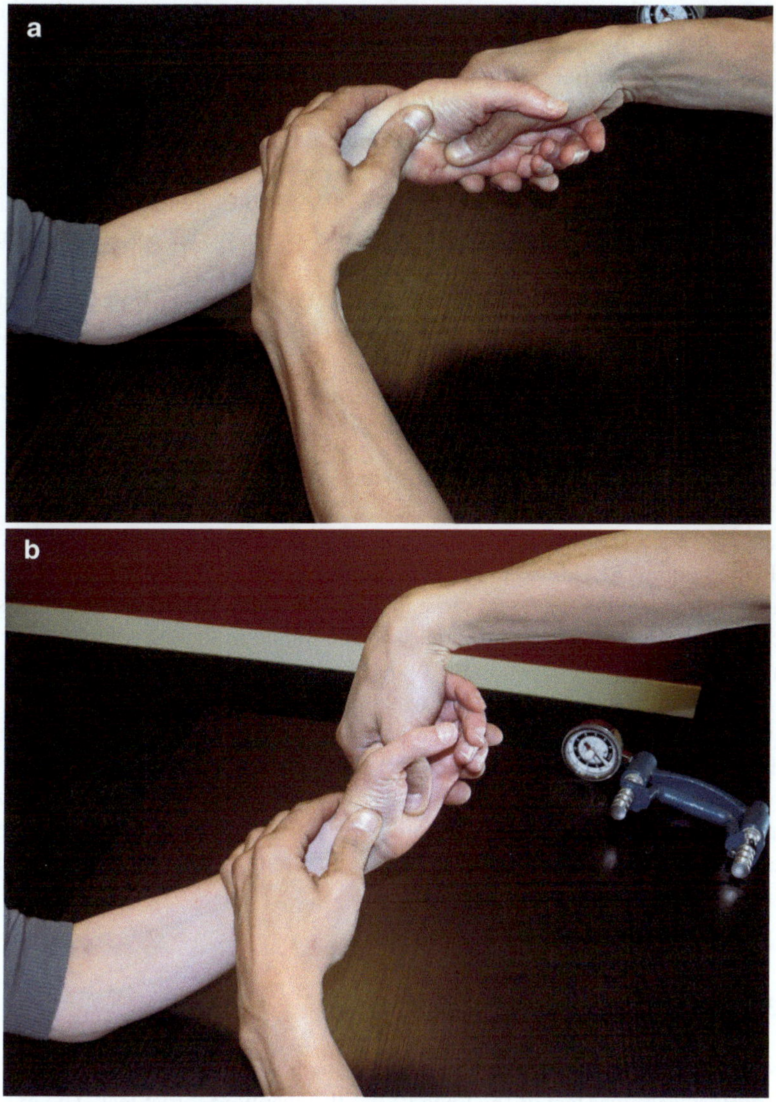

Fig. 16 Watson shift test. The thumb maintains pressure on the scaphoid tubercle. The passage from ulnar (**a**) to radial (**b**) inclination triggers pain

In the years that followed the description of this test by Kirk Watson, many studies evaluated its reliability [15–19], especially radiologically. Most of these studies advocated doing this test under radiological control showing non-pathological clicking in 14–36 % of patients with consensus that pain is necessary and sufficient to declare a positive test. This accentuates the necessity of bilateral comparative examinations especially if a click is found. In partial rupture especially with an intact posterior part (mechanically more competent), the test may produce pain without clicking which is still a positive test indicating SLL lesion.

In 1995, La Stayo et al. [20], compared clinical and arthroscopic findings in 50 painful wrists showing a 69 % sensitivity and 46 % specificity for the test, 48 %positive predictive value (PPV) and 78 % negative predictive value (NPV). Two years after, another methodologically identical study on 37 patients showed better values, 91 % sensitivity, 77 % specificity and 62 % PPV [21]. Both conclude that this test (as the scapholunate test described previously) is important for the examiner to determine the necessity for further investigations.

In our daily practice, this test is performed at the end of the clinical examination because if positive, it triggers intense pain as well a significant click disagreeable to the patient making him/her more apprehensive for the rest of the examination.

11.3.2 The Scaphoid Lift Test of Dobyns (Fig. 17)

The scaphoid lift test or the scapholunate ballottement test is a variant of the Watson test also indicating SLL lesion [11]. The patient places the elbow on the table, the forearm vertical and the hand and wrist in complete supination. The examiner seizes the scaphoid between thumb and index and the lunate in the other hand. A scissoring movement is applied between the two bones from front to back in relation to the wrist axis and high to low in relation to the table axis – hence the name 'lift'. This movement is repeated fixing one bone and moving the other. A certain amount of mobility can be found in the scapholunate joint, and only a painful test is a positive one even without significant hypermobility. The test may be done with a horizontal forearm in pronation. The same study previously cited for the Watson test states that the sensitivity of this test is 64 % with 44 % specificity, a PPV of 24 % and NPV of 81 % [20].

11.3.3 The Scaphoid Thrust Test of Lane

In 1993, Lane described a modification of Watson's test which he compared to the anteroposterior drawer test of the knee [22] – the scaphoid thrust test. The examiner holds the scaphoid between index and thumb but without applying pressure.

To avoid reflex muscular contractions and defensive tensioning, slow small flexion-extension and radioulnar inclination movements are applied. At an instant of neutral wrist position, a sudden strong pressure on the thumb ray onto the tubercle of the scaphoid from front to back is then applied in an attempt to dislocate the scaphoid posteriorly. According to the author, this test can detect moderate even minimal instability by controlling the amplitude of thrusting. This is not possible in the Watson test, which provokes a sudden brutal uncontrollable click. We have found only two publications [11, 19] mentioning this test with no radiological or arthroscopic evaluation having been conducted.

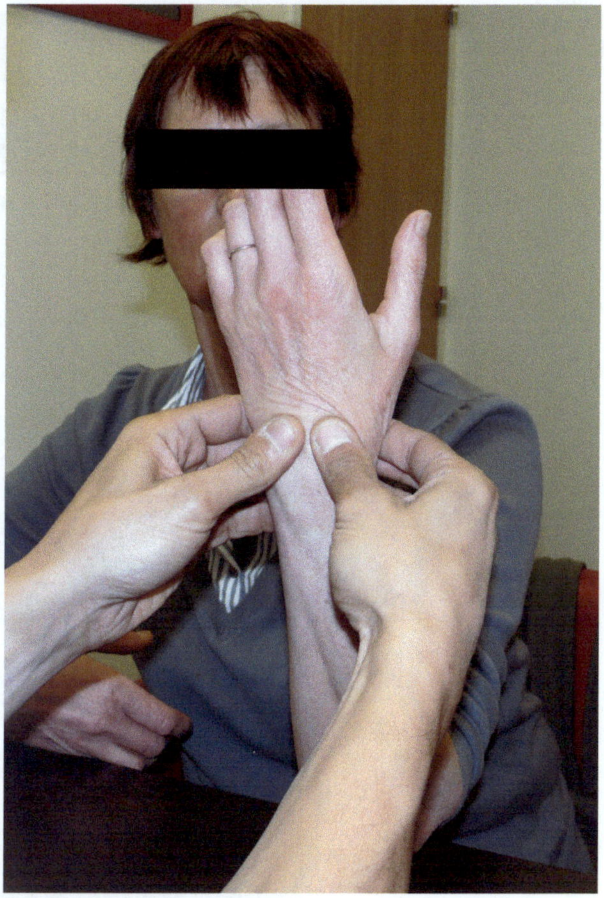

Fig. 17 Scapholunate ballottement test of Dobyns

11.4 Dynamic Lunotriquetral Ligament Test (LTL): Reagan's Test (Fig. 18)

Described in 1984, this is a test of lunotriquetral ballottement as for scapholunate ballottement, seizing the lunate between two fingers and the triquetrum in the other hand. As before, it is the pain and not the mobility that concludes a positive test [23].

11.5 Dynamic Capitolunate Instability Test (Fig. 19)

Ballottement between capitate and lunate is provoked as previously. In neutral wrist position, the lunatum is hidden in the concavity of the radius articular surface and cannot be seized between two fingers. The forearm is therefore laid horizontal in pronation, and the examiner holds the distal forearm with one hand, the capitate with the other and

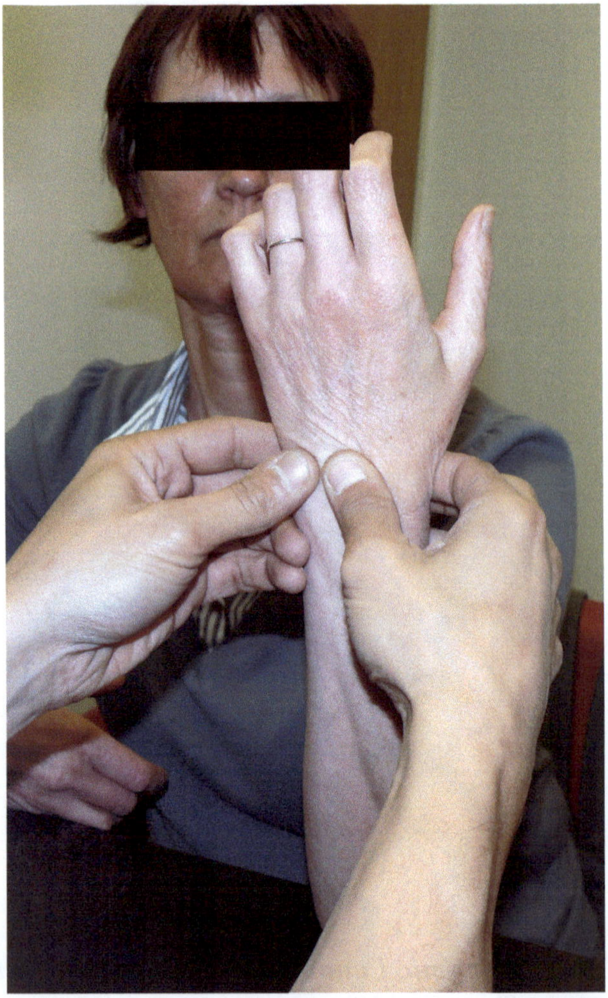

Fig. 18 Lunotriquetral ballottement test of Reagan

attempts ballottement as previously described. Pain indicates a positive test and suspicion of radiocarpal instability due to an anterior radioscaphocapitate lesion [1].

11.6 Dynamic Midcarpal Instability Test: The Forced Extension Manoeuvre (Fig. 20)

Resembling the forced flexion manoeuvre, but starting from neutral position to attain 20° ulnar inclination, a block is reached that 'gives way' suddenly with a painful click and sensation of posterior translation of the carpus. This phenomenon corresponds to the passage of the first carpal row from palmar flexion in neutral position to dorsal flexion in ulnar inclination [1].

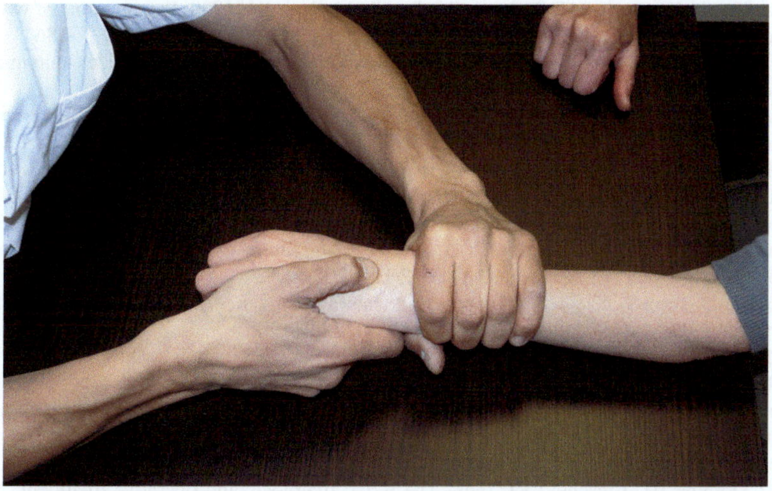

Fig. 19 Capitolunate instability test

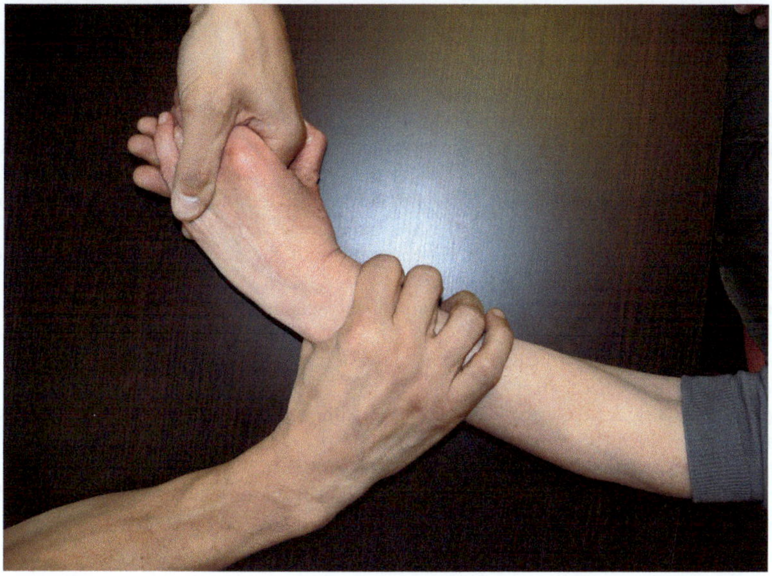

Fig. 20 Midcarpal instability test. From radial inclination, the examiner applies ulnar inclination. After a block that suddenly gives way, a painful click is produced with posterior carpal translation

References

1. Masquelet AC (1994) Examen clinique du poignet. 6e Cahier d'enseignement de la Société Française de Chirurgie de la Main, Paris. Expansion Scientifique Française 6:101–121
2. Institute for Work and Health 2006. The DASH. http://www.dash.iwh.on.ca/system/files/dash_questionnaire_2010.pdf. Accessed on 2010

3. Macdermid JC, Turgeon T, Richards RS, Beadle M, Roth JH (1998) Patient rating of wrist pain and disability: a reliable and valid measurement tool. J Orthop Trauma 12:577–586
4. Firrell JC, Crain GM (1996) Which setting of the dynamometer provides maximal grip strength? J Hand Surg 21A:397–401
5. Haidar SG, Kumar D, Bassi RS, Deshmukh SC (2004) Average versus maximum grip strength: which is more consistent? J Hand Surg 29B:82–84
6. Günther CM, Bürger A, Rickert M, Crispin A, Schulz CU (2008) Grip strength in healthy caucasian adults: reference values. J Hand Surg 33B:558–565
7. Crosby CA, Wehbe MA (1994) Hand strength: normative values. J Hand Surg 19B:665–670
8. Hanten WP, Chen WY, Austin AA et al (1999) Maximum grip strength in normal subjects from 20 to 64 years of age. J Hand Ther 12:193–200
9. Aoki H, Demura S (2008) Characteristics and lateral dominance of hand grip and elbow flexion powers in young male adults. J Phys Anthropol 27:201–206
10. Günther CM, Bürger A, Rickert M, Schulz CU (2008) Key pinch in healthy adults: normative values. J Hand Surg Eur Vol 33B:144–148
11. Young D, Papp S, Giachino A (2007) Physical examination of the wrist. Orthop Clin North Am 38:149–165
12. Cooney WP, Bishop AT, Linscheid RL (1997) Physical examination of the wrist. In: Cooney WP, Dobyns JH, Linscheid RL (eds) The wrist: diagnosis and operative treatment. Mosby, St-Louis, pp 236–261
13. Watson HK, Ryu J, Akelman E (1986) Limited triscaphoid intercarpal arthrodesis for rotary subluxation of the scaphoid. J Bone Joint Surg Am 68A:345–349
14. Watson HK, Ashmead D IV, Makhlouf MV (1988) Examination of the scaphoid. J Hand Surg 13A:657–660
15. Watson HK, Ottoni L, Pitts EC, Handal AG (1993) Rotary subluxation of the scaphoid: a spectrum of instability. J Hand Surg 18B:62–64
16. Easterling K, Wolfe SW (1994) The scaphoid shift in the uninjured wrist. J Hand Surg 19A:604–606
17. Wolfe SW, Crisco JJ (1994) Mechanical evaluation of the scaphoid shift test. J Hand Surg 19A:762–768
18. Wolfe SW, Gupta A, Crisco JJ (1997) Kinematics of the scaphoid shift test. J Hand Surg 22A:801–806
19. Park MJ (2003) Radiographic observation of the scaphoid shift test. J Bone Joint Surg Br 85B:358–362
20. Lastayo P, Howell J (1995) Clinical provocative tests used in evaluating wrist pain: a descriptive study. J Hand Ther 8:10–17
21. Bickert B, Sauerbier M, Germann G (1997) Die klinische untersuchung des verletzten handgelenke. Zentralbl Chir 122:1010–1015
22. Lane LB (1993) The scaphoid shift test. J Hand Surg 18A:366–368
23. Reagan DS, Linscheid RL, Dobyns JH (1984) Lunotriquetral sprains. J Hand Surg 9A:502–514

Imaging of Traumatic Carpal Instability

J.-C. Dosch and T. Moser

Ligaments of the wrist play a fundamental role in the stability of the carpus. Poirier and Charpy [1] and Testut [2] first described this relationship. The works of Mayfield et al. [3] and Taleisnik [4] constitute the basis of the current description. More recently, Berger [5] has contributed some modifications to this classification. Classically, we differentiate between intra-articular or interosseous ligaments and capsular ligaments. The latter group is further classified into intrinsic ligaments, which originate and insert into carpal bones, and extrinsic ligaments, which attach carpal bones to bones of the forearm or the hand [6].

1 Classification of Instability

The classification of carpal instability is complex and variable according to the authors. Larsen proposes an analysis of carpal instability according to six criteria: the duration of evolution, permanent radiographic signs, aetiology, topography, direction and mechanism [7].

J.-C. Dosch (✉)
Hand Surgery Unit, Service de Radiologie, CHU Strasbourg, Hôpital de Hautepierre, Avenue Molière, Strasbourg, Cedex 67098, France

Centre de Chirurgie Orthopédique et de la Main Illkirch, BP 49, Strasbourg, Cedex 67098, France
e-mail: jean-claude.dosch@chru-strasbourg.fr

T. Moser
Département de Radiologie, CHUM, Hôpital St Luc, 1058 rue St Denis, Montréal, QC H2X 3J4, Canada
e-mail: thomas.moser@umontreal.ca

E. Camus, L. Van Overstraeten (eds.), *Carpal Ligament Surgery*,
DOI 10.1007/978-2-8178-0379-1_4,

- Duration: acute being less than 1 week, subacute 1–6 weeks or chronic over 6 weeks. This influences healing of lesions.
- The permanence of the instability is correlated to the severity of the ligamentous lesion. *Static* instability is permanent and visible on static x-rays, whereas *dynamic* instability is only detected on certain movement patterns and is demonstrated only on dynamic radiography (under fluoroscopy). *Predynamic* instability is a subtle anomaly nonapparent on radiography.
- Aetiology is mostly traumatic but may also be congenital or rheumatoid.
- The topography may concern the radiocarpal joint, the proximal row, the midcarpal joint, the distal row or the carpometacarpal joint.
- Directions are variable. Dorsal instability or 'dorsal intercalated segment instability – DISI' is the most common. The lunate is tilted into dorsal flexion and translated anteriorly. The ulnar translation and dorsal subluxation correspond to the sliding of the carpus on the radial slope, medially and posteriorly. We distinguish between type I ulnar translation when the carpus is shifted interiorly and type II when the scaphoid remains in place due to a scapholunate diastasis [6].
- There are several mechanisms. In 'dissociative carpal instability – DCI', there is an imbalance between bones of the same row. The main causes are scaphoid fracture, scapholunate or lunotriquetral ligament rupture [8, 9]. In 'nondissociative carpal instability – NDCI', the instability is radiocarpal (between radius and first carpal row) or midcarpal (between first and second carpal rows). In 'complex carpal instability', elements of both types DCI and NDCI are present. 'Adaptative carpal instability – ACI' is a defect of alignment following an extrinsic anomaly often an epiphyseal nonunion of the radius [10].

2 Mechanisms of Intracarpal Ligament Lesions

2.1 Lesions of the Ligaments of the Radial Side of the Wrist

The mechanism of these traumatic wrist lesions is stereotyped, almost always a fall on the outstretched hand. When the arm is abducted, impact on the thenar eminence induces extension, ulnar deviation and intracarpal supination of the wrist. These displacements are particularly deleterious to the radial ligaments of the wrist.

2.2 Progressive Perilunate Instability

According to Mayfield, this mechanism is the origin of the perilunate instability classification, which is progressive in gravity in function of the energy of the trauma and the number of ligaments ruptured [11]. Pure ligamentous lesions follow the lesser arc of Johnson, first involving the scapholunate junction (scapholunate ligament rupture, stage 1), then the capitolunate junction (rupture of radioscaphocapitate ligament, stage 2), lunotriquetral (stage 3) and radiolunate (rupture of the dorsal radiocarpal ligament, stage 4), leading to the palmar tilt of the lunate [12]. As the energy increases further, lesions progressively involve carpal bones along the greater arc of Johnson, giving the classification table for fracture palmar subluxations of the lunate [13].

2.3 *Progressive Scaphoid Instability*

Watson described the evolution of scapholunate lesions [14, 15]. Stage 1 is a dorsal carpal syndrome – synovitis of the scapholunate interval with moderate ligament injury. Pain is primarily on activity (especially with racquet sports) and its persistence at rest is a sign of aggravation. There is tenderness on the dorsal scapholunate interval and finger extension test is positive.

2.4 *Rotatory Scaphoid Subluxation (RSS)*

This involves more severe ligament injuries causing dorsal displacement with rotation of the proximal pole. The abnormal forces on the radioscaphoid joint cause 'scapholunate advanced collapse SLAC' wrist [16]. There are symptoms of at least 6 months' duration with pain at rest and limitation of range of motion, especially flexion. Tenderness over the scaphoid or on Watson's test is elicited on examination. Watson described five types of RSS. Predynamic RSS (type 1) involves clinical instability with no radiographic abnormality.

Dynamic RSS (type 2): Radiographic abnormality only on stress views: scaphoid shortening with ring sign, superposition of the scaphoid and capitate.

Static RSS (type 3): More severe clinical abnormality and radiographic abnormalities in neutral position: scapholunate gap, increased scapholunate angle with or without DISI. This can be reducible or non-reducible.

Degenerative stage (type 4) or 'SLAC' wrist develops after prolonged evolution. X-rays show radioscaphoid followed by capitolunate arthritis.

The last type of RSS (type 5) is *secondary* to other carpal lesions such as primary necrosis of the lunate (Kienbock's disease) or the scaphoid (Preiser's). When it complicates scaphoid nonunion, it is known as 'scaphoid nonunion advanced collapse – SNAC' wrist.

3 Ulnar-Sided Lesions

Lunotriquetral ligament rupture is encountered in two cases. The first is radial-sided wrist injury as in Mayfield stage 3 where it passes to the next level. Isolated lunotriquetral ligament rupture can occur in ulnar-sided wrist trauma where the mechanism of injury is similar but with arm adduction causing ulnar impact. Trauma to the hypothenar eminence causes extension, radial inclination and intracarpal pronation.

With respect to the Mayfield theory, Viegas et al. described the reversed perilunate instability [17]. Lunotriquetral ligament rupture presents clinically with ulnar-sided wrist pain which is exacerbated by compression tests and lunotriquetral ballottement. X-rays show lunotriquetral diastasis and lunate tilt in VISI.

4 Standard Radiography

Four views are required in any wrist trauma: posteroanterior, lateral, oblique and scaphoid views [18]. Posteroanterior palm down and lateral views are sufficient to show the essential wrist landmarks for assessment of instability. Success criteria for the PA view are (Fig. 1):

1. A continuity between the medial cortex of the ulna and the ulnar styloid
2. ECU gutter in the middle of the fossa [19]

For the lateral view, the criteria are (Fig. 2):

1. Superposition of the radius and ulna
2. Pisiform projects between the anterior cortex of the capitate posteriorly and the distal pole of the scaphoid anteriorly [20]

On these views, we can note:

- Carpal arches described by Gilula to assess the alignment of the two carpal rows. The first arch is formed by the superior convex border of the scaphoid, lunate and triquetrum and the second by their concave borders. The third arch is formed by the proximal borders of the capitate and hamate [21]. These arches delineate harmonious curves in neutral position. In radial or ulnar deviation, we can observe physiological abutment [22].

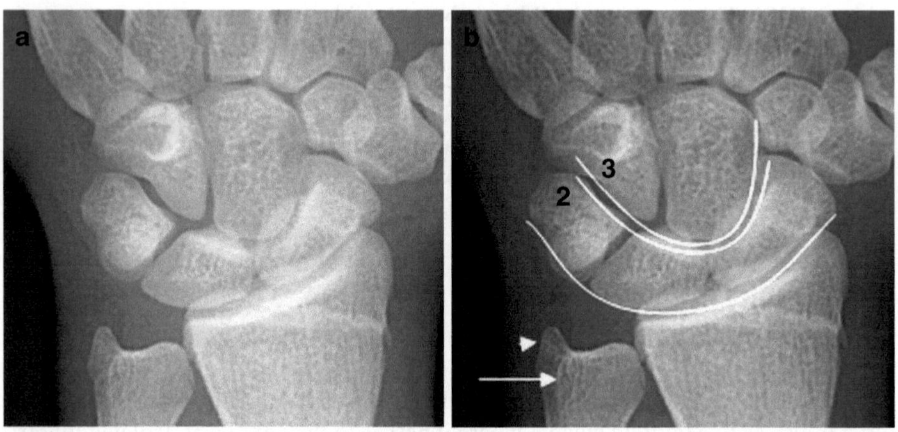

Fig. 1 PA view in neutral position. (**a**) Without marking, (**b**) with marking. Harmonious three Gilula arches, ulnar styloid in the extension of the medial ulnar cortex (*arrow head*), extensor carpi ulnaris groove in relation to fossa (*white arrow*) suppress **2** and **3**

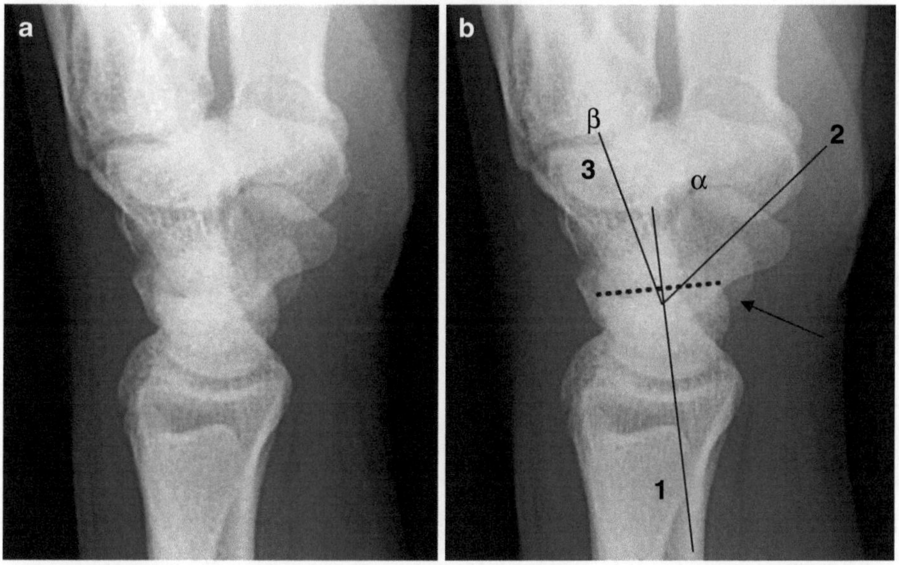

Fig. 2 Lateral view in neutral position. (**a**) Without marking, (**b**) with marking: Superposition of the radius and ulna. Pisiform between scaphoid tubercle and anterior facet of capitate (*arrow*). Lunate axis (*line 1*) perpendicular to the line connecting the anterior and posterior horns (*dotted line*). Scaphoid axis (*line 2*). Capitate axis (*line 3*). Scapholunate *angle alpha*. Capitolunate *angle beta*

- The regularity of these lines (on PA).
- All lines do not normally exceed 3 mm thickness. The opposing articular surfaces are parallel, and in the absence of flexion, any overriding indicates the presence of a fracture or subluxation. The scapholunate space must be carefully scrutinized. In fact, in the axial plane, this interval is parallel in only 80 % and divergent with respect to the anterior and posterior horns of the lunate in 15 % of cases [23]. Thus, the measure of this space must be taken at the middle. Scapholunate diastasis is considered if the interval exceeds 3 mm. This may be physiologic in lunotriquetral synostosis or inherent laxity (bilateral comparative x-rays are recommended), or pathologic in association to ligament rupture (Fig. 3) [24, 25].
- Carpal angles (lateral view).
- The lunate axis is defined by the line perpendicular to the tangent connecting the two horns of the lunate. The scaphoid axis passes through the centre of the tubercle, waist and base of the scaphoid. The axes of the radius and the capitate are calculated by dropping a perpendicular to the line connecting the two equidistant points on the anterior and posterior borders of these two bones. The normal scapholunate angle is between 30° and 70° with a mean value of 55°. It increases in extension instability (DISI) and decreases in flexion instability (VISI). The radiolunate and capitolunate angles range between −15° and +15°. They increase in DISI or VISI (Fig. 4). The theoretical collinearity of the axes of the radius, lunate, capitate and third metacarpal is actually rarely seen (only 11 % normal subjects).

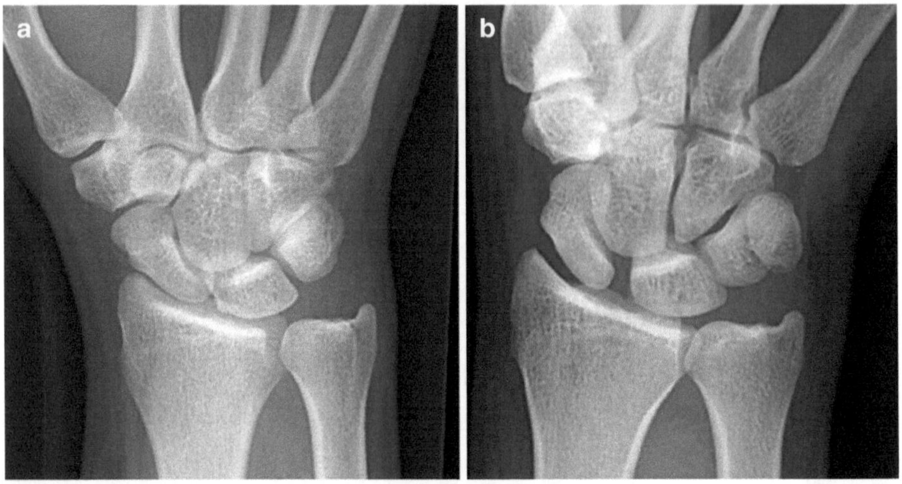

Fig. 3 Scapholunate diastasis. Scapholunate interval is not widened in neutral position (**a**). SL diastasis on AP view with 20° pronation (**b**)

The study of carpal dynamics is usually done to confirm clinical or radiographic suspicion of carpal instability. Gilula proposes PA views in neutral position, ulnar and radial deviation, a clenched fist PA view, lateral views in neutral position, flexion and extension. The clenched fist position increases intra-articular pressure and unmasks scapholunate diastasis [26]. Lawand proposes this test on both sides whilst clenching a pencil [27]. The interpretation of these views requires knowledge of the combined carpal movements in the sagittal and coronal planes (Fig. 5). In radial deviation, the first carpal row flexes. The scaphoid is shortened and shows the ring sign at its distal portion representing the tubercle seen escaping. The lunate follows the movement and appears triangular due to the displacement of its pointed posterior horn. In ulnar inclination, the first carpal row extends. The scaphoid elongates, exposing its waist. The lunate becomes quadrangular due to displacement of its rounded anterior horn which becomes more visible [28].

Radiography remains an investigation of low sensitivity. As repeatedly shown by experimental studies [29], the presence of radiographic signs of instability denotes extensive ligament lesions generally associated with complete or partial intrinsic and extrinsic ligaments, thus the need for complementary investigations [30].

To summarize:

1. Radiographic signs for DISI on PA view in neutral are scapholunate diastasis, superposition of the scaphoid and capitate, ring sign of the scaphoid, quadrangular shape of the lunate. On lateral view, they are the increase of scapholunate, capitolunate and radiolunate angles (Fig. 6).
2. Radiographic signs for VISI are decrease of scapholunate angle and increase of capitolunate and radiolunate angles.

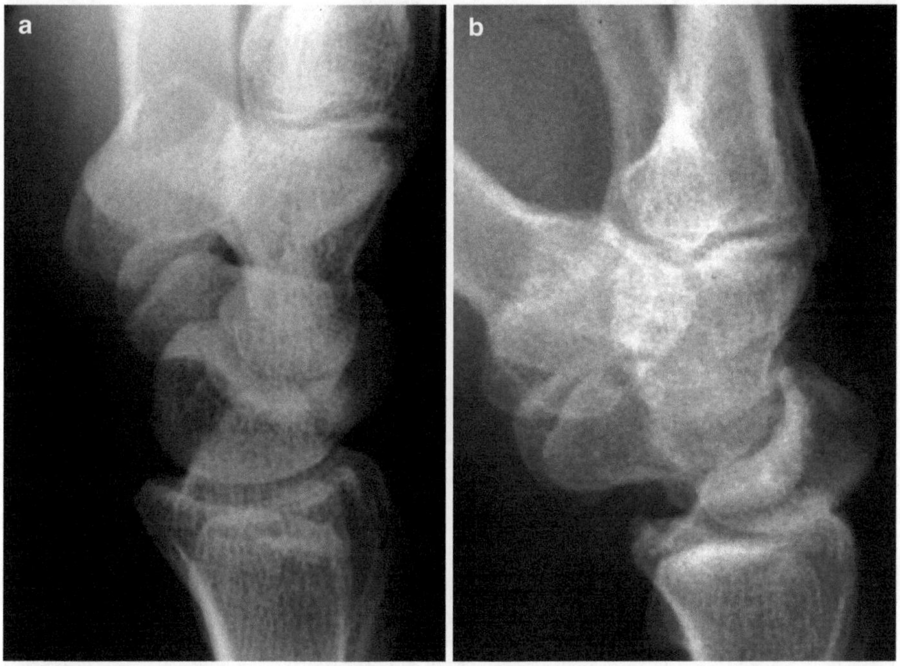

Fig. 4 Carpal instability. *DISI* dorsal tilt of the lunate and increased scapholunate angle, *VISI* ventral tilt of the lunate

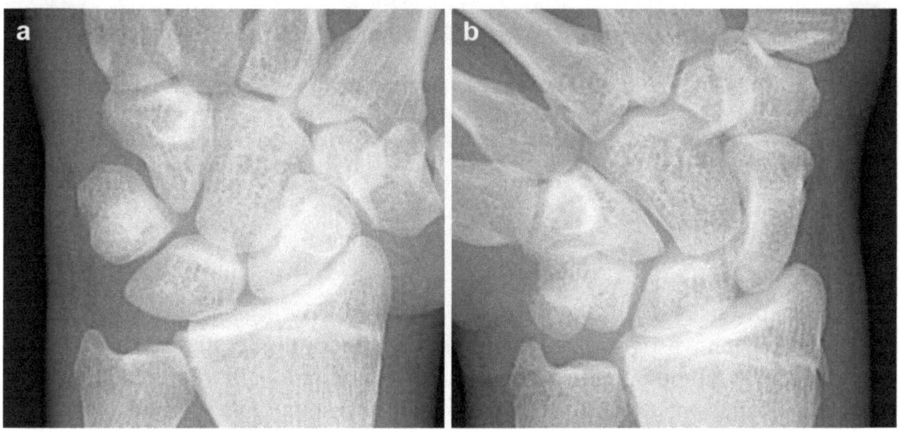

Fig. 5 Carpal dynamics in radial and ulnar inclination. (**a**) Radial inclination: The first carpal row is in flexion. The scaphoid is short and shows the ring sign. Triangular shape of the lunate is due to the pointed shape of its posterior horn. Physiological rupture of Gilula arch 1 regarding the lunotriquetral interval. (**b**) Ulnar inclination: The carpal bones are in extension. The scaphoid is elongated. Quadrangular shape of the lunate due to the large and rounded shape of its anterior horn

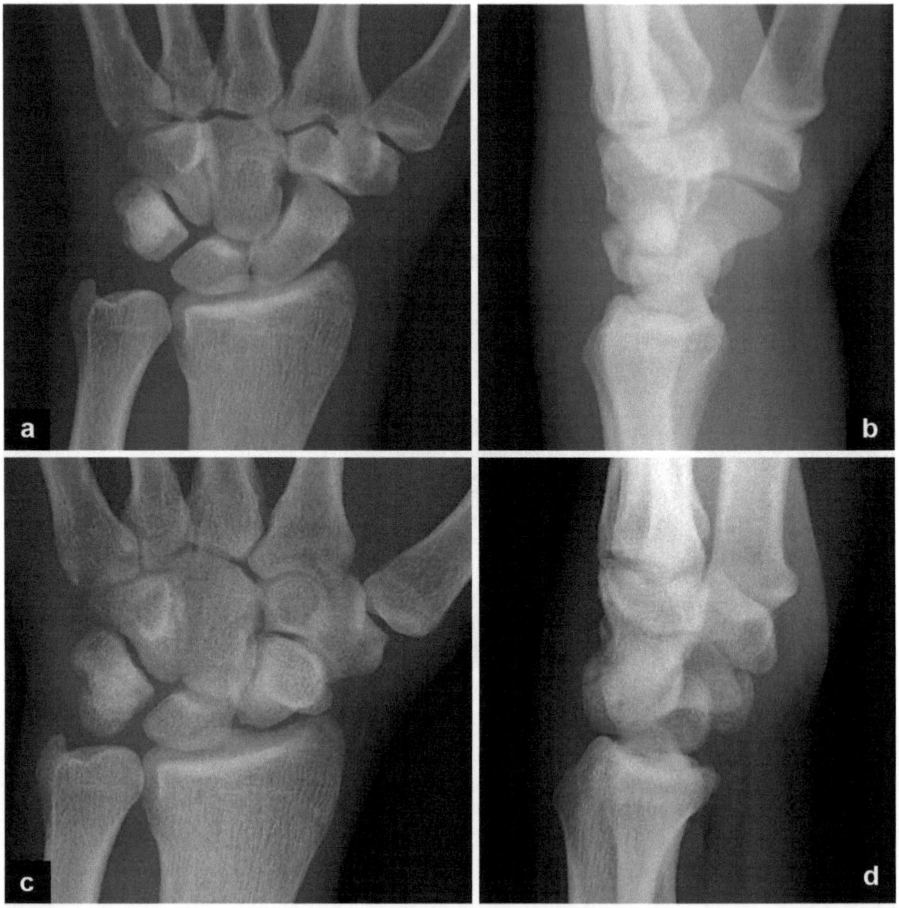

Fig. 6 Dorsal instability (DISI) at 1 month post traumatic. (**a, b**) Radiographs at day 0 showing no abnormality. (**c, d**) Control at 1 month shows a DISI. Pa shows shortened scaphoid with a ring sign, superposition of the scaphoid and capitate denoting rotational displacement, quadrangular lunate. Lateral view confirms the dorsal tilt of the lunate with a widening of the scapholunate angle

5 Ultrasound

The use of ultrasound for diagnosis of lesions of wrist ligaments is very recent [31–33]. It is an investigation of low sensitivity but high specificity which can be a useful cheap complement to the clinical examination. It requires, however, high-quality equipment with high-frequency ultrasound. The dorsal portion of the scapholunate ligament may be seen in most cases, the TFCC in one out of two cases and rarely, the dorsal portion of the lunotriquetral ligament. The interosseous ligaments are examined in transverse cuts from the dorsal side, whilst varying the degree of wrist flexion. The diagnosis of rupture depends on the appearance of the normal fibrous structure which is replaced by a zone of hypoechogenicity (Fig. 7) [34].

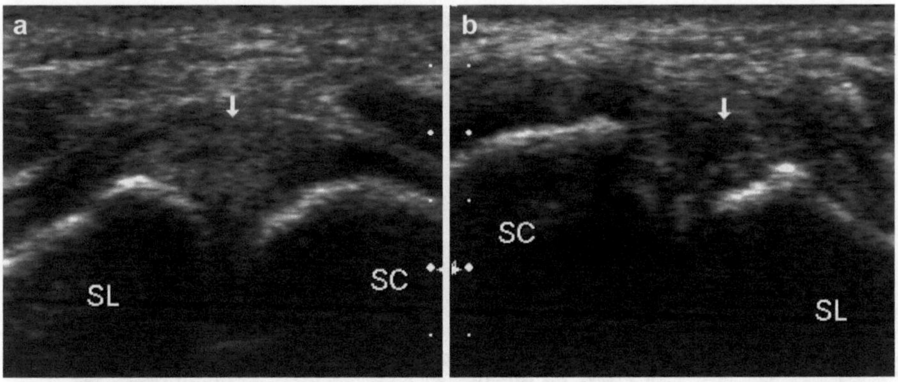

Fig. 7 Ultrasound of the scapholunate ligament. Comparative study of the dorsal portion; *SC* scaphoid, *L* lunate. (**a**) Normal SL (*arrow*), (**b**) Hypoechoic zone denoting rupture (*arrow*)

6 CT Scan

Simple CT scan without injection is not indicated in studying wrist ligaments. However, it shows associated osseous lesions perfectly.

7 MRI

Most studies use the 1.5 T system. A cadaveric study using a low-field machine showed limited results [35]. Several more recent studies compared the same sequences at 1.5 and 3.0 T [36–38]. The subjective quality and signal–noise relation was significantly higher at 3.0 T. The technical considerations of positioning are such that the wrist is seldom in a neutral position and thus the anatomical relations are modified. The most recent 3 T MRI study gives 100 % specificity and 89 and 82 % sensitivity for full-thickness scapholunate and lunotriquetral lesions, respectively [39].

8 Arthrography, Arthro-CT and Arthro-MRI

Opaque arthrography, notably triple arthrography with successive punctures of the midcarpal, radiocarpal and distal radioulnar joints, is but the precursor of CT or MR arthrography. The opacification of these compartments by contrast material – iodides for CT and gadolinium salts for the MRI – allows an exhaustive analysis of the different articular portions of the scapholunate and lunotriquetral ligaments.

The *scapholunate ligament* closes the proximal part of the interval. It is horseshoe-shaped and is formed of three anatomically and functionally distinct portions [40, 41]. The dorsal portion is short, transverse and trapezoidal. Composed of thick and tight collagen bands, it is the strongest part of the ligament. It forms the axis of

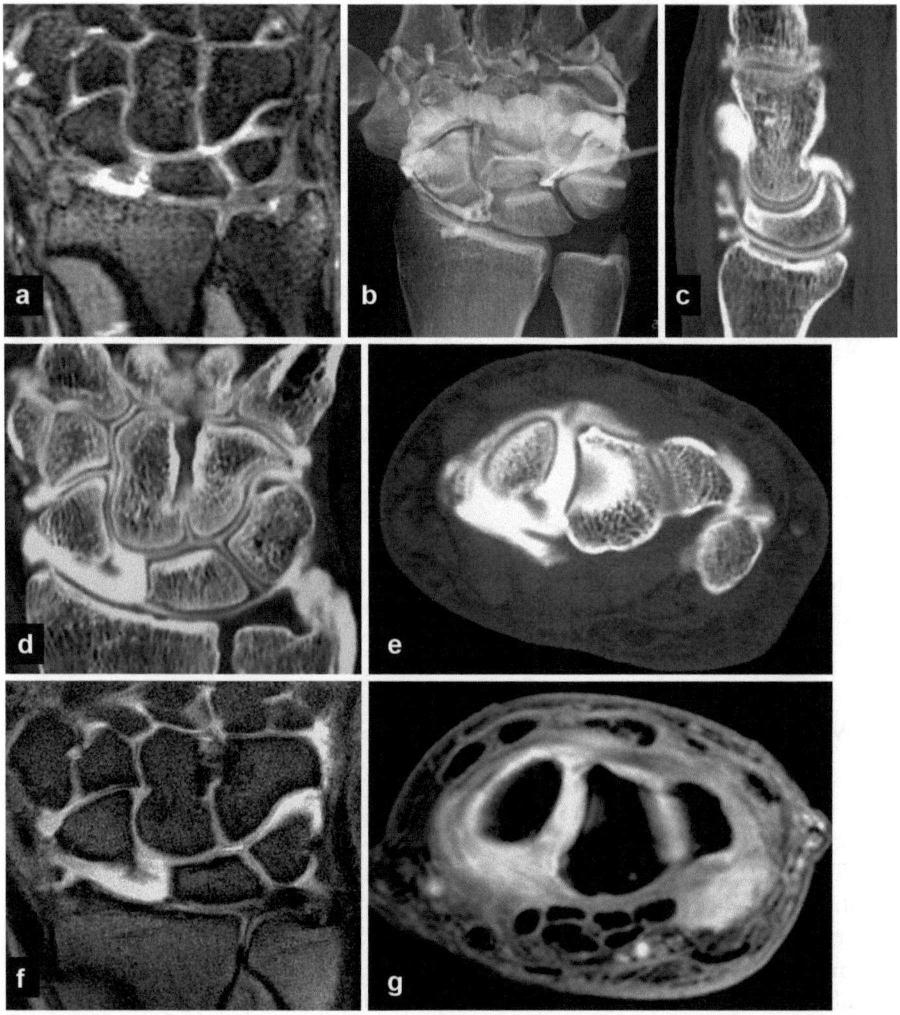

Fig. 8 Complete scapholunate ligament SLL rupture. (**a**) MRI shows scapholunate diastasis with ligament stump outlined by the effusion. (**b**) Midcarpal arthrography with contrast communicating to radiocarpal joint via incompetent SL interval. (**c–e**) CT arthrography showing the SLL stump and dorsal tilt of the lunate in DISI. (**f–g**) MR arthrography. The stump is less visible since soaked with contrast material

rotation between the scaphoid and the lunate. The proximal or intermediate portion resembles a meniscus with its triangular shape and fibrocartilaginous structure. It is proximally attached to the radioscapholunate facet and is the weakest part of the ligament. The palmar portion is long and slopes obliquely below and inwards. It is formed of finer and more loosely arranged collagen bands, allowing an anterior displacement of both bones in flexion. The scaphoid has a greater arc in flexion than the lunate due to a smaller curvature of its proximal pole.

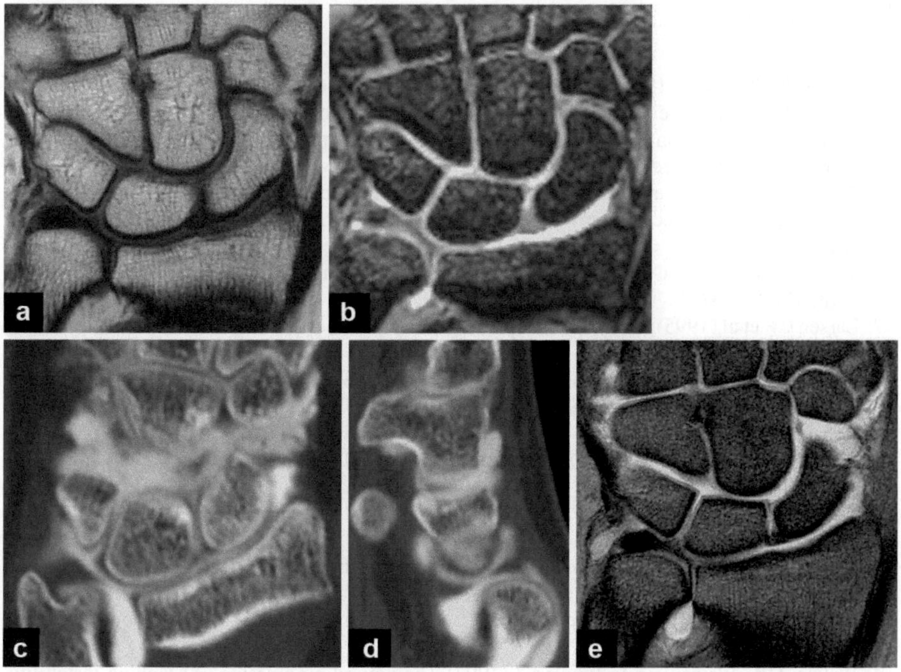

Fig. 9 Partial rupture of the LTL and central portion of the TFCC (type Palmer 2D). (**a**, **b**) MRI shows no visible abnormality. (**c**, **d**) CT arthrography shows the lesion perfectly in coronal and sagittal cuts. (**e**) MR arthrography shows no visible abnormality

The lunotriquetral ligament also has three portions [42, 43]. The dorsal portion is fibrous and is continuous with capsular ligaments posteriorly (radiocarpal and dorsal intracarpal). The proximal portion is fibrocartilaginous and meniscoid like. It is not very strong. The palmar portion is fibrous, strongest and most important functionally.

In arthro-CT [44] and arthro-MRI [30, 45, 46], the intermediate portions of these ligaments can be studied on coronal sections and the dorsal and palmar portions on axial sections. Ligamentous lesions are characterized by their extent and depth. Complete tear involves all three portions, whilst partial tears involve one or two, or even just a segment (punctuate ruptures) of the ligament (Figs. 8 and 9).

Full-thickness tears involve the entire thickness of the ligament whilst partial ones affect the palmar or dorsal aspect only without entailing articular communication. For full-thickness tears, it is important to determine whether the tear is central or peripheral (zone of insertion) for management plan. In a peripheral rupture, the stump retracts and appears thickened.

CT and MRI arthrography performance approaches actual arthroscopy. Associated lesions detected and analysed are primarily state of the cartilage and bone alterations and secondarily bone contusions and occult fractures.

References

1. Poirier P, Charpy A (1911) Traité d'Anatomie Humaine, vol 1. Masson et Cie, Paris
2. Testut L (1904) Traité d'Anatomie Humaine, vol 1. Octave Douin, Paris
3. Mayfield JK, Johnson RP, Kilcoyne RF (1976) The ligaments of the human wrist and their functional significance. Anat Rec 186(3):417–428
4. Taleisnik J (1976) The ligaments of the wrist. J Hand Surg Am 1(2):110–118
5. Berger RA (2001) The anatomy of the ligaments of the wrist and distal radioulnar joints. Clin Orthop 383:32–40
6. Taleisnik J (1988) Current concepts review. Carpal instability. J Bone Joint Surg Am 70(8):1262–1268
7. Larsen CF et al (1995) Analysis of carpal instability: I. Description of the scheme. J Hand Surg Am 20(5):757–764
8. Linscheid RL et al (1972) Traumatic instability of the wrist. Diagnosis, classification, and pathomechanics. J Bone Joint Surg Am 54(8):1612–1632
9. Wright TW et al (1994) Carpal instability non-dissociative. J Hand Surg Br 19(6):763–773
10. Brahin B, Allieu Y (1984) Compensatory carpal malalignments. Ann Chir Main 3(4):357–363
11. Mayfield JK (1984) Patterns of injury to carpal ligaments. A spectrum. Clin Orthop Relat Res 187:36–42
12. Mayfield JK (1984) Wrist ligamentous anatomy and pathogenesis of carpal instability. Orthop Clin North Am 15(2):209–216
13. Johnson RP (1980) The acutely injured wrist and its residuals. Clin Orthop Relat Res 149:33–44
14. Watson HK, Weinzweig J, Zeppieri J (1997) The natural progression of scaphoid instability. Hand Clin 13(1):39–49
15. Watson H, Weinzweig J (2001) The wrist. Lippincott Williams & Wilkins, Philadelphia, p 985
16. Watson HK, Ballet FL (1984) The SLAC wrist: scapholunate advanced collapse pattern of degenerative arthritis. J Hand Surg Am 9(3):358–365
17. Viegas SF et al (1990) Ulnar-sided perilunate instability: an anatomic and biomechanic study. J Hand Surg Am 15(2):268–278
18. Gilula LA et al (1984) Roentgenographic diagnosis of the painful wrist. Clin Orthop Relat Res 187:52–64
19. Levis CM, Yang Z, Gilula LA (2002) Validation of the extensor carpi ulnaris groove as a predictor for the recognition of standard posteroanterior radiographs of the wrist. J Hand Surg Am 27(2):252–257
20. Yang Z et al (1997) Scaphopisocapitate alignment: criterion to establish a neutral lateral view of the wrist. Radiology 205(3):865–869
21. Gilula LA (1979) Carpal injuries: analytic approach and case exercises. AJR Am J Roentgenol 133(3):503–517
22. Peh WC, Gilula LA (1996) Normal disruption of carpal arcs. J Hand Surg Am 21(4):561–566
23. Schimmerl-Metz SM et al (1999) Radiologic measurement of the scapholunate joint: implications of biologic variation in scapholunate joint morphology. J Hand Surg Am 24(6):1237–1244
24. Metz VM et al (1993) Wide scapholunate joint space in lunotriquetral coalition: a normal variant? Radiology 188(2):557–559
25. Gilula LA, Weeks PM (1978) Post-traumatic ligamentous instabilities of the wrist. Radiology 129(3):641–651
26. Moneim MS (1981) The tangential posteroanterior radiograph to demonstrate scapholunate dissociation. J Bone Joint Surg Am 63(8):1324–1326

27. Lawand A, Foulkes GD (2003) The "clenched pencil" view: a modified clenched fist scapholunate stress view. J Hand Surg Am 28(3):414–418; discussion 419–420
28. Schernberg F (1990) Roentgenographic examination of the wrist: a systematic study of the normal, lax and injured wrist. Part 1: the standard and positional views. J Hand Surg Br 15(2):210–219
29. Meade TD, Schneider LH, Cherry K (1990) Radiographic analysis of selective ligament sectioning at the carpal scaphoid: a cadaver study. J Hand Surg Am 15(6):855–862
30. Theumann NH et al (2006) Association between extrinsic and intrinsic carpal ligament injuries at MR arthrography and carpal instability at radiography: initial observations. Radiology 238(3):950–957
31. Dao KD et al (2004) The efficacy of ultrasound in the evaluation of dynamic scapholunate ligamentous instability. J Bone Joint Surg Am 86-A(7):1473–1478
32. Finlay K, Lee R, Friedman L (2004) Ultrasound of intrinsic wrist ligament and triangular fibrocartilage injuries. Skeletal Radiol 33(2):85–90
33. Griffith JF et al (2001) Sonography of the normal scapholunate ligament and scapholunate joint space. J Clin Ultrasound 29(4):223–229
34. Jacobson JA et al (2002) Sonography of the scapholunate ligament in four cadaveric wrists: correlation with MR arthrography and anatomy. AJR Am J Roentgenol 179(2):523–527
35. Ahn JM et al (1998) Evaluation of the triangular fibrocartilage and the scapholunate and lunotriquetral ligaments in cadavers with low-field-strength extremity-only magnet. Comparison of available imaging sequences and macroscopic findings. Invest Radiol 33(7):401–406
36. Anderson ML et al (2008) Diagnostic comparison of 1.5 Tesla and 3.0 Tesla preoperative MRI of the wrist in patients with ulnar-sided wrist pain. J Hand Surg Am 33(7):1153–1159
37. Lenk S et al (2004) 3.0 T high-resolution MR imaging of carpal ligaments and TFCC. Rofo 176(5):664–667
38. Saupe N et al (2005) MR imaging of the wrist: comparison between 1.5- and 3-T MR imaging—preliminary experience. Radiology 234(1):256–264
39. Magee T (2009) Comparison of 3-T MRI and arthroscopy of intrinsic wrist ligament and TFCC tears. AJR Am J Roentgenol 192(1):80–85
40. Berger RA (1996) The gross and histologic anatomy of the scapholunate interosseous ligament. J Hand Surg Am 21(2):170–178
41. Sokolow C, Saffar P (2001) Anatomy and histology of the scapholunate ligament. Hand Clin 17(1):77–81
42. Ritt MJ et al (1998) Lunotriquetral ligament properties: a comparison of three anatomic subregions. J Hand Surg Am 23(3):425–431
43. Ritt MJ et al (1998) The lunotriquetral joint: kinematic effects of sequential ligament sectioning, ligament repair, and arthrodesis. J Hand Surg Am 23(3):432–445
44. Moser T et al (2008) Multidetector CT arthrography of the wrist joint: how to do it. Radiographics 28(3):787–800; quiz 911
45. Maizlin ZV et al (2009) MR arthrography of the wrist: controversies and concepts. Hand (N Y) 4(1):66–73
46. Moser T et al (2007) Wrist ligament tears: evaluation of MRI and combined MDCT and MR arthrography. AJR Am J Roentgenol 188(5):1278–1286

MRI of Normal Anatomy and Injuries of Extrinsic Ligaments

M. Shahabpour, P. Ceuterick, B. Allemon, N. Pouliart, S. Provyn, and M. De Maeseneer

Carpal instability is usually the consequence of a fracture and/or of ligamentous injuries. Sometimes, instability does not evolve and hardly hampers the movements of the wrist or merely provokes a slight pain. But occasionally, on the contrary, instability can lead to functional disability and increasing pain and even result in osteoarthritis [1–3].

MRI and arthroscopy are examinations which allow the direct visualisation and analysis of wrist ligaments. The main goal of the exploration of the ligaments is to recognise and to point out the injuries which can badly evolve and require a specific treatment. They are prescribed to a patient who suffers from a functional discomfort with doubtful radio-clinical results or in case of radio-clinical anomalies, allowing to resort to healing surgery [4, 5].

Most authors agree on the fact that in case of carpal instability, intrinsic and extrinsic ligaments are injured [6]. Nevertheless, interosseous (scapholunate and lunotriquetral) ligaments have to be completely injured to develop a significant carpal instability.

Although some correlation studies between the results of MRI and arthroscopy (often dealing with a limited series of patients) have been mentioned in medical literature on intrinsic ligaments (especially the scapholunate), very few works focus on the comparative study of these techniques to diagnose extrinsic ligamentous injuries.

M. Shahabpour (✉) • B. Allemon • N. Pouliart • M. De Maeseneer
Department of Medical Imaging,
Universitair Ziekenhuis Brussel, Brussels, Belgium
e-mail: maryam.shahabpour@uzbrussel.be

P. Ceuterick
Department of Orthopaedics and Hand Surgery,
Cliniques de l'Europe, Brussels, Belgium

S. Provyn
Department of Experimental Anatomy,
Vrije Universiteit Brussel, Brussels, Belgium

E. Camus, L. Van Overstraeten (eds.), *Carpal Ligament Surgery*,
DOI 10.1007/978-2-8178-0379-1_5, © Springer-Verlag France 2013

This chapter aims at describing the normal and pathological MR appearance of radiocarpal and ulnocarpal extrinsic ligaments. We will go on anatomic descriptions of the literature and personal findings after cadaveric studies and arthroscopic correlations.

Our work is based on the retrospective analysis of 132 wrist MR examinations of 79 patients (from 17 to 57 years old – mean age of 33) who suffer from midpalmar or middorsal chronic pain. These examinations have been performed on a 1.5 T magnet (Symphony-Vision by Siemens) using a wrist coil with four channels. Two-mm-thick slices were obtained in the three orthogonal planes, using spin echo proton density and T2-weighted sequences and proton density sequence with fat saturation as well as 1-mm-thick coronal slices in T2-weighted 3D gradient echo sequence. A detailed arthroscopic correlation has been obtained in 27 cases out of 79 patients (who have systematically been operated by the same hand surgeon) [7].

The anatomy of the extrinsic ligaments is complex. They are intracapsular and link the radius and the ulna to the carpal bones. They gather radiocarpal ligaments (between the radius and the carpal bones) and ulnocarpal ligaments (between the ulna and the carpal bones). All the radiocarpal ligaments are proximally attached to the distal extremity of the radius and distally inserted on one or several carpal bones. They are capsular thickenings which have, for most of them, an oblique direction and thus require several thin adjacent slices to analyse the whole ligaments. They appear as fasciculate and striated structures, presenting bands of low signal intensity alternating with bands of intermediate or high signal intensity on coronal slices [8, 9]. Several extrinsic ligaments are described at the level of the palmar and dorsal parts of the carpus. Palmar ligaments are thicker and stronger than dorsal ligaments. They are important stabilisers of wrist movements [10–12].

Although there are several variations within the nomenclature and the description of the ligaments, we will keep in mind two groups on the palmar side (with a reversed V shape) and a ligamentous group with a transverse direction (with a reversed V shape) on the dorsal side.

1 Palmar Radiocarpal Ligaments

On the palmar side, three strong extrinsic radiocarpal ligaments were clearly identified: the radioscaphocapitate, long radiolunate and short radiolunate ligaments (Fig. 1).

The radioscaphocapitate ligament (*RSC*) extends from the styloid process of the radius; it cravats the scaphoid waist (what enables to maintain the position of the scaphoid as it acts like a seat belt) to insert on the palmar side of the capitate. It acts like a spindle around which revolves the scaphoid and is paramount in the scaphoid stability [13–16].

The radiolunotriquetral ligament (*RLT*) or long radiolunate ligament is paralleled to the radioscaphocapitate ligament, extends from the anterior margin and from the styloid process of the radius to the radial margin of the palmar surface of

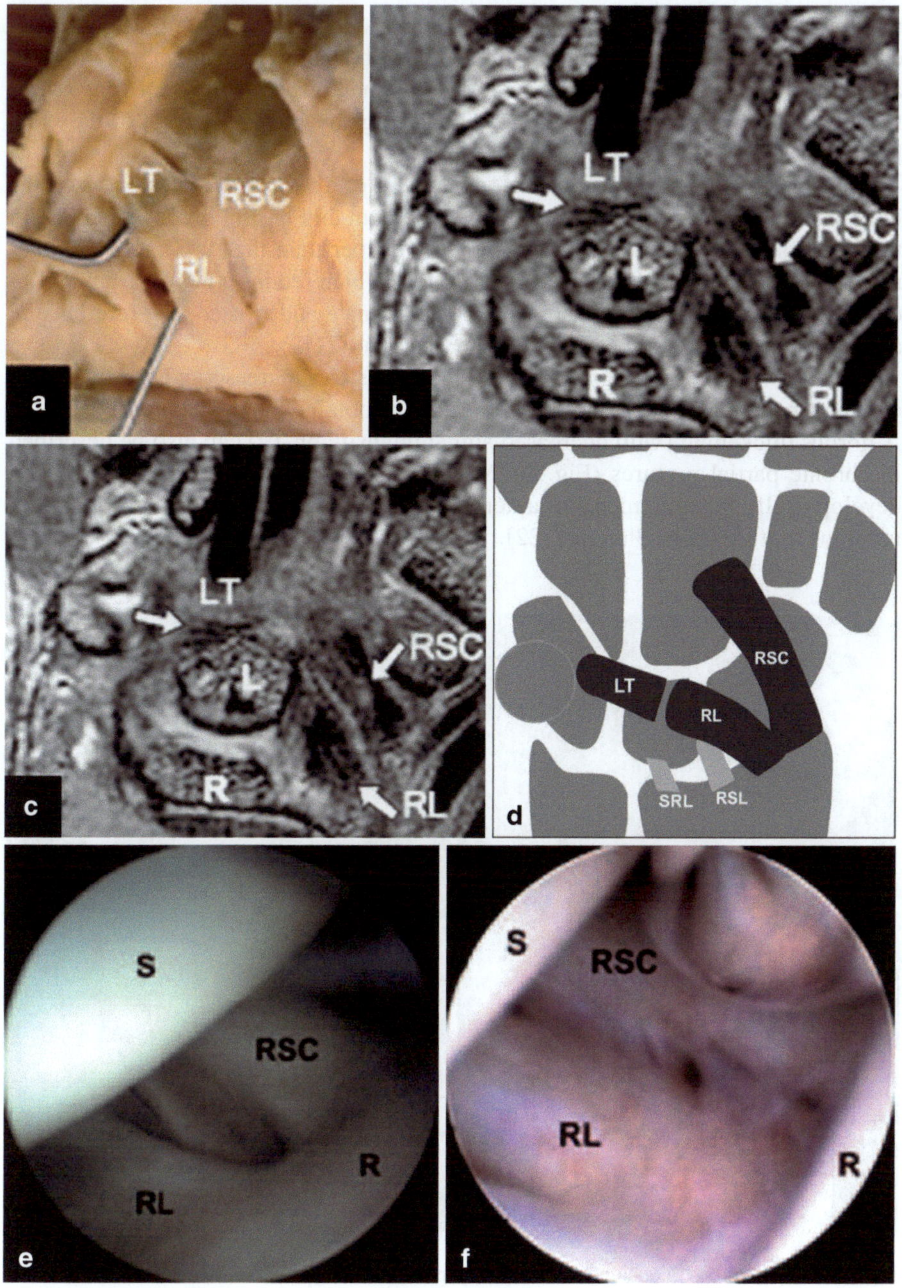

Fig. 1 Palmar extrinsic ligaments : Radioscaphocapitate (*RSC*) and long radiolunate (*RL*) ligaments. Notice the (normal) interruption of the fibres on the lunate attachment with a separated palmar lunotriquetral (*LT*) bundle, which corresponds to an anatomic variation (**a**, **b**). *R* radius, *L* lunate, *S* scaphoid. (**a**) On a cadaveric specimen (Courtesy of David Connell, London), (**b**) normal MR appearance on a thin slice (1 mm thick) obtained in 3D gradient echo sequence, (**c**) partial rupture of the RSC and RL ligaments, (**d**) drawing which shows the trajectory of these two ligaments together with the radioscapholunate ligament (*RSL*) and the inconstant short radiolunate ligament (*SRL*), (**e**) normal arthroscopic view, (**f**) arthroscopic view of the injured RSC and RL ligaments showing synovitis filling the interligamentous sulcus

the lunate and obliquely connects on the palmar side of the triquetrum (where it is covered up by the ulnotriquetral ligament). The fibres of this ligament can interrupt at the lunate attachment and thus create two ligamentous structures, the long radio-lunate and the palmar lunotriquetral. The RLT ligament is the longest of the wrist [17–20].

The radioscapholunate ligament (or ligament of Testut) originates between the long and short portions of the radiolunate ligament and has its fibres embedded in the interosseous scapholunate ligament. It is deeper than the RSC and RLT ligaments. It is rather considered as a synovial fold which retains a neurovascular bundle. It corresponds to the anterior brake of the lunate and is used as a reference in arthroscopy to point out the scapholunate ligament [21].

In case of injury, the signal of these ligaments can increase and the ligaments can lose their sharp outlines on the thin sections obtained in 3D sequence (Fig. 1). A fibrous thickening (with decreased signal intensity on T2) can also be described in chronic partial ruptures (Fig. 2). Moreover a cyst can sometimes appear and develop itself in the ligaments or anterior to it, and be associated to a chronic ligamentous rupture (Figs. 3 and 4) [22].

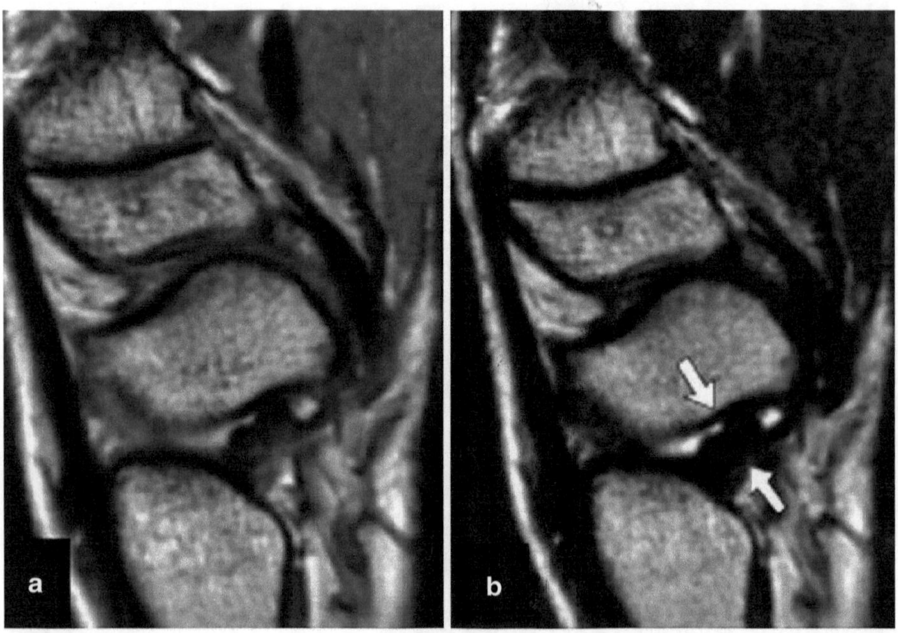

Fig. 2 Chronic fibrous thickening of the radioscaphocapitate ligament (**a**, **b**, *arrows*) of a gymnast who suffered from midcarpal pain. The presence of an associated rupture of the intrinsic scapholunate ligament results in a rotatory subluxation of the scaphoid (with a horizontal orientation of the latter), which is clearly pointed out on the thin sagittal slices (2 mm thick) in proton density (**a**) and T2 (**b**). The ligament seems to be thickened and presents a heterogeneous signal in proton density and weak in T2; it has irregular outlines. Compare with the contralateral wrist (**c**, **d**) where the ligament seems normal (*arrow*), as well as the scaphoid axis

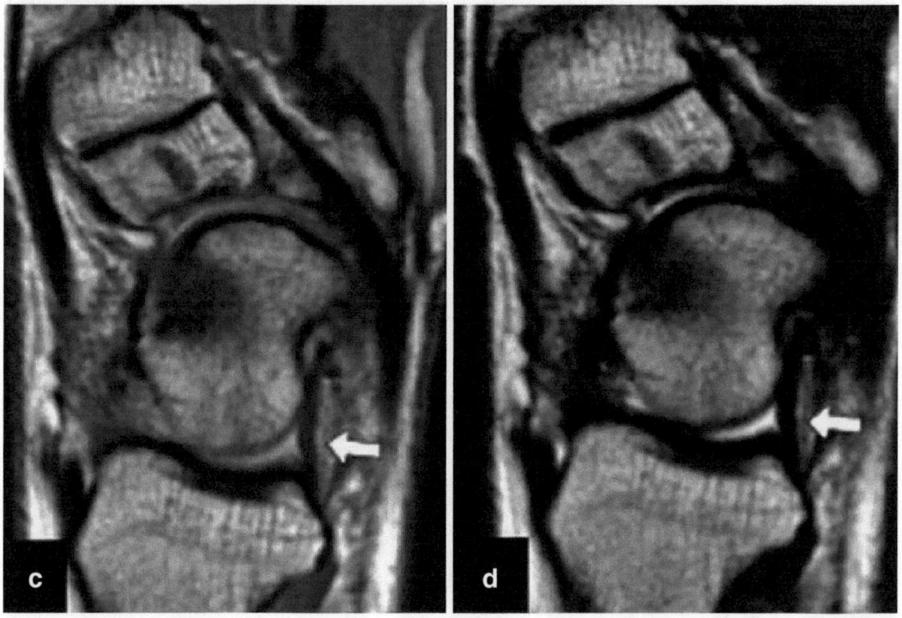

Fig. 2 (continued)

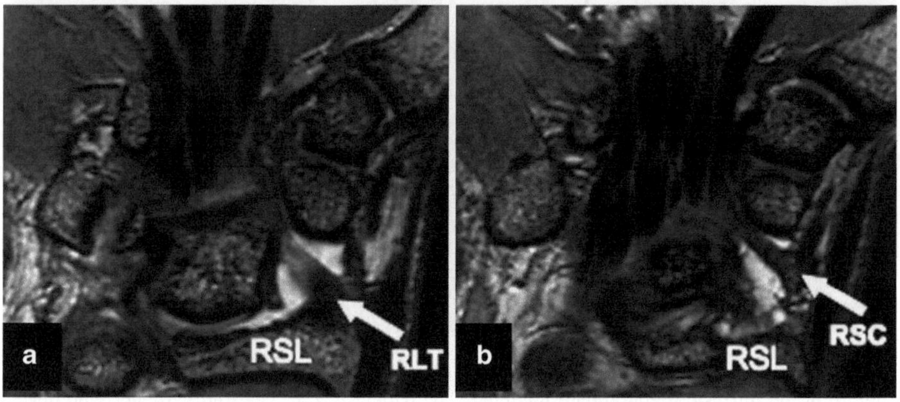

Fig. 3 Synovitis with chronic cystic distension around the radioscapholunate ligament in a patient complaining of palmar radiocarpal pain. On anterior coronal section (of a 3D gradient echo sequence) (**a**, **b**), a cystic distension with a chronic multilobular aspect is put forward at the level of the radioscapholunate ligament (*RSL*). The radiolunotriquetral (*RLT*, **a**) and radioscaphocapitate ligaments (*RSC*, **b**) are continuous

These three palmar ligaments can be visualised by arthroscopy. It is however necessary to precise that the extrinsic ligamentous structures are only reachable during arthroscopic examination for their very short intra-articular part.

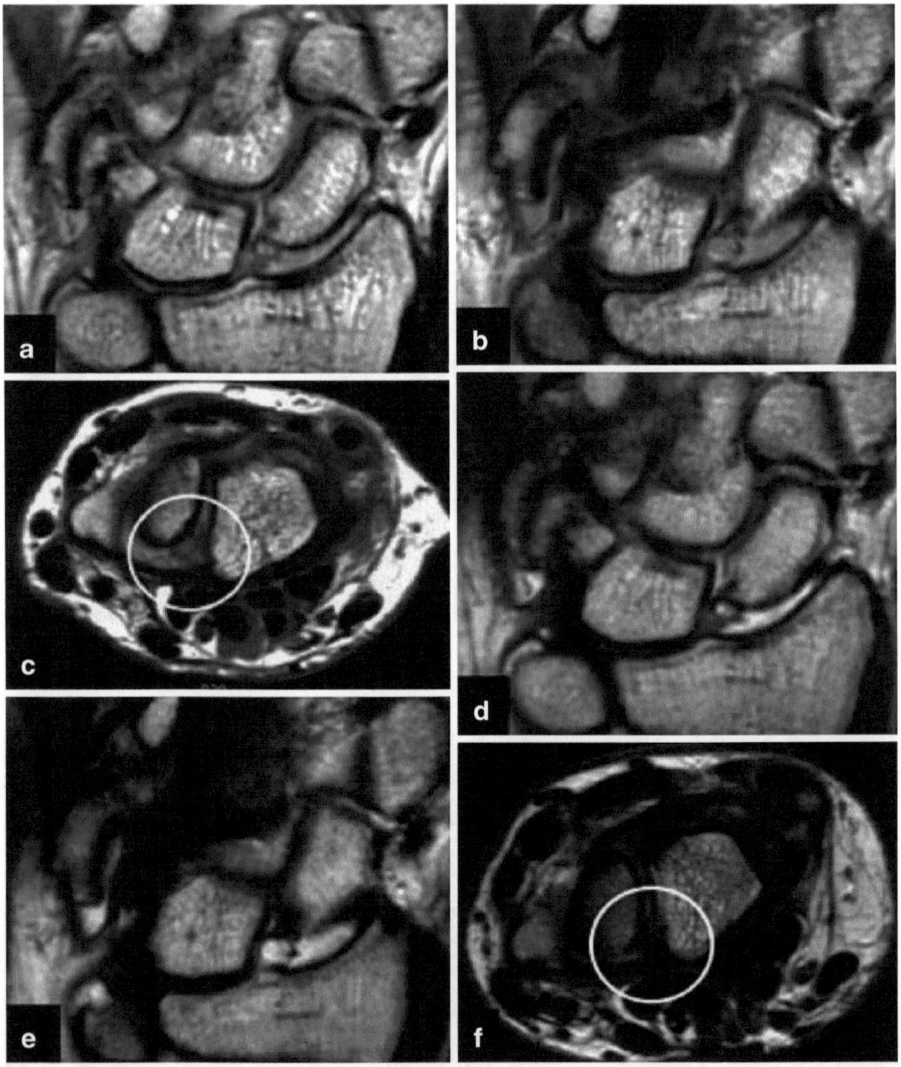

Fig. 4 Thickening of the radioscapholunate ligament and surrounding synovitis associated with a rupture of the intrinsic scapholunate ligament. The patient is a 40-year-old gardener who developed a localised palmar distension after he had pruned trees; he had already fallen from a ladder 4 years before as his wrist was in dorsal hyperflexion. The coronal slices in proton density (**a**, **b**) and T2 (**d**, **e**) reveal the presence of a fluid distension with a cystic aspect at the level of the palmar fibres of the scapholunate and the radioscapholunate ligament with a widening of the scapholunate space. The rupture of the palmar bundle of the intrinsic ligament is confirmed on the transverse section (**c**) on which the ligament has an increased signal intensity, is thickened and has blurred contours in comparison with the normal ligament of the contralateral uninjured wrist (**f**); the dorsal bundle was also torn (not shown) (**c** *circle*, torn palmar bundle of scapholunate ligament; **f** *circle*, normal palmar bundle of scapholunate ligament). The radioscapholunate ligament appears thickened with a heterogeneous signal on the sagittal section (**h**) (*arrow*), whereas the contralateral sagittal section is normal (**g**). Arthroscopy (**i**) reveals the presence of an important synovitis associated with a rupture of the palmar fibres of the scapholunate ligament with partly detached strips. These strips can also be seen on the sagittal section (**h**) at the level of the anterior radiocarpal space, ahead of the tilted lunate (compare to the normal contralateral sagittal section) (**g**). *R* radius, *L* lunate, *S* scaphoid

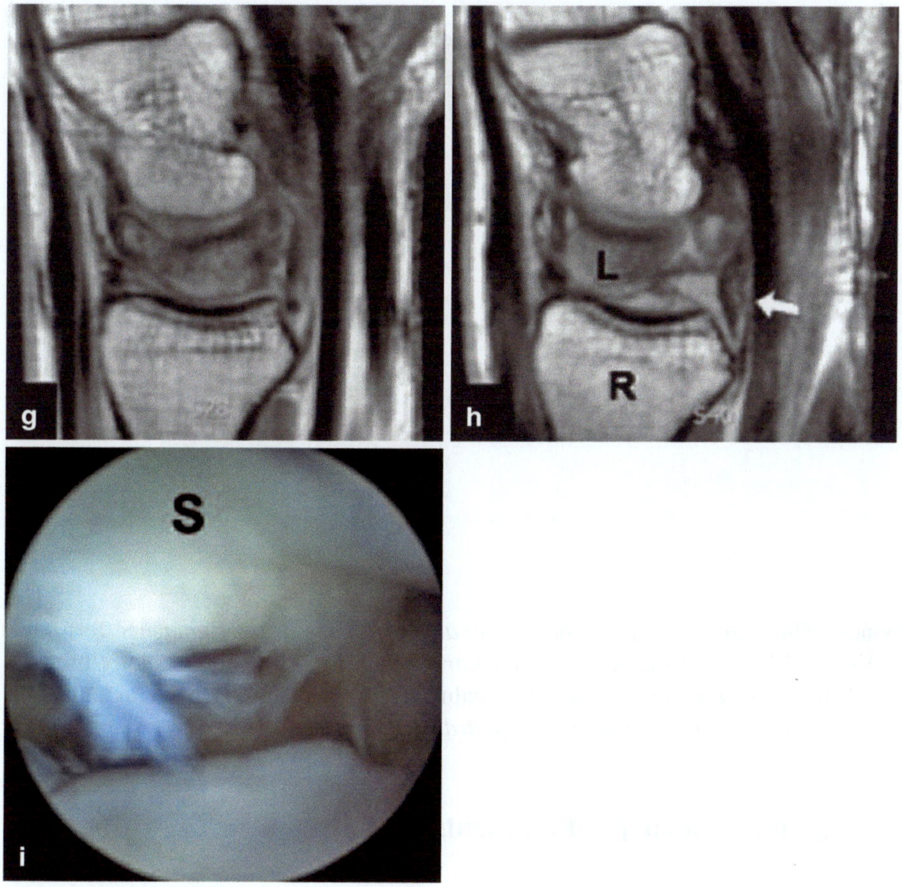

Fig. 4 (continued)

The general configuration of the palmar ligaments has a "V" structure which is weaker at one point, a triangular area in the capsule, so-called space of Poirier. This space is situated between the two palmar arcs with a V shape, above the lunocapitate joint where the lunate can dislocate [23].

The short radiolunate ligament, which is not described by all the researchers, is close to the palmar fibres of the triangular fibrocartilaginous complex. It is an anterior capsular thickening. Its origin is usually described on the palmar and ulnar rim of the distal part of the radius and the ligament inserts at the proximal part of the palmar surface of the lunate. This ligament stabilises the lunate [23] (Fig. 1).

The *distal palmar* ligamentous group (with a reversed V shape) is composed of the intrinsic triquetrocapitate ligament on the medial side and of the extrinsic radioscaphocapitate ligament and of the intrinsic scaphocapitate ligament on the lateral side. This group stabilises the capitate and thus the distal row of the carpal

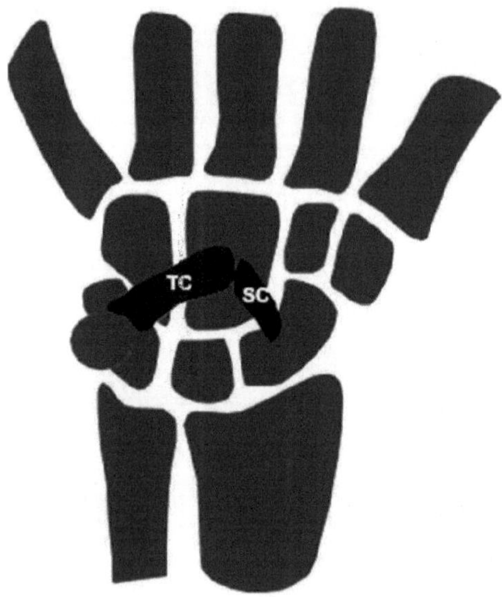

Fig. 5 Image showing the components of the arc-shaped (intrinsic midcarpal): triquetrocapitate (*TC*) and scaphocapitate (*SC*) ligaments

bones. The *intrinsic triquetrocapitate and scaphocapitate ligaments* form the arc-shaped ligament of the wrist or *volar arcuate ligament* (terminology used by hand surgeons) which is an important palmar midcarpal stabiliser. Theumann et al. identified it as the *palmar scaphotriquetral ligament* [7, 24] (Fig. 5).

2 Palmar Ulnocarpal Ligaments

The *proximal palmar* ligamentous group (with a reversed V shape) is made of the extrinsic ulnotriquetral and ulnolunate ligaments, on the medial side and of the extrinsic radiolunotriquetral ligament on the lateral side. This group stabilises the lunate and thus the proximal row of the carpal bones.

The ulnocarpal ligaments originate on the anterior rim of the palmar radioulnar ligament or of the triangular fibrocartilage or the base of the styloid process of the ulna (according to the different authors). The ulnolunate ligament is situated next to the short radiolunate ligament following the same direction and then is inserted on the palmar side of the lunate. The ulnotriquetral ligament originates medial to the former and inserts on the triquetrum [25] (Fig. 6).

3 Dorsal Radiocarpal Ligaments

Dorsal ligaments are thinner and biomechanically less important than palmar ligaments. The *dorsal radiolunotriquetral ligament* (radiocarpal ligament) is the main extrinsic ligament, extending from the distal radius (at the level of the Lister tubercle and/or the styloid process of the radius) to the lunate and the triquetrum.

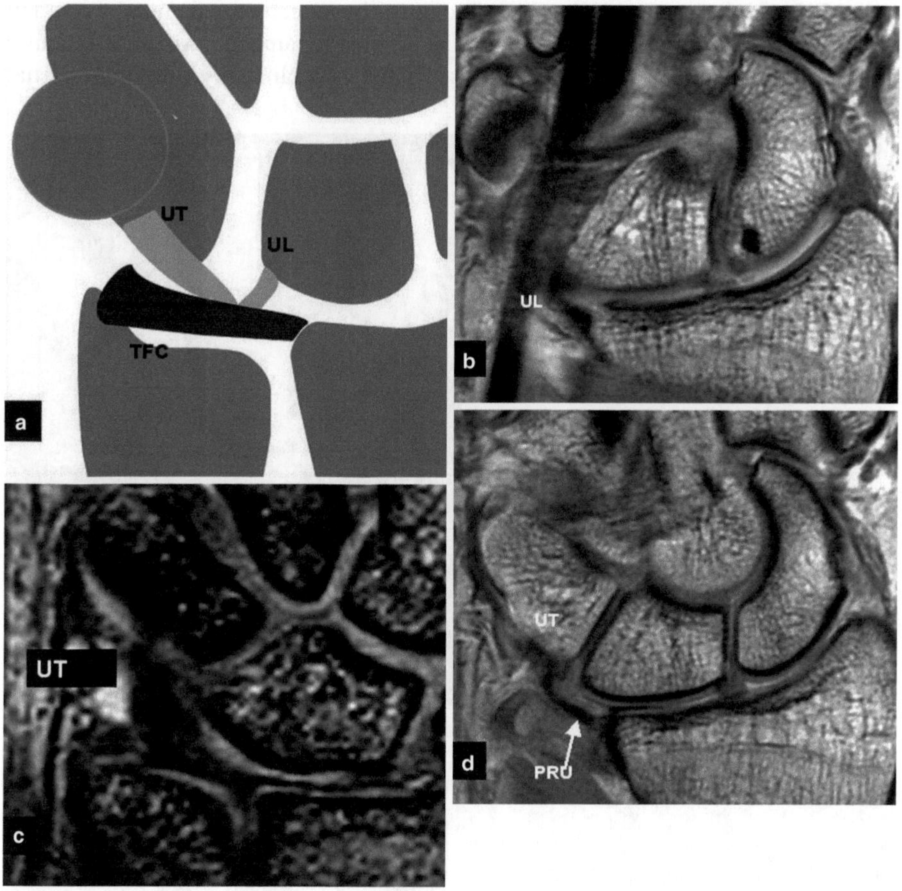

Fig. 6 Normal palmar ulnocarpal ligaments: (**a**) Drawing demonstrating the palmar ulnotriquetral (*UT*) and ulnolunate ligaments (*UL*) attached to the triangular fibrocartilage (*TFC*). (**b**) Normal ulnolunate ligament (*UL*) on an anterior coronal section (2 mm thick) obtained in proton density spin echo sequence. (**c**) Ulnotriquetral ligament (*UT*) on the triangular fibrocartilage observed on a thin section (1-mm-thick) 3D gradient echo image. (**d**) Ulnotriquetral ligament (*UT*) attached on the palmar radioulnar ligament (*PRU*) on an anterior coronal section obtained in proton density spin echo sequence (posterior to (**b**) and anterior to (**c**))

Several dorsal midcarpal ligaments link the carpal bones. Among these ligaments are the *dorsal intercarpal ligament*, which includes the triquetroscaphoidal and the triquetro-trapezoido-trapezial ligaments [23, 26–28] (Figs. 7 and 8).

The dorsal ligamentous group which has a transverse orientation (with a reversed V shape) is composed by these ligaments. They also participate in the stability of the proximal row of the carpus.

According to the arthroscopic correlation study performed by Scheck et al. dealing on 20 patients who were operated and examined by MRI and by MR arthrography, radiocarpal ligaments cannot be accurately analysed on a MRI, even with thin slices [29, 30]. According to our experience, ligamentous injuries could be suspected on a MRI with intravenous injection of contrast, by detecting oedematous reaction and granulation tissue at the level of the injured ligaments. An intra-articular injection of contrast might hide signs associated to a clinically important partial

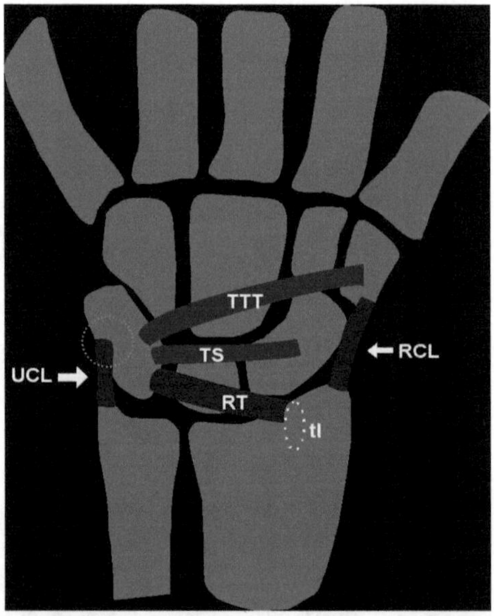

Fig. 7 Image indicating the dorsal radiotriquetral ligament (*RT*) with its proximal insertion on the tubercle of Lister (*tl*). The other two ligaments are midcarpal ligaments: the triquetroscaphoidal (*TS*) and the triquetro-trapezoido-trapezial (*TTT*), also called "dorsal intercarpal ligament." *RCL* radial collateral ligament, *UCL* ulnar collateral ligament

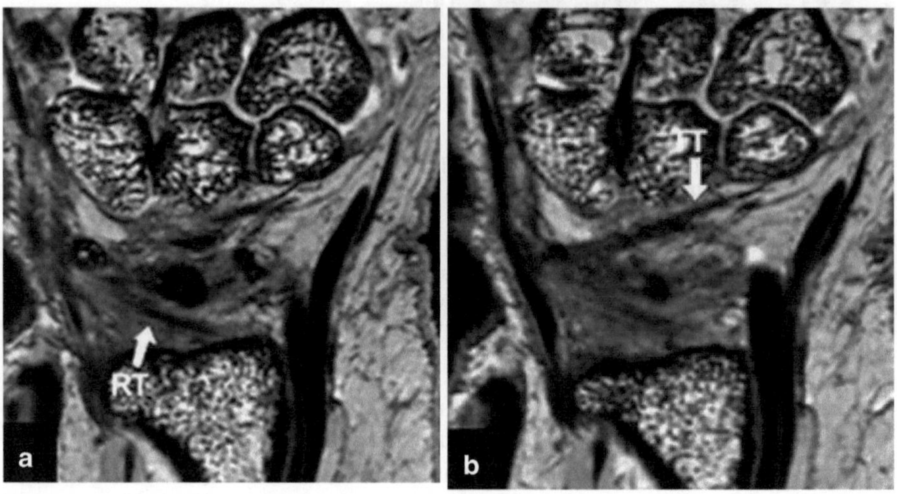

Fig. 8 Normal extrinsic dorsal radiotriquetral ligament (*RT*), normal midcarpal triquetroscaphoidal (*TS*) and triquetro-trapezoido-trapezial ligaments (*TTT*). (**a, b**) Thin coronal slices (1 mm) in 3D gradient echo sequence obtained on a cadaveric specimen. (**c**) Thin coronal slice (1 mm) in 3D gradient echo sequence on a patient whose dorsal ligaments were normal. (**d, f**) Coronal slices (2 mm) in STIR sequence on a gymnast presenting clinical signs of dorsal impingement, whose triquetroscaphoidal ligament was thinned but continuous (**d**) with cystic distension between the dorsal ligaments. (**e**) Photograph of the cadaveric specimen

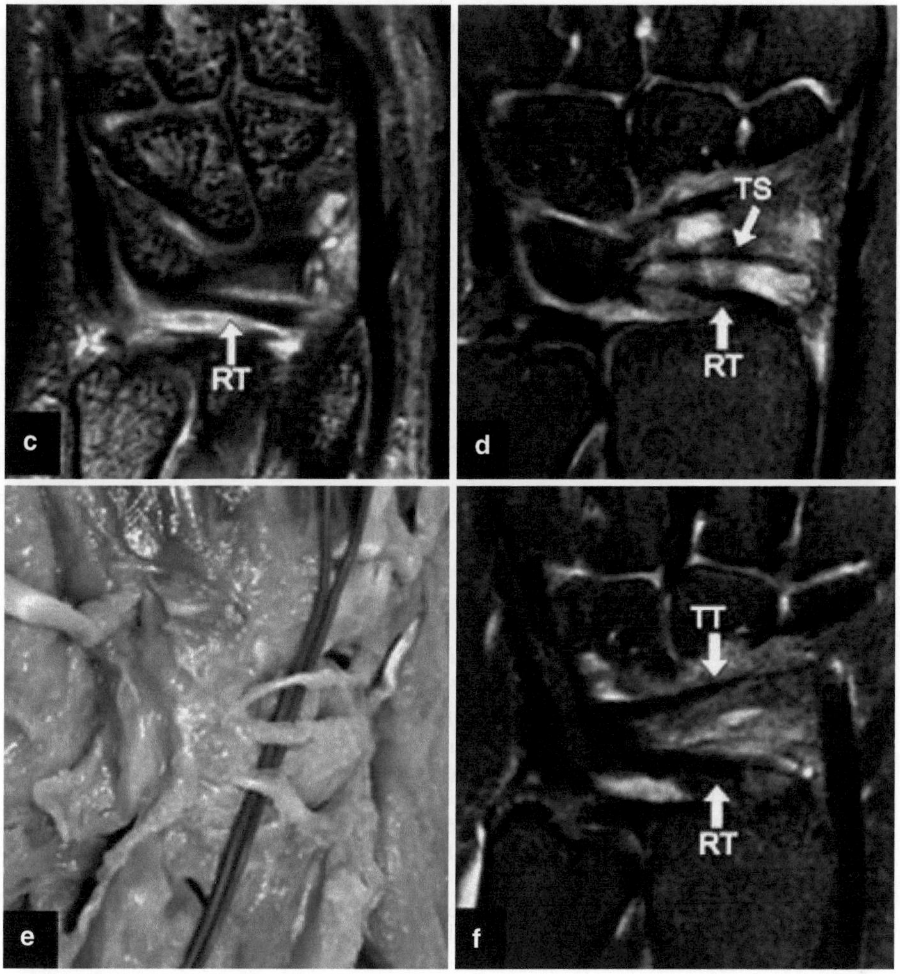

Fig. 8 (continued)

ligamentous rupture. These signs could be the presence of a native cyst, a local fluid reaction or an associated osseous oedema, which could often be useful to diagnose the injuries.

4 Collateral Ligaments

Collateral ligaments of the wrist are thickenings of the fibrous capsule; their function is less important than those of the knee or the elbow. The *radial collateral ligament* is a dorsal extension of the palmar radioscaphoidal ligament and extends from the apex of the styloid process of the radius to insert on the scaphoid waist (Fig. 7).

The *ulnar collateral ligament* reinforces the palmar ulnotriquetral ligament and is proximally connected to the basis and to the body of the styloid process of the ulna (with an extension towards the triangular fibrocartilage). It is distally connected to the triquetrum and to the pisiform [23] (Fig. 7).

On the basis of this preliminary retrospective study of MR images compared to arthroscopic findings, it is possible to notice that if we use magnets with high magnetic fields (from 1.5 to 3 T) and dedicated wrist coils, MRI could become a supplementary paramount help to the imaging methods already used to detect carpal instabilities (dynamic radiographs, CT arthrography etc.). It may in the future even replace diagnostic arthroscopy of the wrist. Nevertheless, the positive aspect of arthroscopy is to give a dynamic approach which cannot be given by high resolution MRI. Moreover, numerous injuries of the ligamentous structures of the wrist detected, thanks to MRI, will always have to be interpreted with caution and associated with clinical findings to avoid excessive surgical treatments.

Acknowledgements To Eddy Broodtaerts, Filip, Bart, Els and Yasmina for their precious collaboration in the elaboration of MR images.

References

1. Linscheid RL, Dobyns JH, Beabout JW et al (1972) Traumatic instability of the wrist: diagnosis, classification and pathomechanics. J Bone Joint Surg Am 54A:1612–1632
2. Trail IA, Stanley JK, Hayton MJ (2007) Twenty questions on carpal instability. J Hand Surg Eur Vol 32(3):240–255
3. Schmitt R, Frochner S, Coblenz G et al (2006) Carpal instability. Eur Radiol 16:2161–2178
4. Roulot E (2001) Arthroscopie du poignet. In: Godefroy D et al (eds) Intérêt diagnostique et thérapeutique dans Imagerie du poignet et de la main. Sauramps Médical, Paris
5. Dautel G, Et Blum A (2001) In: Godefroy D et al (eds) Place de l'arthroscanner et de l'arthroscopie dans le diagnostic des instabilités du poignet dans Imagerie du poignet et de la main. Sauramps Médical, Paris
6. Theumann NH, Etechami G, Duvoisin B (2006) Association between extrinsic and intrinsic carpal ligament injuries at MR arthrography and carpal instability at radiography: initial observations. Radiology 238:950–957
7. Shahabpour M, Van Overstraeten L, Ceuterick P, Milants A, Goubau J, Boulet C, De Mey J, Demaeseneer M (2012) Pathology of extrinsic ligaments: a pictorial essay. Semin Musculoskelet Radiol 16(2):115–128
8. Totterman SM, Miller R, Wasserman B, Blebea JS, Rubens DJ (1993) Intrinsic and extrinsic carpal ligaments: evaluation by three-dimensional Fourier transform MR imaging. AJR Am J Roentgenol 160:117–123
9. Brown RR, Fliszar E, Cotten A, Trudell D, Resnick D (1998) Extrinsic and intrinsic ligaments of the wrist: normal and pathologic anatomy at MR arthrography with three-compartments enhancement. Radiographics 18:667–674
10. Viegas SF, Patterson RM, Hokanson JA, Davis J (1993) Wrist anatomy: incidence, distribution, and correlation of anatomic variations, tears, and arthrosis. J Hand Surg Am 18: 463–475
11. Viegas SF, Patterson RM, Ward K (1995) Extrinsic wrist ligaments in the pathomechanics of ulnar translation instability. J Hand Surg Am 20A:312–318

12. Feipel V, Rooze M (1999) The capsular ligaments of the wrist: morphology, morphometry and clinical applications. Surg Radiol Anat 21:175–180
13. Taleisnik J (1976) The ligaments of the wrist. J Hand Surg Am 1:110–118
14. Berger RA, Landsmeer JM (1990) The palmar radiocarpal ligaments: a study of adult and fetal human wrist joints. J Hand Surg Am 15:847–854
15. Reicher M (1990) Normal wrist anatomy, biomechanics, basic imaging protocol, and normal multiplanar MRI of the wrist. In: Reicher MA (ed) MRI of the wrist and hand. Raven Press, New York, pp 17–48
16. Theumann NH, Pfirrmann CW, Antonio GE, Chung CB, Gilula LA, Trudell DJ (2003) Extrinsic carpal ligaments: normal MR arthrographic appearance in cadavers. Radiology 226:171–179
17. Smith DK (1993) Volar carpal ligaments of the wrist: normal appearance on multiplanar reconstructions of three-dimensional Fourier transform MR imaging. AJR Am J Roentgenol 161:353–357
18. Rominger MB, Bernreuter WK, Kenney PJ, Lee DH (1993) MR imaging of anatomy and tears of wrist ligaments. Radiographics 13:1233–1246
19. Timins ME, Jabnke JP, Krah SF, Erickson SJ, Carrera GE (1995) MR imaging of the major carpal stabilizing ligaments: normal anatomy and clinical examples. Radiographics 15: 575–587
20. Boutry N, Lapegue F, Masi L et al (2005) Ultrasonographic evaluation of normal extrinsic and intrinsic carpal ligaments: preliminary experience. Skeletal Radiol 34:513–521
21. Berger RA, Kauer JM (1991) Radioscapholunate ligament: a gross anatomic and histologic study of fetal and adult wrists. J Hand Surg Am 16:350–355
22. Connell D, Page P, Wright W, Hoy G (2001) MRI of the wrist ligaments. Australas Radiol 45(4):411–422
23. Resnick D, Kang HS, Pretterklieber ML (2007) Wrist and hand in internal derangements of joints, vol 1, 2nd edn. Saunders, Philadelphia, pp 1218–1418
24. Chang W, Peduto AJ, Aguiar RO, Trudell DJ, Resnick DL (2007) Arcuate ligament of the wrist: normal MR appearance and its relationship to palmar midcarpal instability: a cadaveric study. Skeletal Radiol 36:641–645
25. Tanaka T, Ogino S, Yoshioka H (2008) Ligamentous injuries of the wrist. Semin Musculoskelet Radiol 12:359–378
26. Smith DK (1993) Dorsal carpal ligaments of the wrist: normal appearance on multiplanar reconstructions of three-dimensional Fourier transform MR imaging. AJR Am J Roentgenol 161:119–125
27. Mitsuyasu H, Patterson RM, Shah MA, Buford WL, Iwamoto Y, Viegas SF (2004) The role of the dorsal intercarpal ligament in dynamic and static scapholunate instability. J Hand Surg Am 29:279–288
28. Sarazin L, Godefroy D, Rousselin B, Drapé JL, Chevrot A (2005) Imagerie par résonance magnétique du poignet et de la main dans les situations normales. Atlas anatomique. Encycl Méd Chir. Elsevier SAS, Paris
29. Scheck RJ, Romagnolo A, Hierner R, Pfluger T, Wilhelm K, Hahn K (1999) The carpal ligaments in MR arthrography of the wrist: correlation with standard MRI and wrist arthroscopy. J Magn Reson Imaging 9:468–474
30. Maizlin ZV, Brown JA, Clement JJ, Grebenyuk J, Fenton DM, Smith DE, Jacobson JA (2008) MR arthrography of the wrist: controversies and concepts. Hand (N Y) 4(1):66–73

Definition and Classification of Carpal Instability

E. Camus

1 Introduction

Although the study of the different types of carpal instability goes back to 1905 with Destot's [1] publication, the word "instability" itself was first used in 1967 [2]. In 1972, Linscheid et al. came up with the first classification of the different types of wrist instability, among which are the notions of dorsal flexion and palmar flexion instability [3]. But the definition, in order to be complete, had to be revised several times. The classification of these lesions requires the analysis of many criteria.

2 Definition

In a way, a wrist may be considered as unstable if there is a malalignment of the carpal bones [4]. But this description is limited in the sense that certain hyperlax wrists present a carpal malalignment without being symptomatic and that some radiographically normal wrists are symptomatic and cannot bear loads [5]. Therefore, the definition of instability cannot be restricted to a loss of alignment of the carpal bones visible on plain X-rays. Instability could be defined as the inability of the wrist to transmit physiologic loads. But this definition does not render the "snapping" phenomena which certain patients sometimes feel while grasping. The IFSSH wished to clarify this definition published in 1999 [5]. A wrist is considered to be unstable "when it is not capable of bearing loads without sudden changes of cartilaginous pressure or when its kinematics is perturbed, including brutal changes in the alignment of the carpal bones."

E. Camus
Hand Surgery Unit, SELARL Chirurgie de la Main,
Polyclinique du Val de Sambre,
162, route de Mons, 59600 Maubeuge, France
e-mail: ejcamus@wanadoo.fr, emmanuel.camus@wanadoo.fr

E. Camus, L. Van Overstraeten (eds.), *Carpal Ligament Surgery*,
DOI 10.1007/978-2-8178-0379-1_6, © Springer-Verlag France 2013

3 Classification

In fact, instability can be classified according to different criteria brought together in 1995 by Larsen et al. [6, 7]. In this way, six categories appear; these may be combined in order to add more precision to the description.

I Chronicity

(a) Acute (<1 week; maximum healing potential)
(b) Subacute (1–6 weeks; healing potential)
(c) Chronic (>6 weeks; little healing potential)

II Variability

(a) Static, visible on standard pictures (reducible or irreducible)
(b) Dynamic, visible on stress or fluoroscopic radiographies
(c) Predynamic, or occult [8], invisible on radiographies but visible in arthroscopy

III Etiology

(a) Congenital
(b) Traumatic
(c) Inflammatory
(d) Arthritis
(e) Osteonecrosis (Kienböck's disease, necrosis of the capitate)
(f) Neurological
(g) Iatrogenic

IV Location

(a) Radiocarpal
(b) Intercarpal
(c) Midcarpal
(d) Carpometacarpal
(e) Particular bones or ligaments

V Direction of the Instability

(a) VISI
(b) DISI
(c) Ulnar
(d) Radial
(e) Volar
(f) Dorsal
(g) Proximal
(h) Distal
(i) Rotatory
(j) Combined

VI Types

(a) Carpal instability dissociative (CID): intra-row instability, proximal most of the time, if not, distal
(b) Carpal instability nondissociative (CIND): inter-row instability, generally visible through a shift of the first row, can be of radiocarpal or midcarpal origin
(c) Carpal instability combined or complex (CIC): association of an intra-row (CID) and inter-row [5] (CIND) instability
(d) Carpal instability adaptive (CIA): of extracarpal origin, most of the time due to the adaptation of the carpus to a vicious callus of the radius

These type descriptions were detailed in "Terminology and Definitions" works of the IWIW (International Wrist Investigators' Workshop), published in 2002 [9].

4 Discussion

None of these classification categories is sufficient to give an idea of the variety of different types of instability, of circumstances in which these may appear, of diagnostics, of possible evolutions and of treatments. The cross-checking of these classifications also enables one to understand that several evolutive or lesional aspects may correspond to a similar clinical or radiographic aspect. Finally, a normal use of these classification systems leads to answering various questions.

The aim is to help the practitioner select the most suitable treatment. Certain categories (I, II, VI) contain exclusive choice possibilities, with only one possible item being retained. In categories III, IV, and V, several items may simultaneously correspond to the lesional description [6, 7]. Finally, even if all the descriptive categories are useful to the therapeutic discussion, categories I, II, III, and VI have specific implications in the evaluation of the lesion, and categories III, IV, and V have specific implications in envisaging the therapeutic options.

5 Conclusion

Thanks to these works of clarification and lesional description, the practitioner now has at his/her disposal a tool enabling a theoretical analysis of the situation. It is all about a language in the process of becoming adopted by all which will enable one to better compare populations and treatments. Of course, for each clinical case, one still has to put to good use the diagnostic tools necessary to answer in the best way possible the different questions brought to light by this classification.

References

1. Destot E (1905) Lésions du poignet et accidents du travail. Vigot, Paris
2. Dobyns JH, Perkins JC (1967) Instability of the carpal navicular. J Bone Joint Surg 49 A:1014
3. Linscheid R, Dobyns JH, Beabout JW, Bryan RS (1972) Traumatic instability of the wrist: diagnosis, classification, and pathomechanics. J Bone Joint Surg 54-A:1612–1632
4. Ruby LK (1995) Carpal instability. J Bone Joint Surg 77A:476–487
5. The Anatomy and Biomechanics Committee of the International Federation Societies for Surgery of the Hand (IFSSH) (1999) Definition of carpal instability. J Hand Surg 24A:866–867
6. Larsen CF, Amadio PC, Gilula LA, Hodge JC (1995) Analysis of carpal instability: I. Description of the scheme. J Hand Surg Am 20(5):757–764
7. Hodge JC, Gilula LA, Larsen CF, Amadio PC (1995) Analysis of carpal instability: II. Clinical applications. J Hand Surg Am 20(5):765–776
8. Nathan R, Blatt G (2000) Rotary subluxation of the scaphoid. Revisited. Hand Clin 16:417–430
9. Gilula LA, Mann FA, Dobyns JH, Yin Y, IWIW Terminology Committee (2002) Wrist terminology as defined by the International Wrist Investigators' Workshop (IWIW). J Bone Joint Surg 84A(suppl 1):1–67

Normal Wrist Arthroscopy

G. Dautel

The appearance of wrist arthroscopy as a diagnostic tool in the armamentarium of wrist investigations and treatment is relatively recent [1, 2], probably due to the technical constraints imposed by such a small joint interval involved. However, this technique has become inevitable today for diagnosis as well as management of wrist pathology [3], even as noninvasive imaging has continued to progress in performance as well as in definition. Arthroscopy remains the gold standard for evaluation of wrist ligament lesions by the direct vision it provides as well as the dynamic testing which makes it possible to detect even very early stages of dissociative instability [4, 5].

1 Performing a Wrist Arthroscopy

1.1 Anaesthesia

Wrist arthroscopy is performed under locoregional anaesthesia as a day case procedure. The patient may follow the procedure on screen if he/she wishes.

1.2 Setup

Arthroscopy necessitates joint distraction which is obtained by setting up the hand on a traction tower with the forearm vertical and a counter traction support applied to the arm above the elbow. The Chinese finger traps are placed on the index and middle fingers (Fig. 1).

G. Dautel
Service de Chirurgie Plastique et Reconstructrice de l'Appareil Locomoteur,
Centre Chirurgical Emile Gallé, 49 rue Hermite, 54000 Nancy, France
e-mail: gilles.dautel@wanadoo.fr

E. Camus, L. Van Overstraeten (eds.), *Carpal Ligament Surgery*,
DOI 10.1007/978-2-8178-0379-1_7, © Springer-Verlag France 2013

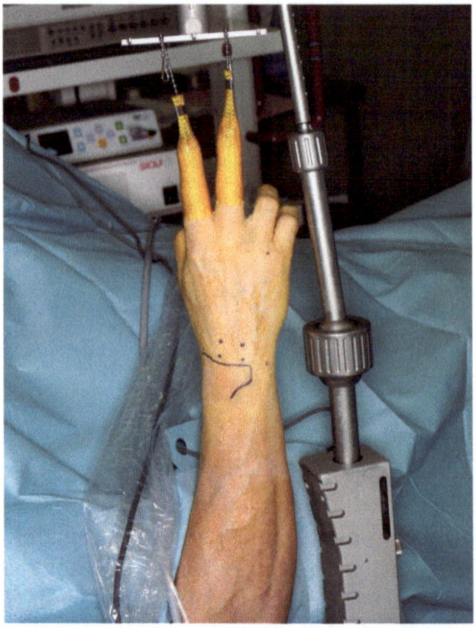

Fig. 1 Arthroscopy tower. This type of tower provides distraction whilst allowing repositioning and wrist orientation as required

The scope used is 2.7-mm calibre oriented at 30°. This scope is adequate for exploration of the radiocarpal and midcarpal joints. The 'needle' 1.9-mm scope is only rarely used for exploration of the distal radioulnar joint. The trocar is smooth-tipped to avoid cartilaginous lesions during introduction. It bears the connection for the light source, and the irrigation. Once in place, the light connects to the video camera where the joint is visualized on a monitor screen and not by direct vision. The probe is an indispensable instrument in this set. Its size and the smoothness of its tip must be adapted to the size of the joint explored. A set of two graspers (straight and curved) as well as a single-use knife are useful for debridement of the TFCC when necessary. The use of powered instruments (shavers and burrs) for arthroscopic surgery for the TFCC is quite common practice now [6].

1.3 Access Portals

The portals of access are designated by the corresponding dorsal extensor compartments (Fig. 2). We recommend defining all the portals that will be needed at the beginning of the operation. The development of a 'hydroma' due to diffusion of the irrigation fluid renders it difficult to identify bone and tendon landmarks later throughout the course of the procedure. For all portals, a small calibre needle is used for identification. If elastic resistance is encountered at the point of entry, it is easy to reposition the needle to avoid tendons. A hard resistance is characteristic of bone. Correct penetration into the joint interval is denoted by a suction sound due to the

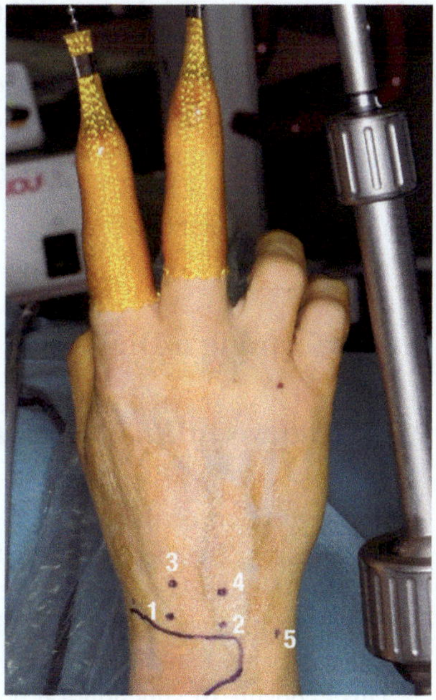

Fig. 2 Portals for exploration of the wrist. The current portals for wrist exploration are identified in relation to the extensor compartments. Portal 3/4 is on the radial border of the extensor communis EDC (*1*) and portal 4/5 on the ulnar border of EDC (*2*). Portals for the midcarpal joint are RMC (*3*) and UMC (*4*). Portal 6U (*5*) is commonly used as drainage outlet for the irrigation

intra-articular negative pressure resulting from the distraction. Once the interval is marked by the needle, portal access can be established using an N°15 blade perpendicular to the surface. The scope or probe can then be introduced.

To explore the radiocarpal joint, three portals are usually sufficient.

Portal 3/4 is the first point of introduction of the scope. This portal is situated at the radial border of extensor communis tendon. The tubercle of Lister is the bony landmark for this portal. It is found by palpating with the thumb along the posterior border of the radial glenoid.

The depression indicating the joint interval can be palpated about 1 cm above (distal) this point. The needle should be introduced obliquely on account of the radial slope in the sagittal plane. The knife should be held sharp facing downward to avoid iatrogenic lesion of the scapholunate interosseous ligament.

Portal 4/5 is between the EDC and EDM and serves for probe introduction for exploration of the radiocarpal joint. The depression between the two tendons is readily palpable and introduction is more proximal than the previous portal on account of the radial slope in the frontal plane. These portals 3/4 and 4/5 are the least risky for sensory nerve branches [7].

Portal 6U is situated on the ulnar border of the ECU. This is the site for the needle for drainage of the irrigation fluid.

Other portals. The 6U portal is seldom used. It is useful for arthroscopic surgery of the TFCC. Palmar portals are only used for arthroscopically assisted reduction of distal radius fractures. Introduction of the scope through the FCR has been proposed as a secure method of exploring the most palmar portion of the scapholunate ligament [8, 9].

1.3.1 Portals for Exploration of the Midcarpal Joint

The radial midcarpal RMC is situated on the radial border of the EDC, about 1 cm distal to the 3/4 portal (Fig. 2). This corresponds to the scaphocapitate interval more difficult to palpate than the radiocarpal interval. The ulnar midcarpal portal UMC is situated on the ulnar border of EDC about 15 mm from 4/5 and corresponds to the triquetrohamate interval.

2 Performing a Diagnostic Arthroscopy

2.1 Analysis of Radiocarpal Chondral Lesions

Simple inspection of the articular surfaces is followed by probing any cartilage defect or lesion. The topography, extent and severity of the lesion is appreciated and noted. Healthy cartilage feels firm and elastic when palpated using the probe. The probe does not leave an imprint on healthy cartilage, and a full-thickness cartilaginous lesion is hard on probing.

This exposure of subchondral bone is synonymous to arthritis even if the lesion is of limited extent and does not show on X-ray. All other chondral lesions without bone exposure are grouped under the generic term 'chondritis'. A precise description of the lesion must specify if it is simple cartilage oedema (the cartilage bears the imprint of the probe), a fibrillary chondritis (associated with cartilaginous flaps) or a partial defect not exposing the underlying bone (without arthritis).

2.2 Study of the Radiocarpal Articular Surfaces

Diagnostic arthroscopy begins by visualization of the scaphoid and lunate fossae of the radius, separated by a blunt anteroposterior ridge (Fig. 3). Through the same portal, the scope is oriented ulnar to explore the horizontal portion of the TFCC.

The radial insertion, central portion and the anterior border of the TFCC must be systematically palpated as they are often the site of traumatic or degenerative lesions. An intact healthy TFCC gives a firm elastic resistance to probing – described as the 'trampoline effect'. When pushed to the ulnar side of the radiocarpal interval, the probe may access the prestyloid recess and penetrate it. This is a physiologic extension of the radioscaphoid joint. A radial traction motion must be applied as if to pull the full thickness of the TFCC laterally. This can depict a peripheral (ulnar) disinsertion of the TFCC. If no lesion, the peripheral TFCC insertion stays taut resisting probing and no wave effect is elicited. Examination of the carpal surfaces follows. Scaphoid convexity is examined until the styloscaphoid space and then the lunate dome is inspected. The 3/4 portal does not allow easy access to the triquetrum; thus, the scope must be reintroduced through the 4/5 portal to complete the radiocarpal examination.

Fig. 3 Exploration of the radiocarpal joint. Scaphoid (S), Scaphoid fossa (*fs*) and Lunate fossa of the radius (*fl*) separated by a blunt ridge

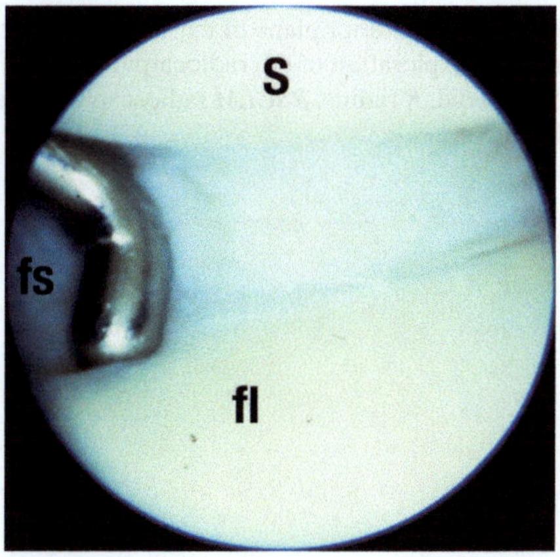

2.3 Study of Ligamentous Structures in the Radiocarpal Joint

Extrinsic ligaments: Due to the dorsal entry point of the scope, the only extrinsic ligaments accessible are those of the anterior plane. The posterior plane cannot be studied – a minor inconvenience since they have a minor role in intracarpal stability. Arthroscopy gives quite a clear intra-articular view of these ligaments [10]. Heated controversy exists as to the nomenclature of these ligaments. We have adopted those best suited to this arthroscopic intra-articular view.

- *The most radial is the radioscaphocapitate ligament* (Fig. 4):
  This ligament arises from the anterior border of the radial glenoid and wraps around the waist of the scaphoid to reach the waist of the capitate. There is a distinct space between it and the radiolunotriquetral which the probe can penetrate and which Berger and Landsmeer named the *interligamentary sulcus* [11]. Thus positioned, the probe can be used to test the tension of the radioscaphocapitate ligament.
- *The second ligament of the anterior extrinsic plane is the radiolunotriquetral ligament*:
  It is distinguished from the previous ligament by the obliquity of its fibres. This ligament arises from the anterior border of the radius facing the scaphoid fossa and directing obliquely towards the triquetrum, to insert on the anterior horn of the lunate and onto the anterior portion of the scapholunate interosseous ligament. As above it can be inspected and tested during the radiocarpal examination.
- *The radioscapholunate ligament* (*ligament of Testut*):
  This ligament is easily identified in arthroscopic examination; its fibres are strictly vertical, inserting onto the radius at the level of the anteroposterior ridge separating the scaphoid and lunate fossae of the radius. The previous two ligaments had oblique fibres. From its radial insertion, this ligament diverges in a T shape where each limb inserts into either part of the interosseous ligament. On palpation, it seems less tense than the other two ligaments whatever the degree of articular

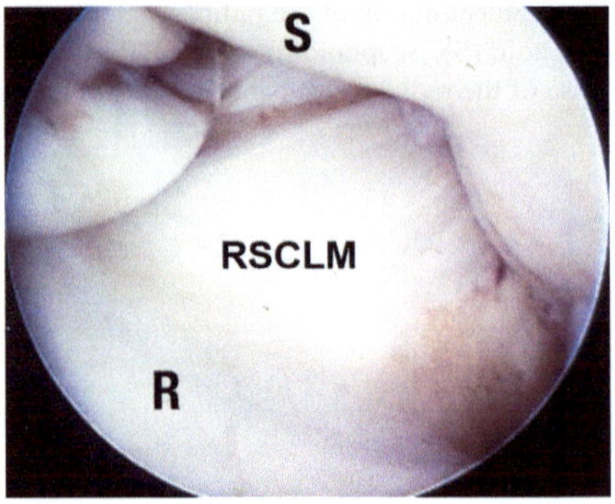

Fig. 4 The anterior plane of extrinsic ligaments seen on exploration of the radiocarpal joint. *S* scaphoid, *R* radius, *RSCLM* radioscaphocapitate ligament

distraction. These arthroscopic findings confirm the accessory biomechanical role played by this ligament, which is otherwise considered as a vessel bearing matrix – an intra-articular extension of the anterior interosseous pedicle [11].

- The radial half of the radiocarpal joint is thus lined at its palmar aspect by three easily distinguished ligaments; the ulnar half is sealed palmarly by a continuous sheet of ligament consolidating with the anterior border of the TFCC. Classic descriptions report two principal ligaments (ulnolunate and ulnotriquetral). Both arise from the ulnar styloid but their respective limits cannot be distinguished by arthroscopy. It is still possible to test this ligament curtain using the probe to appreciate its tension and verify continuity with the anterior border of the TFCC.

3 Intrinsic Ligaments

The scapholunate and lunotriquetral interosseous ligaments must be assessed.

Their posterior two-thirds are accessible to inspection and palpation due to the posterior entry points of the scope.

3.1 The Scapholunate Interosseous Ligament

It is identified at the 'ceiling' of the carpus through the 3/4 portal. Covered by a layer of articular cartilage continuous with that of the scaphoid and the lunate, it may be difficult to identify when healthy; it is palpated as a zone of attenuated tension vertically above the anteroposterior ridge separating the scaphoid and lunate fossae and the deep radioscapholunate ligament (of Testut) (Fig. 5). The entire extent of the ligament should be assessed in search of lesions of the middle or anterior thirds. Traumatic lesions affect the insertion onto the scaphoid, the body of the ligament or less frequently, the lunate insertion.

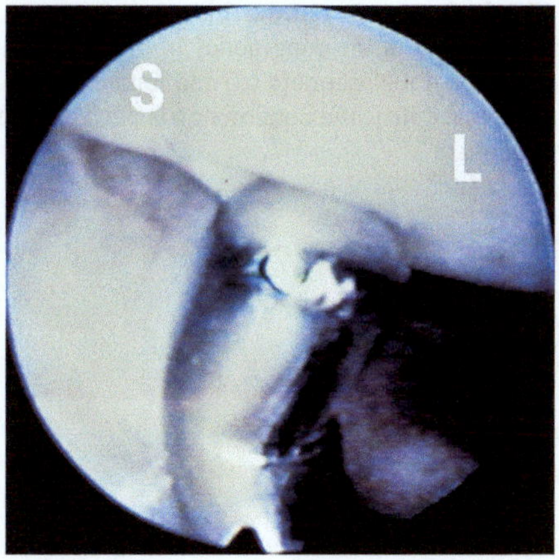

Fig. 5 The scapholunate interosseous ligament. It is identified by the probe as an area of attenuated tone between scaphoid (*S*) and lunate (*L*). It is entirely covered by cartilage

3.2 The Lunotriquetral Interosseous Ligament

It is more difficult to localize due to the absence of anatomical landmark. The scope should be reintroduced through the 4/5 portal, and often probe palpation is necessary.

4 Midcarpal Examination

4.1 Examination of Articular Surfaces

The scope is introduced through the RMC which is generally sufficient for complete exploration of the midcarpal joint including its ulnar corners. The use of a probe is indispensable through the UMC portal. During introduction, the first image seen is the scaphocapitate space. The distal scaphoid fossa and the scapholunate interval are examined at this point. With no ligament lesion, these fossae are perfectly congruent (Fig. 6) and the space between the two bones admits only the tip of the probe.

The slope of this interval is then followed apically and radially to reach the distal pole of the scaphoid and the STT joint. The scope is then pushed ulnarly assessing the capitate head on the way as well as the tip of the hamate and the capitohamate junction. The lunotriquetral interval is also hereby assessed with the same criteria of congruency and cohesion as for the scapholunate interval.

In most cases, it is possible to extend the examination following the helicoidal slope of the hamate to the ulnar corner of the midcarpal joint.

Different morphological types of the midcarpal joint have been described; we have adopted the terminology of Viegas [12] who described type I lunate with a single midcarpal facet and type II when a second facet is present, separated from the

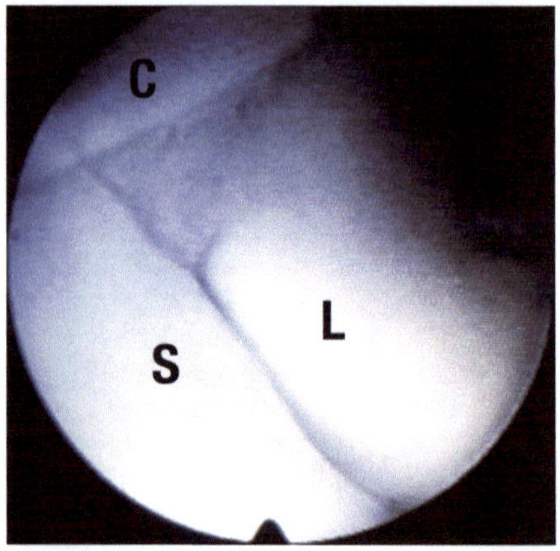

Fig. 6 Assessment of the midcarpal joint. Assessment of the congruency of distal articular surfaces of the scaphoid (*S*) and lunate (*L*). If no instability, the congruency is perfect at rest. *C* capitate

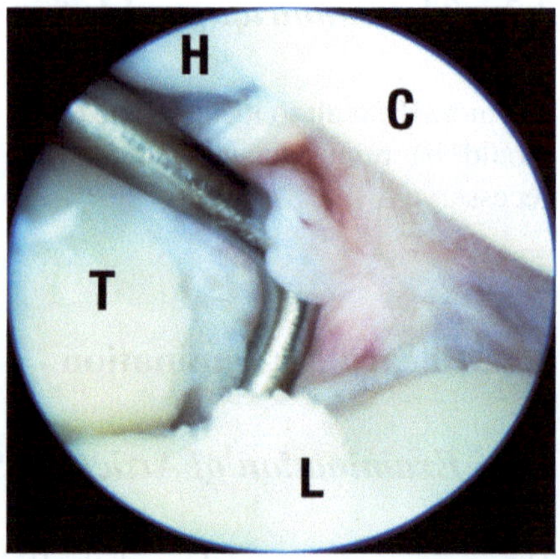

Fig. 7 Examination of the midcarpal interval. Junction of the four bones. The four internal bones are seen on this midcarpal view: *L* lunate, *T* triquetrum, *C* capitate, *H* hamate. The medial branch of the deltoid V is also seen (V)

first by an anteroposterior ridge. The second type appears to predispose to late degenerative midcarpal lesions [12, 13]. As will be further discussed, arthroscopy has a decisive role in the diagnosis and management of these lesions in the ulnar confines of the midcarpal joint which are not detected by X-ray (Fig. 7).

4.2 Examination of Ligamentous Structures in the Midcarpal Joint

Only two extrinsic ligamentous structures are accessible during midcarpal examination.

The first is the midcarpal segment of the radioscaphocapitate ligament. It is sometimes seen as a ligamentous structure barring the scaphocapitate space. In fact, this tough ligament firmly closes this space, preventing access to the anterior capsule and ligaments. The second is the medial branch of the deltoid V, a ligament stretching between the hamate and capitate. Lesions of this ligament are incriminated in the development of midcarpal instability.

5 Dynamic Tests During Arthroscopy

In diagnostic arthroscopy, it is possible to mobilize the bones in the carpal range to detect instability. These dynamic tests are adapted to the diagnosis of the so-called dissociative instability which is denoted by a modification of spatial coherence (or dissociation) between two adjacent bones. Practically, these dynamic tests are most relevant for the scapholunate and lunotriquetral instability, with the first being by far the most commonly encountered.

It is established that the generation of this type of instability does not follow an 'all or none' law but comes in a wide spectrum of lesions. During the early stages of scapholunate instability, static and dynamic radiography may not detect any lesions. The clinical suspicion evoked is thus confirmed by arthroscopy [4]. The next chapter is dedicated to the use of arthroscopy for the diagnosis of dissociative instability.

References

1. Chen YC (1979) Arthroscopy of the wrist and finger joints. Orthop Clin North Am 10:723–733
2. Whipple TL, Marotta J, Powell J (1986) Techniques of wrist arthroscopy. Arthroscopy 2:244–252
3. Slutsky DJ, Nagle DJ (2008) Wrist arthroscopy: current concepts. J Hand Surg Am 33(7):1228–1244
4. Dautel G, Goudot B, Merle M (1993) Arthroscopic diagnosis of scapholunate instability in the absence of X-ray abnormalities. J Hand Surg 18B:213–218
5. Dautel G, Merle M (1993) Tests dynamiques arthroscopiques pour le diagnostic des instabilités scapholunaires – note de technique. Ann Chir Main 12:206–209
6. Whipple L (1988) Powered instruments for wrist arthroscopy. Arthroscopy 4(4):290–294
7. Abrams RA, Petersen M, Botte MJ (1994) Arthroscopic portals of the wrist: an anatomic study. J Hand Surg Am 19(6):940–944
8. Abe Y, Doi K, Hattori Y, Ikeda K, Dhawan V (2003) Arthroscopic assessment of the volar region of the scapholunate interosseous ligament through a volar portal. J Hand Surg Am 28(1):69–73
9. Abe Y, Doi K, Hattori Y, Ikeda K, Dhawan V (2003) A benefit of the volar approach for wrist arthroscopy. Arthroscopy 19(4):440–445
10. North ER, Thomas S (1988) An anatomic guide for arthroscopic visualisation of the wrist capsular ligaments. J Hand Surg 13A:815–822
11. Berger RA, Landsmeer JMF (1990) The palmar radiocarpal ligaments/a study of adult and fetal human wrist joints. J Hand Surg 15A:847–850
12. Viegas SF (1990) The lunato-hamate articulation of the midcarpal joint. Arthroscopy 6(1):5–10
13. Viegas SF, Wagner K, Patterson R, Peterson P (1990) Medial (hamate) facet of the lunate. J Hand Surg 15A:564–571

Application of Wrist Arthroscopy to the Study of the Intrinsic Ligaments

G. Dautel and F. Delétang

The so-called intrinsic ligamentous structures, scapholunate and pyramido-lunate are implied in the instabilities which are said to be dissociative. Just like 'noninvasive' imagery (MRI and arthroscanner), arthroscopy is a means to study these ligamentous structures. It has even been reported that the arthroscanner has an excellent 'sensitiveness' to detect breaches in the interosseous ligaments [1]. Nevertheless, arthroscopy's superiority is to be found in the dynamic aspect of this exam, which not only enables to study the mechanical qualities of these ligaments but also to analyse the consequences of a ligamentous lesion resorting to dynamic tests. Only one diagnostic stage is enough to prove a ligamentous injury and, even more important, to demonstrate the consequences of this injury on the dynamics of the carpal bones, asserting or invalidating the existence of an instability or a dissociation. To end up, the same exam enables to accurately analyse the chondral impact of the instability and thus contributes to evaluate how long it has been lasting. The quality of the ligamentous stumps can also be studied to judge whether a fixing by direct suture is possible or not. For all these reasons, arthroscopy remains the gold standard to diagnose dissociative instabilities.

G. Dautel (✉)
Service de Chirurgie Plastique et Reconstructrice de l'Appareil Locomoteur, Centre Chirurgical Emile Gallé, 49 rue Hermite, 54000 NANCY, France
e-mail: gilles.dautel@wanadoo.fr

F. Delétang
SOS Mains Orléans Val de Loire, Polyclinique des Longues Allées, 25 rue Mondésir, 45800 Saint-Jean-de-Braye, France
e-mail: fabiendeletang@me.com

E. Camus, L. Van Overstraeten (eds.), *Carpal Ligament Surgery*,
DOI 10.1007/978-2-8178-0379-1_8, © Springer-Verlag France 2013

1 Anatomic Reminder: Intrinsic Ligaments

1.1 The Scapholunate Ligament

The scapholunate ligament [2, 3] is a ligament covered up with synovial tissue and tensed between the scaphoid and the lunate. It is divided into three sections: the posterior, the proximal and the anterior section. The posterior section, which is made of transverse conjunctive fibres, is the strongest. This section links the radial side of the posterior horn of the lunate to the dorso-ulnar part of the proximal pole of the scaphoid. Some fibres, which come from the extrinsic intercarpal ligament and from the radiocarpal articular capsule, are getting into it. The proximal section is avascularized and has little conjunctive tissue. A fibrocartilage is unequally dispatched on its length. The absence of fibrocartilage makes this part of the ligament thin, and degenerative perforations are possible. The anterior section is stronger as it has more conjunctive tissue. It is as strong as the posterior section.

1.2 The Triquetrolunate Ligament

The triquetrolunate ligament links the lunate to the triquetrum. The constitution of the ligament is more or less the same as that of the scapholunate ligament: it is divided into three parts and one-third of it has a real subordinate mechanical role.

2 The Role of the Intrinsic Ligamentous Structures in the Etiopathogeny of Dissociative Instabilities

2.1 Scapholunate Dissociative Instability

Most authors agree on the fact that the apparition of a dissociative instability needs the combination of an intrinsic and an extrinsic ligamentous injury. However, opinions still diverge on the nature of the extrinsic injuries which must be combined to the rupture of the interosseous ligament. For some authors, it is the ligamentous complex of the STT joint which plays the main role. Indeed, it maintains the distal pole of the scaphoid in place [4, 5]. Other authors underlined the role of the volar or dorsal extrinsic ligamentous structures [6]. Short and Werner [7], after an experimental study consisting in sequential ligamentous sections followed by cyclic and repetitive motions of the wrist, assert that the scapholunate interosseous ligament is the ‘primary’ stabilising structure of the scapholunate couple while the extrinsic structures (radioscaphocapitate ligaments and STT ligamentous complex) are the ‘secondary’ stabilisers. The same authors also mentioned that the dorsal ligamentous plane plays a part in the stabilisation of the scapholunate couple and thus assert the alteration of the scapholunate kinematic in case of capsulotomy which gets over this dorsal extrinsic ligamentous plan [8]. If nowadays it is difficult to accurately define which extrinsic ligaments are responsible for the apparition of an instability, it is partly because it is difficult to reproduce the effects of a traumatic rupture in an experiment. On the contrary, retrospective clinical studies are faced with the methodological difficulty which consists in separating the ligamentous injuries at the origin of the instability from those which are associated to it by chance [9].

2.2 Pyramido-Lunate Dissociative Instability

Once again, the triquetrolunate interosseous ligament embodies the 'main ligamentous bolt' as it maintains the spatial cohesion between the semilunate and the triquetrum. The anterior third of this ligament plays the most important part [10].

3 Practice of a Diagnostic Arthroscopy in Search of a Scapholunate Dissociative Instability (Study of Intrinsic Ligaments)

3.1 Portals for the Diagnostic Exploration of Dissociative Instabilities

The usual portals which are used to make a diagnostic arthroscopy of the wrist are enough to estimate the intrinsic ligaments and to make dynamic tests. The SLIOL is correctly analysed by the combination of the 3/4, 4/5 and 6u portals. The arthroscope is first placed in the 3/4 portal and the hook palpator in the 4/5 portal. The 6u portal is used to let the washing fluid go out. To explore the triquetrolunate joint space, you will just have to exchange the instruments and to place the arthroscope in the 4/5 portal. The resort to a volar portal has been evoked to allow a more complete exploration of the SLIOL. Abe et al. [11, 12] insists on the interest of such a volar portal to explore the anterior third of the SLIOL.

3.2 Study and Palpation of the Intrinsic Ligamentous Structures

3.2.1 Intrinsic Ligaments

The scapholunate and pyramido-lunate interosseous ligaments must be explored. For each of these ligaments, only the anterior two-thirds will be reachable to study and palpation, considering the posterior point of penetration of the arthroscope.

3.2.2 The Scapholunate Interosseous Ligament

It is looked for in the 'roof' during the exam of the carpal condyle and the arthroscope is introduced by the 3/4 portal. When it is healthy, it can be difficult to find since it is covered up with a layer of articular cartilage which is the continuity of the scaphoid and the semilunate. Palpation is the best means to locate it as it is in a zone where tonus is diminished at the level of the anteroposterior crest of separation from the scaphoidal and lunar fossas and the deep radioscapholunate ligament (ligament of Testut) (Fig. 1). The whole ligament has to be analysed in search for injuries of the mid-third or the anterior third. Traumatic injuries lie in the insertion zone on the scaphoid, right inside the ligament or, more rarely, where the lunate inserts itself. Apart from typical ligamentous breaches and tears (Fig. 2), it is also necessary to recognise a healed ligament, which takes the shape

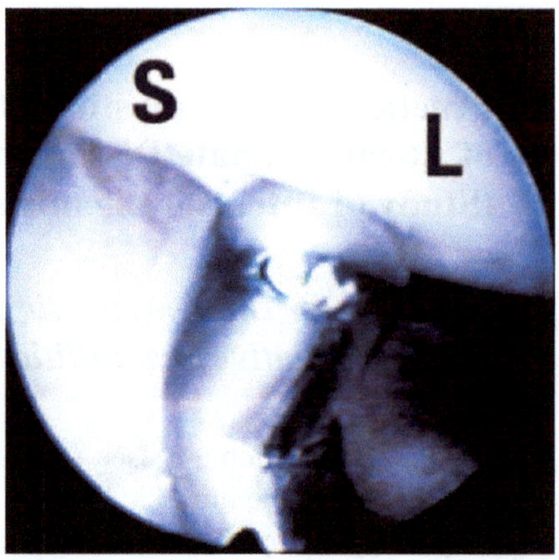

Fig. 1 Localisation of the scapholunate interosseous ligament thanks to palpation. The ligament is found during the exam of the radiocarpal interval: tonus in the interval between the scaphoid and semilunate is diminished. *S* scaphoid, *L* lunate

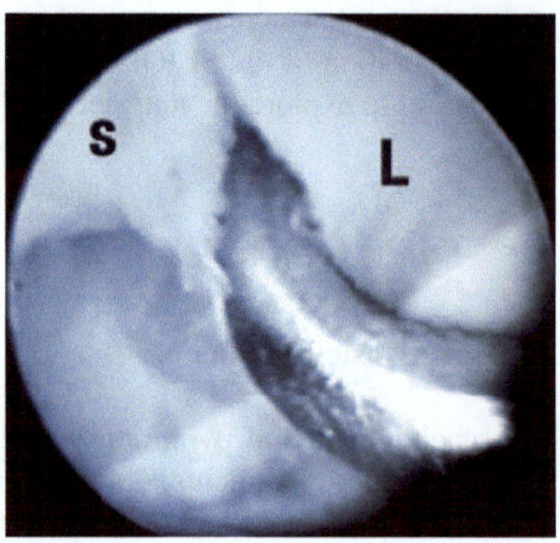

Fig. 2 Breach of the scapholunate interosseous ligament: the hook is introduced in the breach inside the ligament. *S* scaphoid, *L* lunate

of a zone of fibrous continuity, where it is not possible to introduce the hook but where the tonus and the normal consistency of the interosseous ligament are not restored.

3.2.3 The Pyramido-Lunate Interosseous Ligament

It is more difficult to locate than the previous one as there is no topographic reference. To locate it, the arthroscope has to be reintroduced by the 4/5 portal, and once again, palpation with the hook is often necessary.

3.3 Practice of Arthroscopic Dynamic Tests [13]

3.3.1 Dissociative Scapholunate Instabilities

Before any dynamic test, it is necessary to reduce the tension on the finger traps so as not to distort the interpretation by the artificial tension impressed on the extrinsic ligamentous structures induced by distraction. At the beginning of our experiment, we systematically used *dynamic tests in the radiocarpal joint.* The examining hook was introduced in a ligamentous breach and moved axially to try and separate the scaphoid from the semilunate, or the lunate from the triquetrum. In the same way, we made an 'arthroscopic test of Watson' as we dorsally pushed on the tubercle of the scaphoid to try and put forward a rotatory subluxation of the proximal pole of the scaphoid. Retrospectively, it becomes obvious that the analysis of these tests' results is difficult, especially when the interval contains post-traumatic ligament remnants. Thus, these tests have now been abandoned and replaced by *the midcarpal dynamic tests* which interpretation is far easier.

In the midcarpal space, it is also possible to use the hook to estimate the stability of the scapholunate or the pyramido-lunate couples. To make these tests, the arthroscope is introduced by one of the midcarpal portals (RMC or UMC), and it visualises the junction of the scapholunate or pyramido-lunate distal facets. Normally, it is impossible to slip the hook in the interosseous scapholunate and pyramido-lunate intervals. When there is no instability, the hook can definitely not penetrate into the interosseous interval. If there is an instability, the hook can be pushed into the interosseous interval, towards the midcarpal. The axial movements that are impressed on it manage to move both osseous pieces apart (Figs. 3 and 4). The interosseous interval opens and makes the remnants of the interosseous ligament visible at the floor.

At a further stage of instability, these dynamic manoeuvres with the hook even allow an opening which is wide enough to let the arthroscope go from the radiocarpal to the midcarpal space, through the ligamentous breach (Figs. 5, 6 and 7). However, this is only possible when the instability is further in the spectrum of injuries and can usually be established by a radiographic diagnosis.

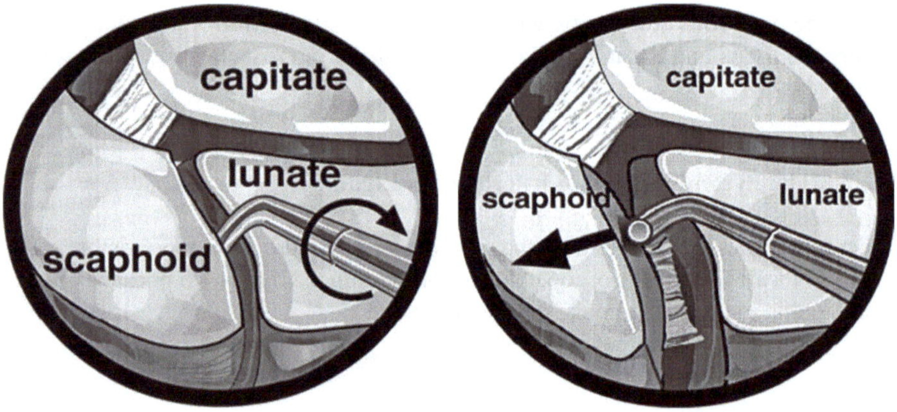

Figs. 3 and 4 Practice of dissociative dynamic tests in the scapholunate interval: the hook is introduced by the UMC portal and pushed towards the scapholunate interval. Axial movements are created to try and create a diastasis in the scapholunate interval. In the case of dissociative instability, the opening of the interval becomes clearly visible (see text)

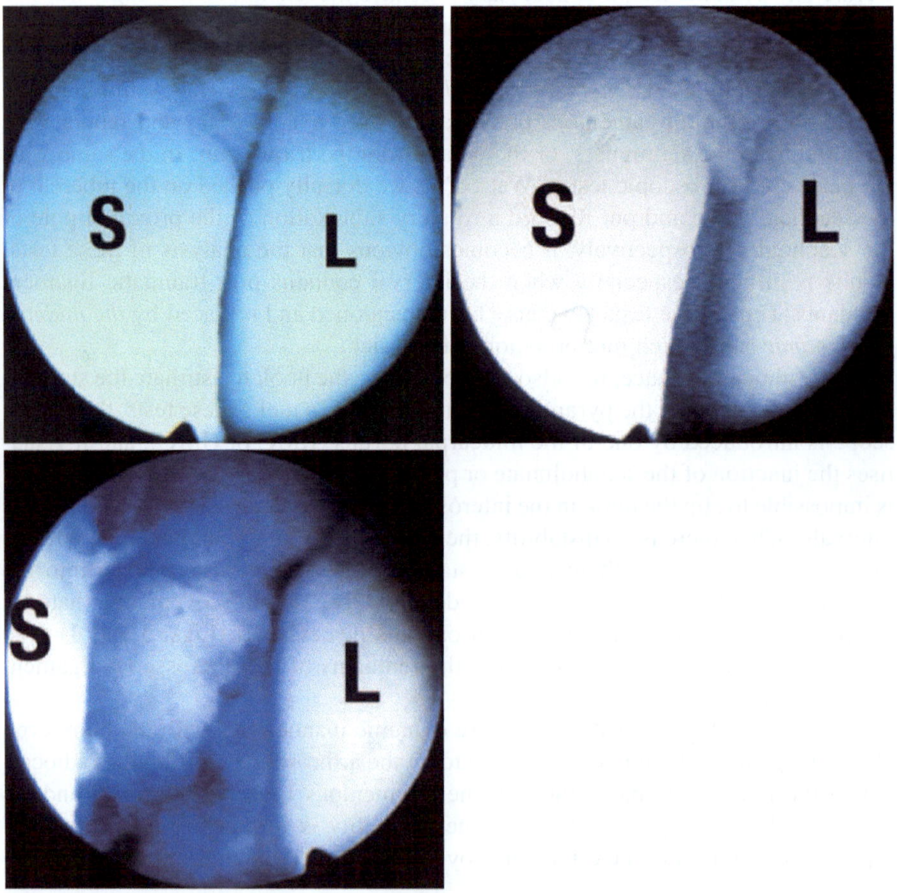

3.4 *Meaning of the Dynamic Arthroscopic Tests in the Dissociative Scapholunate Instabilities*

These manoeuvres and dynamic tests thus enable to put forward a deficiency in the ligamentous devices. The surgeon indirectly analyses the effects of intrinsic and/or extrinsic possible ligamentous injuries on the carpal stability. Throughout our experiment, thanks to these dynamic arthroscopic tests, it has been made possible to point out an early instability before it creates abnormalities in the dynamic or a fortiori static radiographic results [14, 15]. It is easy to understand the higher 'sensitiveness' of arthroscopy as far as dissociative instabilities are concerned since this exam enables to make a test of direct dissociation and impress constraints on the bones (under the effect of the twisting motion applied to the hook). On the contrary, in a dynamic radiographic study, the component of dissociation is indirectly induced under the effect of axial compression which is itself induced by fist clenching. Scapholunate dissociative instability is probably an entity with various declinations following a vast spectrum of injuries. The distinction between a static and a dynamic instability only is not sufficient to make the vastness of this spectrum clear. If the conditions in which radiographic images are made are perfectly standardised, correlations can be established between the severity of ligamentous injuries seen in arthroscopy and their radiographic interpretation [16].

3.5 *Dynamic Arthroscopic Tests in Pyramido-Lunate Dissociative Instabilities*

The practice of these tests has been deduced from what was observed in the scapholunate interval. In that case, the absence of ligamentous injury does not let the hook penetrate into the triquetrolunate interosseous interval. Instability is established after an abnormal opening of the interosseous interval impressed by the twisting motion applied to the hook (Fig. 8).

3.6 *Other Ligamentous Structures*

During a diagnostic arthroscopy, our clinical practice systematically consists in the inspection and the palpation of the extrinsic ligamentous structures. Through the

Figs. 5, 6 and 7 Midcarpal view of the scapholunate base during dissociative tests: (Fig. 5) The scapholunate interval is perfectly congruent and 'continent'. If there is a breach in the SLIOL, there is no instability. (Fig. 6) Moderate opening of the interval under the twisting motion applied to the hook. (Fig. 7) The interval is clearly opened and leaves the remnants of the SLIOL visible at the floor. The arthroscope easily goes from the midcarpal to the radiocarpal joint, through the ligamentous breach (see text). *S* scaphoid, *L* lunate, *T* triquetrum, *H* hamate, *RSCL* radioscaphocapitate ligament

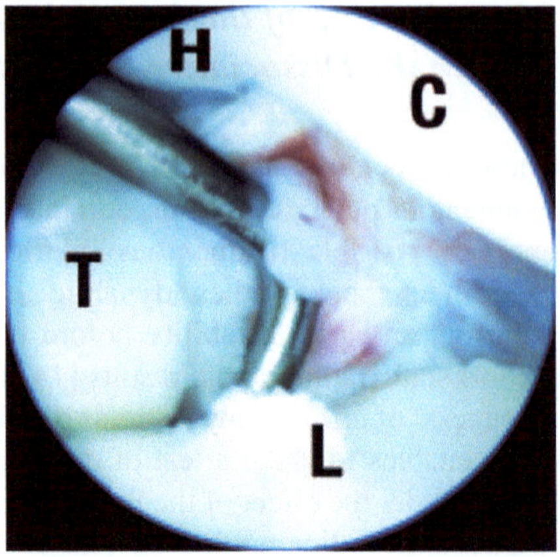

Fig. 8 Dynamic testing in the interval between lunate and triquetrum (midcarpal joint). *L* lunate, *T* triquetrum, *H* hamate, *C* capitate

classic dorsal portals, it is possible to inspect and palpate the short intra-articular section of the extrinsic anterior ligamentous plane, while the dorsal plane escapes from a 'normal' arthroscopy (that is to say, by a dorsal portal). Despite this systematic testing, the information we have is not sufficient to confirm or to contradict one or other etiopathogenic theories relating to the participation of these structures in the birth of dissociative instabilities.

3.7 Study of the Chondral Effect of the Instability

The initial diagnostic arthroscopy is also the best moment to establish an assessment of the chondral effect of a dissociative instability. If this method is not really interesting on the triquetrolunate side as the TL dissociative instability is not said to be very arthrogen, it is paramount on the scapholunate side. The inspection and the accurate palpation of the stylo interval or radioscaphoidal joint enable to detect an early chondrite or arthrosis which testifies to the oldness of the instability. As a matter of fact, deep radioscaphoidal chondral injuries have sometimes been diagnosed while the patient just mentioned a unique and recent trauma. The search for the chondral effect is useful to detect ruptures with multiple stages which are classic phenomena of scapholunate instabilities.

4 Arthroscopy to Analyse the Severity and the Oldness of a Scapholunate Instability

Considering the performances of arthroscopy as far as diagnostic evaluation is concerned, it became obvious to use it to establish a score of severity, especially in the case of scapholunate instability which is now known to be a vast spectrum of injuries and not a binary entity. The arthroscopic classification of instabilities that we use is reproduced below [15, 17]. The other existing classification was made by Geissler [18, 19].

5 Arthroscopy to Treat Early Stages of Scapholunate Instability

A mere arthroscopic debridement has often been mentioned as a means to treat the isolated injuries of the scapholunate or pyramido-lunate interosseous ligaments [20, 21]. However, it is still difficult to make a distinction between what can be granted to the debridement itself and what is the consequence of the effects of immobilisation which is associated to it or the mid-term spontaneous evolution towards indolence, which is often observed in the context of scapholunate dissociation, a fortiori when a scapholunate and/or scaphocapitate broaching has also been made. Most of the studies published refer to the development of a mere functional score (Mayo wrist score or else) to judge of the efficiency of arthroscopy on the long term.

Arthroscopic severity score for scapholunate instability (Dautel)
Stage 0: Absence of instability, normal wrist as far as the scapholunate kinetics is concerned. This stage is a means to list the SLIOL breaches without instability
Stage 1: The tip of the hook can be introduced in the scapholunate interval. Normal radiography
Stage 2: Moderate opening of the scapholunate interval with the use of the twisting motion applied to the hook
Stage 3: Clear opening of the scapholunate interval, possibility to introduce the arthroscope from the radiocarpal to the midcarpal space

This type of scoring can judge the global function and the comfort but remains unable to analyse the consequences of arthroscopy on wrist stability. The same can be said of the ligamentous electro-thermocoagulation techniques which are still used but for which there is no proof of real efficiency.

References

1. Bille B, Harley B, Cohen H (2007) A comparison of CT arthrography of the wrist to findings during wrist arthroscopy. J Hand Surg Am 32(6):834–841
2. Berger RA, Blair WA, Crowninshield RD, Flatt AE (1982) The scapholunate ligament. J Hand Surg 7A:87–91
3. Berger RA (1992) Update, scapholunate ligament. EMB 2:19–23
4. Drewniany JJ, Palmer AK, Flatt AE (1985) The scaphotrapezial ligament complex: an anatomic and biomechanical study. J Hand Surg 10A:493–497
5. Jantea CL, An KN, Lindscheid RL, Cooney WP (1994) The role of the scaphotrapezial-trapezoidal ligament complex in scaphoid kinematics. In: Schuind F (ed) Advances in the biomechanics of the hand and wrist. Plenum Press, New York, pp 345–361

6. Elsaidi GA, Ruch DS, Kuzma GR, Smith BP (2004) Dorsal wrist ligament insertions stabilize the scapholunate interval: cadaver study. Clin Orthop Relat Res 425:152–157
7. Short WH, Werner FW, Green JK, Masaoka S (2002) Biomechanical evaluation of ligamentous stabilizers of the scaphoid and lunate. J Hand Surg Am 27(6):991–1002
8. Short WH, Werner FW, Green JK, Weiner MM, Masaoka S (2002) The effect of sectioning the dorsal radiocarpal ligament and insertion of a pressure sensor into the radiocarpal joint on scaphoid and lunate kinematics. J Hand Surg Am 27(1):68–76
9. Slutsky DJ (2005) Arthroscopic dorsal radiocarpal ligament repair. Arthroscopy 21(12):1486
10. Ritt MJ, Linscheid RL, Cooney WP 3rd, Berger RA, An KN (1998) The lunotriquetral joint: kinematic effects of sequential ligament sectioning, ligament repair, and arthrodesis. J Hand Surg Am 23(3):432–445
11. Abe Y, Doi K, Hattori Y, Ikeda K, Dhawan V (2003) A benefit of the volar approach for wrist arthroscopy. Arthroscopy 19(4):440–445
12. Abe Y, Doi K, Hattori Y, Ikeda K, Dhawan V (2003) Arthroscopic assessment of the volar region of the scapholunate interosseous ligament through a volar portal. J Hand Surg Am 28(1):69–73
13. Dautel G, Merle M (1993) Tests dynamiques arthroscopiques pour le diagnostic des instabilités scapholunaires. Note de technique. Ann Chir Main 12:206–209
14. Dautel G, Goudot B, Merle M (1993) Arthroscopic diagnosis of scapho-lunate instability in the absence of X-ray abnormalities. J Hand Surg Br 18(2):213–218
15. Dautel G, Merle M (1993) Dynamic arthroscopic tests for the diagnosis of scaphoid-lunar instabilities. Ann Chir Main Memb Super 12(3):206–209
16. Kwon BC, Baek GH (2008) Fluoroscopic diagnosis of scapholunate interosseous ligament injuries in distal radius fractures. Clin Orthop Relat Res 466(4):969–976
17. Dreant N, Dautel G (2003) Development of a arthroscopic severity score for scapholunate instability. Chir Main 22(2):90–94
18. Geissler WB (2006) Arthroscopic management of scapholunate instability. Chir Main 25(Suppl 1):S187–S196
19. Geissler WB, Freeland AE, Savoie FH, Mcintyre LW, Whipple TL (1996) Intracarpal soft-tissue lesions associated with an intra-articular fracture of the distal end of the radius. J Bone Joint Surg Am 78(3):357–365
20. Earp BE, Waters PM, Wyzykowski RJ (2006) Arthroscopic treatment of partial scapholunate ligament tears in children with chronic wrist pain. J Bone Joint Surg Am 88(11):2448–2455
21. Chloros GD, Wiesler ER, Poehling GG (2008) Current concepts in wrist arthroscopy. Arthroscopy 24(3):343–354

Arthroscopic Anatomy and Lesions of the Extrinsic Ligaments

L. Van Overstraeten

1 Introduction

The anatomy of the extrinsic ligaments of the wrist is quite complex as is the understanding of their kinematics involved in wrist stabilization [6–8, 15, 23–25].

Arthroscopy has allowed a different approach to these extrinsic ligaments compared to conventional diagnostic methods. The morphological study remains restricted to the intraarticular zones but may be complemented by specific and precise testing of each ligament group.

2 Arthroscopic Anatomy of Extrinsic Ligaments

To facilitate understanding, we have distinguished three groups of extrinsic ligaments:

- Anterior proximal carpal plane: RSC – RLT (LRL, SRL) – RSL – UL – UT
- Anterior midcarpal plane: STq – SC – ST – CTz – TqC
- Dorsal plane: DRC – DIC

Each group is assessed through a certain arthroscopic approach with a possible specific approach that may be needed.

Only the anterior proximal plane of carpal ligaments is accessible to direct arthroscopic vision.

L. Van Overstraeten
Hand and Foot Surgery Unit SPRL,
Rue Pierre Caille N° 9, B-7500 Tournai, Belgium
e-mail: l.v.o@skynet.be

E. Camus, L. Van Overstraeten (eds.), *Carpal Ligament Surgery*,
DOI 10.1007/978-2-8178-0379-1_9, © Springer-Verlag France 2013

Even if the arthroscope can only examine the intraarticular portion of these extrinsic ligaments, the data collected can be used to assess the stability of the wrist and orient the choice of technique for potential surgical repair.

3 The Anterior Proximal Carpal Plane

It is composed of two subgroups, the radiocarpal and ulnocarpal, and is explored essentially through dorsal radiocarpal portals.

The classic portals 3–4 and 4–5 allow direct visualization of the scapholunate and lunotriquetral interosseous ligaments. They also give access to the intraarticular portions of the extrinsic ligaments of the anterior radiocarpal and ulnocarpal planes [28–30]. The SRL, UL and UT can also be approached.

3.1 The Anterior Radiocarpal Plane

The radioscaphocapitate ligament (RSC) is a large strong ligament which inserts onto the radial styloid and is directed radially and obliquely towards the capitate. It runs along the proximal half of the scaphoid where it inserts at the level of the waist distal to the tubercle [19] and is fixed distally on the palmar tubercle of the capitate (Fig. 1) [22]. According to Berger, only 10 % of the fibres insert into the capitate [19]. The RSC is intimately related to the distal fibres of the lunocapitate (LC) and the palmar scaphotriquetral (STP) ligaments [19]. The RSC crosses two articular chambers (radiocarpal and midcarpal). Its role is to 'fix' the scaphoid preventing dorsal tilting of its proximal pole. In ulnar deviation, it helps the verticalization of the scaphoid acting as a secondary stabilizer of the scapholunate complex [11], and its injury may be the cause of scaphoid instability with DISI and scapholunate diastasis [12].

On arthroscopic examination of the radiocarpal joint, the RSC is most radial (Fig. 2). Its fibres are obliquely oriented from radial to ulnar, and it is separated from its neighbouring radiolunotriquetral by a hiatus – the interligamentary sulcus which allows testing of both ligaments using the hook palpation (Fig. 3).

The radiolunotriquetral ligament (RLT) is also very strong and usually composed of two bands: the long radiolunate (LRL) radially and the short radiolunate (inconstant) (SRL) separated by the radioscapholunate (Fig. 1). It is almost parallel to the RSC and usually divided into two parts: a proximal purely radiolunate half and the distal palmar lunotriquetral. The SRL fibres cross with those of the ulnotriquetral.

It traces a proximal inverted 'V' with the anterior ulnocarpal where the apex of the V represents the triquetral and lunate insertions.

It forms the palmar part of the triquetral sling [21] and contributes to the stabilization of the lunate, preventing its dorsal flexion and palmar translation. It prevents

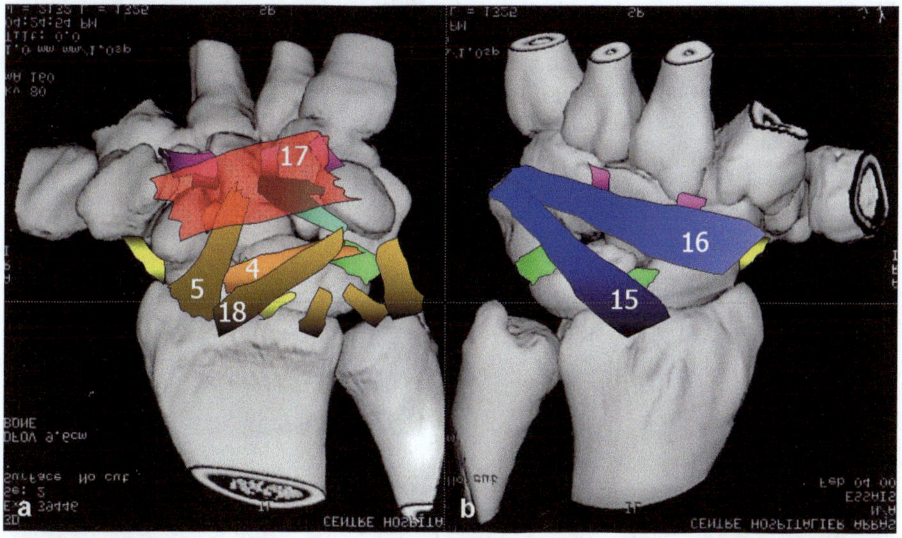

Fig. 1 The plane of extrinsic wrist ligaments, (**a**) palmar and (**b**) dorsal views. *4* Scaphotriquetral ligament, *5* Radioscaphocapitate ligament, *15* dorsal radiocarpal ligament, *16* dorsal intercarpal ligament, *17* annular anterior carpal ligament, *18* long radiolunate ligament

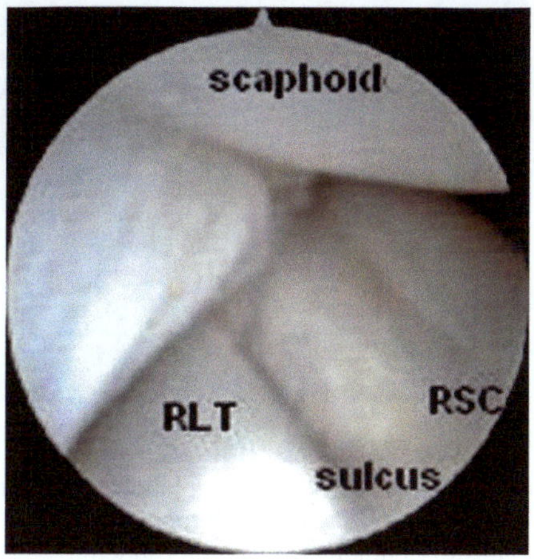

Fig. 2 Arthroscopic view of the radiocarpal interval left wrist. *Right* to *left*: *RSC ligament*, interligamentary sulcus and *RLT* ligament

the ulnar translation of the carpus, and its injury destabilizes the perilunate region. On arthroscopic assessment, the radiolunotriquetral ligament RLT is the ulnar neighbour of the RSC. It links the anterior border of the scaphoid fossa of the radius to the triquetrum, and its fibres are more oblique than those of the RSC (Fig. 2). On its way, it also inserts onto the anterior horn of the lunate.

The radioscapholunate ligament (RSL) or ligament of Testut is quite a lax fibrous structure (Fig. 4). According to Berger, 'the RSL ligament is not a real ligament in the biomechanical or the histological sense of the term'. It can be considered as a

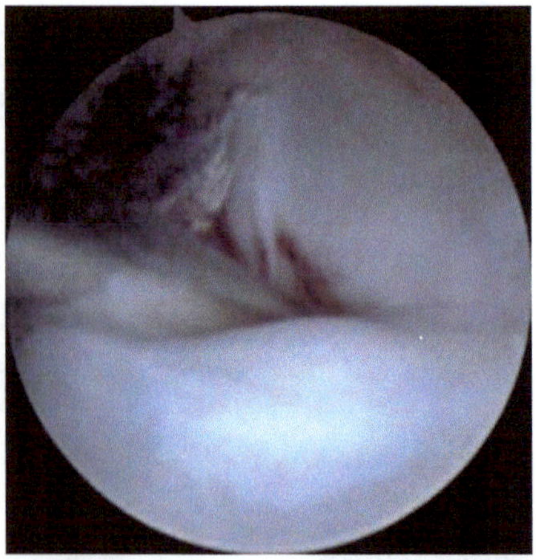

Fig. 3 Arthroscopic view of the left radiocarpal interval. Probing RLT (which is lax stage 2). Probe is in the interligamentary sulcus. Hemorrhagic synovitis in the radial part of the RSC ligament

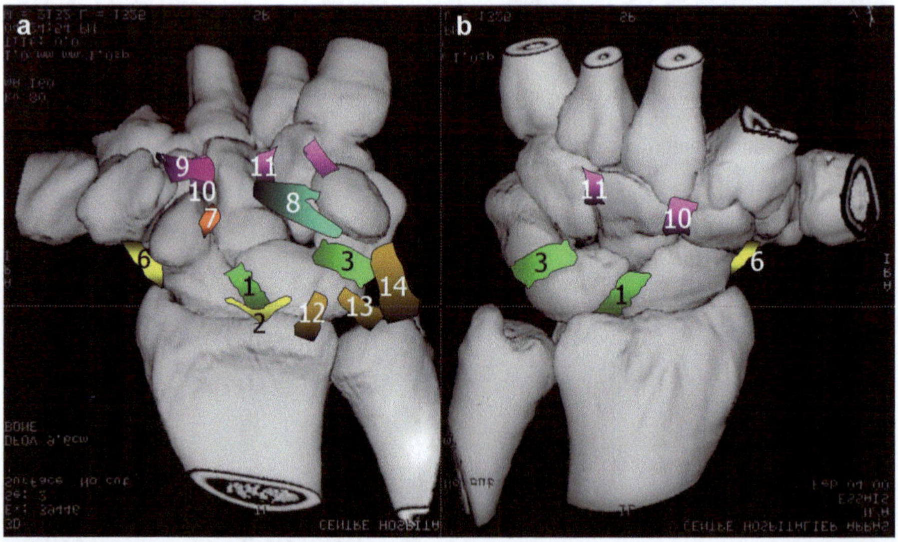

Fig. 4 The plane of extrinsic and intrinsic wrist ligaments, (**a**) palmar and (**b**) dorsal views. *1* Scapholunate, *2* radioscapholunate, *3* lunotriquetral, *6* scaphotrapezial, *7* scaphocapitate, *8* triquetrohamatocapitate, *9* capitotrapezial, *10* capitotrapezoidal, *11* capitohamatal, *12* short radiolunate, *13* ulnolunate, *14* ulnotriquetral

mesocapsule. It contains terminal branches of the anterior interosseous nerve and rami from the radial arcade [19, 20].

It serves as an arthroscopic landmark for the scapholunate ligament which is sometimes difficult to identify without probing which depresses it (Fig. 4). It is characterized by its vertical fibres which extend along the scapholunate crest of the radius. It is the most superficial from the scope and can sometimes obscure the anterior part of the radiocarpal joint like a veil (Fig. 5).

It is more lax than the previous ligaments and feels always more so on probe palpation.

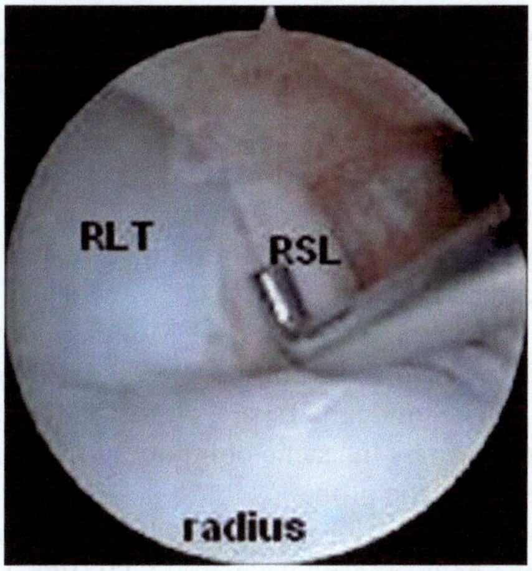

Fig. 5 Arthroscopic view of the right radiocarpal interval. *Left* to *right*: LRTL (long radiotriquetral) and hemorrhagic synovitis on the *RSL* ligament

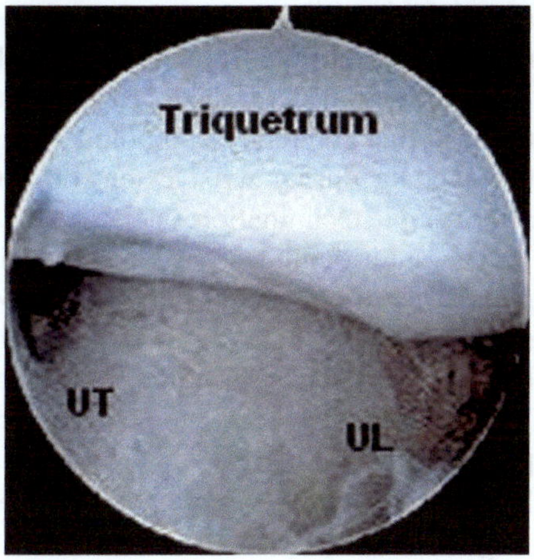

Fig. 6 Arthroscopic view of the left ulnocarpal interval: 3 years after shortening osteotomy described by Milch, 'scarring' chondritis triquetrum. Ulnocarpal ligaments stretched with no clear separation between the *UT* and the *UL*

3.2 The Anterior Ulnocarpal Plane

This is formed by the RLT ligament, the proximal palmar 'V' ligament (Fig. 1), which is formed of the ulnolunate UL and lunotriquetral LT ligaments. It inserts on the proximal part of the anterior portion of the TFCC and the ulnar styloid. It contributes to the stabilization of the lunotriquetral complex and TFCC tension. The ulnolunate ligament may sometimes share fibres with the short RL ligament.

Ulnarly, the anterior floor is composed of less distinctly individualized ligaments (Fig. 6). The difference in obliquity distinguishes between the UL and UT ligaments which appear to be intimately attached to the TFCC and represent an extension of this structure. They are also palpated by the probe.

4 The Anterior Midcarpal Plane and the Scaphotrapeziotrapezoid Complex

The anterior midcarpal plane is formed of a combination of extrinsic and intrinsic ligaments. It includes the distal part of the RSC ligament; the intraarticular midcarpal part of the RSC forming the distal palmar 'V' is visible through the standard arthroscopic portals.

Thus, the RMC and UMC classic midcarpal portals give direct access to the intraarticular part of the RSC and TC ligaments.

The midcarpal part of the radioscaphocapitate ligament is easily identified (Fig. 7) by the same obliquity of fibres as its radiocarpal portion. It is easily accessible to the probe.

The anterior midcarpal plane also includes the triquetrocapitate TC (Fig. 4) and the palmar scaphotriquetral STP (Fig. 1) ligaments.

The TC extends from the distal radial angle of the triquetrum to the ulnar cortex of the capitate [19]. It forms the distal and ulnar part of the palmar midcarpal 'V' and is the palmar ulnar stabilizer of the midcarpal joint. On arthroscopic examination, it is discernible from the RSC by the inverted obliquity of its fibres.

Described in 1994, the STP ligament prevents scaphotriquetral palmar dissociation and thus indirectly scapholunate dissociation. It probably supports the head of the capitate during wrist extension [20]. It is extraarticular and inaccessible to arthroscopic examination.

The anterior midcarpal plane also includes the scaphotrapeziotrapezoid complex. It is strictly palmar and is composed of three distinct exclusively intrinsic structures: the palmar scaphotrapezial ligament (STz) and radially a scaphocapitate ligament (SC) and a capitotrapezoid ligament (CTzo) distal to the scaphoid (Fig. 4). The STz ligament seems to act as a secondary stabilizer to the scapholunate complex along with the RSC and the dorsal intercarpal ligament (DIC) [11–13]. The two ligaments materialize the flexion-extension axis of the scaphoid (Fig. 8). This axis

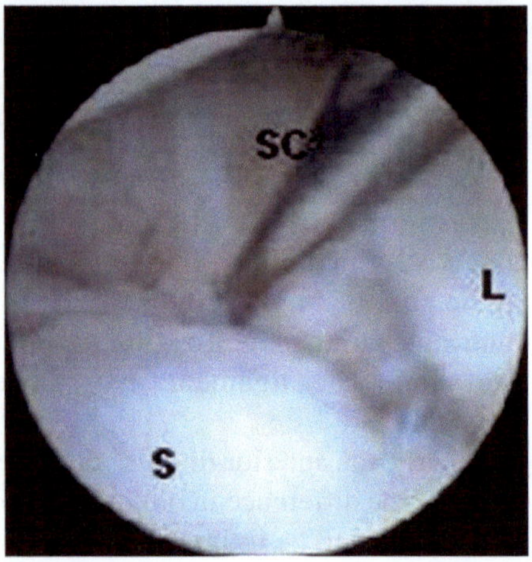

Fig. 7 Arthroscopic view of the right midcarpal interval: stage 1 laxity of the midcarpal portion of the RSC

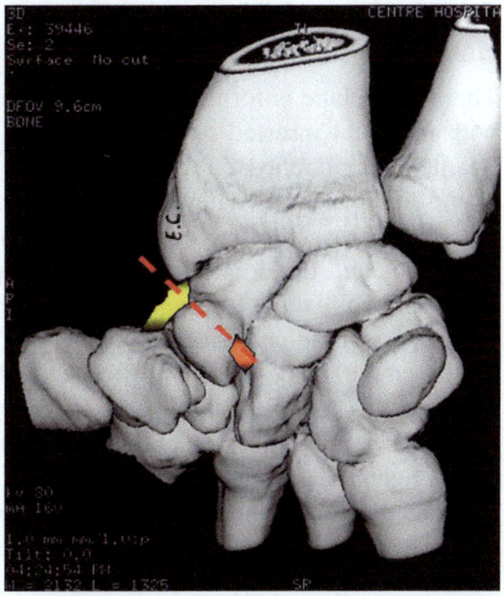

Fig. 8 Plate of extrinsic wrist ligaments: the scaphotrapezial STz and scaphocapitate SC tracethe axis of flexion-extension of the scaphoid

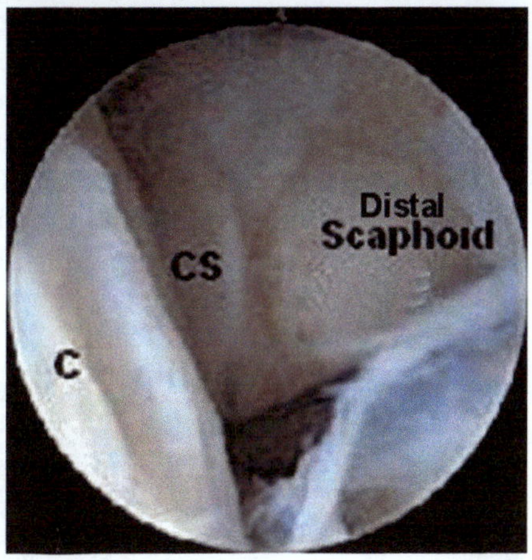

Fig. 9 Arthroscopic view of left midcarpal interval. Scope through RMC, probe through MC 1–3. Enlarged distal scaphocapitate interval allowing palpation of SC ligament

passes through the waist of the capitate [16, 17]. The SC ligament is also an important stabilizer of the scaphoid [19].

The SC ligament is accessible only when the distal scaphocapitate interval is open, i.e., in a pathological situation of instability (Fig. 9).

The CTz ligament is inaccessible to arthroscopic examination, and the STz is not accessible through the dorsal midcarpal ptortals. It is possible to introduce the probe through an MC 1–3 portal in the distal anatomical snuffbox taking care to avoid the dorsal recurrent branch of the radial artery. Recently, we use standard portals (scope through RMC and probe through MC). The probe crosses up the scope into the midcarpal joint and goes to palpate the STz ligament in the STT joint. The scope is slid through the MCR along the scaphoid to visualize the scaphotrapeziotrapezoid junction.

5 The Dorsal Plane

The dorsal plane is formed by two ligaments forming a sloping 'V' open radially with the point inserted on the triquetrum. Viegas describes it as a radioscaphoid ligament which relays on the triquetrum [4]. It is distinguished by the constant tension of its branches whatever the opening angle of the 'V' and whatever the movement of the wrist (in the sagittal or the frontal plane). Thus, in ulnar inclination, the 'V' opens and the dorsal ligament plane participates in the verticalization of the scaphoid, while the triquetrum passes under the hamate (Fig. 10) [26].

The dorsal radiocarpal ligament (DRC) unites the radius and the triquetrum and inserts on the lunate (Fig. 1). It forms the dorsal component of the Khulman's sling [21] and is a secondary stabilizer of the carpus [12, 13]. A lesion here is as destabilizing to the carpus as a lesion of the palmar bands of the scaphocapitate and scaphotrapezial ligaments [13]. It is ruptured in 50 % of cases of carpal instability usually associated with scapholunate ligament injury but may also be a solo ligament injury [27]. The pain occurs more rapidly with the existence of associated lesions.

The ceiling of the joint space may only be visualized through lateral portals 1–2 and 6U. Care should be taken with approaches through these portals to protect the dorsal sensory branch of the ulnar nerve as well as the radial artery. The dorsal synovium is thick and its folds often obscure the dorsal ligaments. However, careful probing through 3–4 and 4–5 portals – across the synovium – gives a fair appreciation of the tension of the dorsal radiocarpal ligament.

The dorsal intercarpal ligament (DIC) unites the triquetrum and distal scaphoid sometimes extending onto the trapezium and trapezoid [5, 33] (Fig. 1). It is the 3rd secondary stabilizer of the carpus [13, 18].

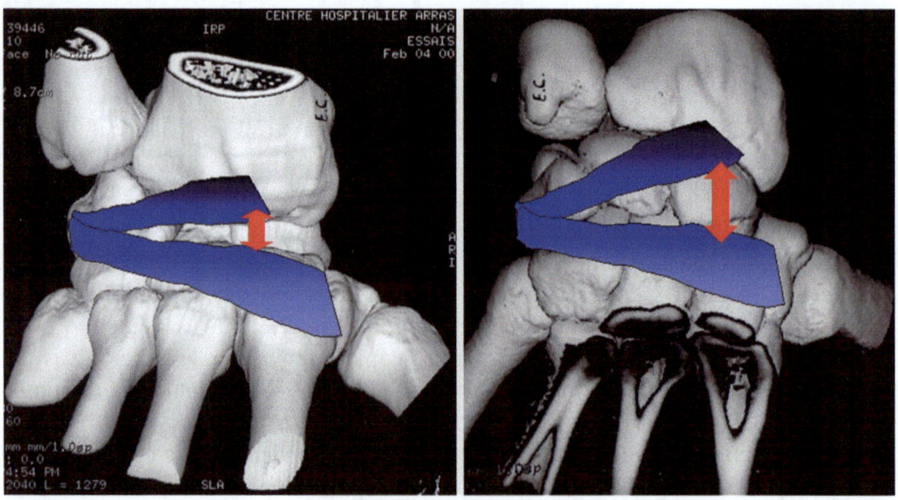

Fig. 10 Plate of extrinsic dorsal wrist ligaments: the 'V' opens in ulnar inclination

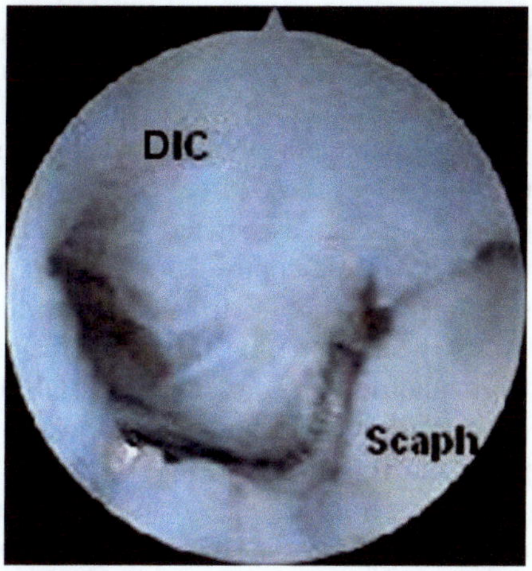

Fig. 11 Arthroscopic view of left midcarpal interval. Scope through MC 1–3, probe through RMC. After synovial débridement using a shaver, the dorsal intercarpal *DIC* ligament is palpated

The DIC ligament may be seen through MC 1–3 and palpated through UMC; it is likewise possible to estimate the tension of the dorsal intercarpal ligament (Fig. 11).

6 Pathologic Arthroscopy of the Extrinsics

6.1 Genesis of Perilunate Dissociative Instability: Nebulous? Biokinematic and Pathologic Hypothesis

Most authors appear to accept that responsibility for dissociative scapholunate or lunotriquetral is shared by intrinsic and extrinsic ligaments [2, 3, 4, 11, 12, 14, 23–25]. The majority of authors also agree on the primacy of the scapholunate and lunotriquetral ligament lesions as essential for carpal destabilization [1, 11–13].

In the analysis of scapholunate dissociative instability, some consider that in addition to the interosseous ligament, the proximal palmar ligament is essentially involved. Others have incriminated essentially the distal extrinsics or the scaphotrapeziotrapezoid complex [31, 32].

Short et al. consider that the scapholunate ligament is the principal stabilizer of the scapholunate complex, and the extrinsics RSC, DIC and STz are secondary stabilizers [11–13]. For them, the carpus destabilizes progressively under phasic stresses [9, 10].

We propose the following biokinematic theory. The scapholunate complex is stabilized by the scapholunate ligament which is the fundamental intrinsic restrain and also by three extrinsic locks: the distal (STz, CTz, SC), the palmar proximal radial (RSC) and the dorsal (DIC) ligaments. For the stability of the complex to be preserved, the scapholunate ligament as well as two of the three restrains must be intact. If the scapholunate ligament is completely ruptured (Dautel 3; Geissler 4), dissociative instability is clear. We have never witnessed isolated scapholunate ligament rupture without associated extrinsic laxity. If the scapholunate ligament is partially ruptured (Dautel 1 or 2; Geissler 3) and one extrinsic restrain is loosened, the instability process has begun and – without treatment – will inevitably progress to adaptative decompensation.

In the management of an acute sprain (more recent than 6 weeks) we must verify the integrity of these three restrains and systematically repair all partial SL lesions (Dautel 1), when associated with a lesion of at least one extrinsic restrain. It is also necessary in the control of a chronic prearthritic dissociative lesion to assess the state of these three extrinsic locks which will modulate our choice of technique. This will substitute for the broken restrain.

In lunotriquetral dissociative instability, the role of the lunotriquetral interosseous ligament seems fundamental [10], and this interval is systematically tested in our protocol.

As for extrinsics, their responsibility seems even more complex than in scapholunate instability. We test the palmar and dorsal (RLT and DRC) planes of the Khulman's sling and the palmar ulnocarpal (UT) and the DIC ligaments. We have never witnessed frank lunotriquetral instability (combining Dautel 2 with triquetral hypermobility and marginal chondritis of the lunotriquetral interval and the tip of the hamate) without laxity of the components of the triquetral sling. Up to now, we do not modulate the technique of management of instability to any such extrinsic ligament lesion.

7 Approach to Extrinsics

The arthroscopic approach to the extrinsics involves both modalities of assessment: direct vision inspection and testing by probing. Analysis is completed by clinical examination using special tests such as Watson and interosseous ballottement, intraarticular interosseous gaping and hypermobility of the bones.

7.1 Direct Vision Inspection

Radiocarpal through portals 3–4, 4–5, 6U and 1–2 (RSC – LRL – RSL – (SRL inconstant) – UL – UT)
Midcarpal through portals MC 1–3, RMC, UMC, RSC and TC

7.2 Probe Palpation Assessment

For lesions of the extrinsic ligaments in the proximal palmar plane, we propose the following staging:

- Stage 0: Perfect tension: harp string effect.
- Stage 1: Ligament laxity: possible mobility, corresponding to the thickness of the probe 1 mm (Fig. 10).

- Stage 2: Partial ligament degeneration as seen by fibrillary appearance, thinning and blurred edges.
- Stage 3: Complete disappearance of the extrinsic ligament, only remnants may be seen.

This testing may be applied to the distal palmar plane (the scaphotrapezotrapezoidal complex) where only the scaphotrapezial STz ligament can be tested, since – as previously mentioned – the CTz and SC are only accessible in pathological situations.

The palmar plane assessment is completed by probing of the distal scaphocapitate interval. We propose extending the Dautel scapholunate staging [28–30] to the distal scaphocapitate interval (Fig. 11).

We consider stage 2 (easy probe penetration and opening of the interval by torsion) and 3 (spontaneously open interval) to signify a severe lesion of the extrinsic lock, the distal scapholunate.

This testing may be applied to the dorsal plane. It is difficult and needs the use of special portals 1–2, 6U and MC 1–3. It is sometimes necessary to debride the bulky dorsal synovium using the shaver to optimize palpation under visual control. It is also sometimes necessary to use the second probe.

8 Other Arthroscopic Signs of Instability

In recent trauma, hemorrhagic synovitis pigments the stretched extrinsic ligament and is an indicator of the lesion in arthroscopy [34].

Hypermobility of one of the proximal carpal bones, better visualized through the midcarpal, is a better sign especially if the interosseous ligament testing is equivocal.

Chondritis of the borders of the scapholunate or lunotriquetral intervals is a sign of an old instability [34].

Watson's test and interosseous ballottement are of anecdotal importance.

9 Conclusion

The extrinsic ligaments – intimately related to the intrinsics – seem to play a role much more significant than that originally described in the genesis of perilunate dissociative instability.

Arthroscopy allows a descriptive and kinematic study of wrist ligament pathology. It presents an inevitable stage in the assessment of wrist instability.

We systematically assess the extrinsic locks through a lateral approach (portals 1–2, 6U, MC 1–3) to complete the classical examination.

We propose a staging for extrinsic lesions and an application of the Dautel staging to the distal scaphocapitate interval.

We propose the hypothesis that SL dissociative instability is due to SL ligament lesion associated with a lesion of at least one of the three extrinsic locks.

We think that the extrinsic locks' lesion should modulate the choice of technique for treatment of chronic scapholunate instability.

References

1. Mayfield JK (1984) Pattern of injury to carpal ligaments. Clin Orthop Relat Res 187:36–42
2. Berger RA (1999) Constraint and material properties of the subregions of the scapholunate interosseous ligament. J Hand Surg Am 24:953–962
3. Berger RA, Linscheid RL (1998) Lunotriquetral properties: a comparison of three anatomic subregions. J Hand Surg Am 23:425–431
4. Viegas SF (1999) The dorsal ligaments of the wrist: anatomy, mechanical properties and function. J Hand Surg Am 24:456–468
5. Viegas SF (2004) The role of the dorsal intercarpal ligament in dynamic and static scapholunate instability. J Hand Surg Am 29:279–288
6. Camus EJ, Dumontier C (2006) A quoi sert la biomécanique du carpe ? Face à face. Paris 57th meeting of French Hand Surgery Society
7. Camus (2004) Biomécanique du scaphoide. In: Lussiez, Rizzo, Lebreton (eds.) Le scaphoide. Sauramps Paris, pp 45–54
8. Oberlin C (1990) Les instabilités et désaxations du carpe. Bases anatomiques Etude clinique et radiologique. Conférence d'enseignement SOFCOT 38:235–50
9. Short WH (2002) The effect of sectioning the dorsal radiocarpal ligament and insertion of a pressure sensor into the radiocarpal joint on scaphoïd and Lunate kinematics. J Hand Surg Am 27:68–76
10. Cooney WP, An KN, Linscheid RL, Berger RA (1998) The lunotriquetral joint: kinematic effects of sequential ligament sectioning, ligament repair, and arthrodesis. J Hand Surg Am 23:432–445
11. Short WH, Werner FW (2002) Biomechanical evaluation of ligamentous stabilizers of the scaphoid and lunate. J Hand Surg Am 27:991–1002
12. Short WH, Werner FW (2005) Biomechanical evaluation of ligamentous stabilizers of the scaphoid and lunate. J Hand Surg Am 30:24–34
13. Short WH, Werner FW (2007) Biomechanical evaluation of ligamentous stabilizers of the scaphoid and lunate. J Hand Surg Am 32:297e1–297e18
14. Short WH, Werner FW (1995) A dynamic biomechanical study of scapholunate ligament sectioning. J Hand Surg Am 20:986–999
15. Ishiko T, Puttlitz CM, Lotz JC, Diao E (2003) Scaphoid kinematic behavior after division of the transverse carpal ligament. J Hand Surg Am 28:267–271
16. Moritomo H, Viegas SF, Patterson RM, Da Silva MF, Nakamura K (2000) The scaphotrapezio-trapezoidal joint. Part 1: an anatomic and radiographic study. J Hand Surg Am 25:899–910
17. Moritomo H, Viegas SF, Patterson RM, Da Silva MF, Nakamura K (2000) The scaphotrapezio-trapezoidal joint. Part 2: kinematic study. J Hand Surg Am 25:911–920
18. Viegas SF, Patterson RM (2005) Three-dimensional description of ligamentous attachments around the lunate. J Hand Surg Am 30:685–672
19. Berger RA (2001) The anatomy of the ligaments of the wrist and distal radioulnar joints. Clin Orthop Relat Res 383:32–40
20. Sennwald GR, Zdravlovic V, Oberlin C (1994) The anatomy of the palmar scaphotriquetral ligament. J Bone Joint Surg Br 76:147–149
21. Kuhlman JN (2002) La stabilité et les instabilité radio- et médio-carpienne. Montpellier: Sauramps Médical

22. Oberlin C (1990) Les instabilités et désaxations du carpe. Bases anatomiques. Etude clinique et radiologique Conférence d'enseignement de la SOFCOT, Paris 38:235–250
23. Larsen CF, Amadio PC, Gilula LA (1995) Analysis of carpal instability: 1. Description of the schema. J Hand Surg Am 20:757–764
24. Larsen CF, Amadio PC, Gilula LA (1995) Analysis of carpal instability: 2. Clinical applications. J Hand Surg Am 20:765–776
25. Trial IA, Stanley JK, Hayton MJ (2007) Twenty questions on carpal instability. J Hand Surg Eur Vol 32(3):240–255
26. Camus Emmanuel J (2009) MD Biomécanique du carpe. Application aux lésions ligamentaires. Congrès franco-belge, Tournai
27. Slutsky DJ (2008) The incidence of dorsal radiocarpal ligament tears in patients having diagnostic wrist arthroscopy for wrist pain. J Hand Surg 33A:332–334
28. Dreant N, Dautel G (2003) Development of a arthroscopic severity score for scapholunate instability. Chir Main 22(2):90–94
29. Dautel G (2009) Arthroscopie normale du poignet. Congrès franco-belge, Tournai
30. Dautel G, Deletang F (2009) Application de l'arthroscopie à l'étude des ligaments intrinsèques. Congrès franco-belge, Tournai
31. Drewniany JJ, Palmer AK, Flatt AE (1985) The scaphotrapezial ligament complex: an anatomic and biomechanical study. J Hand Surg 10A:493–497
32. Jantea CL, An KN, Lindscheid RL, Cooney WP (1994) The role of the scapho-trapezial-trapezoidal ligament complex on scaphoid kinematics. In: Schuind F (ed) Advances in the biomechanics of the hand and wrist. Plenum Press, New York, pp 345–361
33. Elsaidi GA, Ruch DS, Kuzma GR, Smith BP (2004) Dorsal wrist ligament insertions stabilize the scapholunate interval: cadaver study. Clin Orthop Relat Res 425:152–157
34. Van Overtsraeten L (2009) Critères arthroscopiques de datation du traumatisme Congrès franco-belge, Tournai

Dynamic Arthroscopic Testing: False Positives and False Negatives

N. Dréant

This chapter is a short technical note which completes the 'Application of wrist arthroscopy to the study of intrinsic ligaments' written by Gilles Dautel. It aims at quantifying the causes of false positives and false negatives during the dynamic testing of scapho- and pyramidolunate instabilities at the midcarpal space.

1 False Positives

In these situations, the arthroscopic dynamic testing tends to overestimate the score of severity of a scapho- or triquetrolunate instability.

1.1 The Examining Hook and the Optic

Although it can seem trivial, an undersized examining hook can engender a misinterpretation of the testing. It becomes impossible to make real dynamic testing if the hook is too thin and its tip small. The examining hook should be 2 mm thick and the tip with a right angle should be at least 3 mm deep. In stage 1 of Dautel's classification, it is possible to introduce the tip of the hook in the interosseous space. In stage 2, the hook must be long and strong enough to test the interosseous laxity with the use of a twisting motion applied to the hook. In stage 3, the optic easily passes from the midcarpal to the radiocarpal space through the diastasis. It can be understood that the use of an optic for small joints (1.9 mm) can distort the results.

N. Dréant
Pole Urgence Main Nice,
10 Bd Pasteur, 06000 Nice, France
e-mail: ndreant@sfr.fr

E. Camus, L. Van Overstraeten (eds.), *Carpal Ligament Surgery*,
DOI 10.1007/978-2-8178-0379-1_10, © Springer-Verlag France 2013

1.2 Natural Ligamentous Laxity

It is difficult to understand the degree of physiologic laxity of these interosseous ligaments. However, two elements can be useful:

First of all, the pre-operating clinical exam gives us information about the degree of laxity which can be expected if we are, as described by Christophe Rizzo, systematically bilateral and comparative. This exam is always completed by a dynamic radiographic report which is bilateral too.

Then, if we are lucky enough to use arthroscopy to test a wrist with one of the two interosseous ligaments which is sane in the midcarpal space, it is possible to trust its behaviour in the radiocarpal space. It is as if the sane couple was the reference to the injured couple. In other words, if the laxity detected in the testing of the scapholunate couple, which has an injured radiocarpal ligament, is the same as the one of the healthy triquetrolunate couple, we can come to the conclusion that this is a physiologic laxity.

2 False Negatives

These are situations when the arthroscopic dynamic testing tends to underestimate the score of severity of a scapho- or triquetrolunate instability.

2.1 The Tension Applied on the Finger Traps

It is necessary to insist on the fact that when the tension impressed on the extrinsic ligaments during wrist arthroscopy is too important, there can be a misinterpretation. Once the hook and the optic are in place in the midcarpal space, tension has to be relaxed. Moreover, the wrist has to be in a neutral position in prono-supination. Indeed, too many constraints in twisting motion have the same indirect effect on the extrinsic ligaments and can modify the interpretation of the arthroscopic testing.

2.2 The Position of the Examining Hook

It is essential that the hook is introduced in the axis of the interval to be tested. Indeed, for a testing of the scapholunate couple, the hook must be introduced by the radial midcarpal portal (RMC). The hook is thus parallel to the scapholunate interval, and the twisting motion becomes easy and natural. Once the hook is deeply introduced in the scapholunate space, until its right angle is inserted, a strong and progressive twisting motion is axially applied to the hook.

For the testing of the triquetrolunate couple, the hook must be parallel to the triquetrolunate interval, and thus it must be introduced by the ulnar midcarpal portal (UMC).

The previous elements can lead to a misinterpretation of the results of the dynamic testing. However, these inconveniences can be easily avoided if the surgeon has the adequate material, a good technique of arthroscopic palpation and if he takes care to get rid of the variations induced by the elements of extrinsic stabilization.

Arthroscopic Criteria to Date Traumas

L. Van Overstraeten

As already mentioned, the dating of radio- and intracarpal sprains often raises a therapeutic and forensic question.

Is the trauma reported as being the causal element the only one to be responsible?

This question has a therapeutic impact since, as we know it, the stabilization of unstable injuries within 6 weeks allows to get an anatomic and functional healing to prevent adaptive decompensation.

This question also has a forensic impact.

In common law (for instance, when an accident on the public highway implies the third party responsibility), the previous state erases the damage, and except if the victim can prove a worsening of his/her previous state, the damage will not be repaired.

The author puts forward three criteria to estimate when the trauma first appeared and to argue anamnestic information given by the victim.

1 The Turbidity of the Synovial Fluid

At the beginning of an arthroscopy, after the tourniquet has been inflated, needles are placed in the usual portals. Most of the time, the 3/4 portal easily allows to get synovial fluid.

The author himself always injects 5 cc of physiologic fluid he gets back in a white bottle or on a compress.

This fluid is scarcely translucent when the trauma is less than 6 weeks old!

This idea has come to estimate the turbidity following a score of colouration.

L. Van Overstraeten
Hand and Foot Surgery Unit SPRL,
Rue Pierre Caille N° 9, B-7500 Tournai, Belgium
e-mail: l.v.o@skynet.be

E. Camus, L. Van Overstraeten (eds.), *Carpal Ligament Surgery*,
DOI 10.1007/978-2-8178-0379-1_11, © Springer-Verlag France 2013

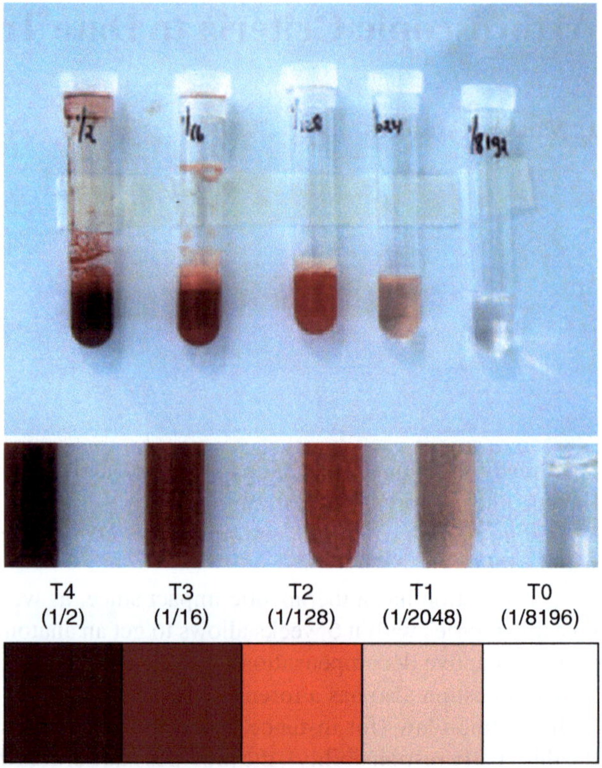

Fig. 1 Turbidity: scale of reference (from 0 to 4); dilutions

At first, there were three scores: transparent, rosy and bloody.

For a short time, the author has been estimating turbidity on a scale from 0 to 4, reproduced by dilution 1/2 (dilutions from 1/2 to 1/8196) (Fig. 1).

A colourful fluid (T3–T4) testifies to a recent trauma which happened less than 2 weeks before (usual delay for hemarthroses to disappear).

A rather clear fluid (T1–T2) testifies to a trauma of less than 6 weeks old.

A transparent fluid (T0) testifies to a trauma of more than 6 weeks old.

Be careful of the variations linked to some microcrystalline or rheumatoid arthritides.

2 The Presence of Hematic Synovitis

We all noticed the presence of hematic synovitis in wrists that have just been injured. It shows the extrinsic ligamentous zone implied in the injury. It gives a real topography of the zone.

In recent traumas, less than 2 weeks old, the whole ligamentous zone is red from the proximal to the radial ligament.

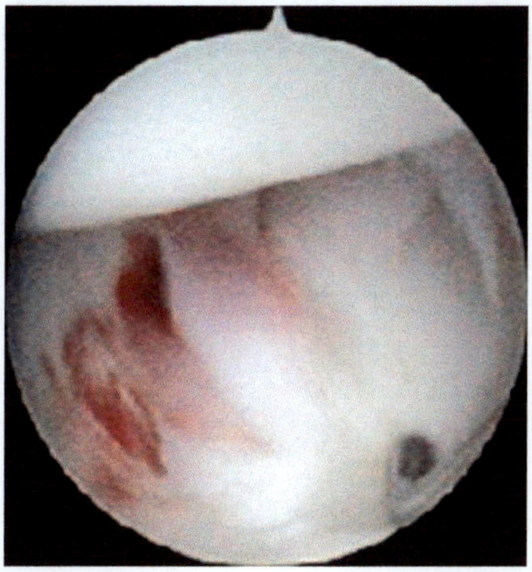

Fig. 2 Hematic synovitis at the foot of the radioscaphocapitate ligament: S1

When traumas are older, from 3 weeks to 6 months, the hematic synovitis probably concentrates itself in the disinsertion zone (Fig. 2) in radiocarpal and in midcarpal.

A recent pathological wrist which has no hematic synovitis but a scapho- or triquetrolunate instability, or a laxity of the extrinsic ligamentous apparatus, has necessarily been previously injured. The trauma is often reported to be superior to 6 months.

3 The Scoring of the Associated Chondrite

This is Outerbridge's scoring of chondrites [1]:

- *Stage 1*: soft chondrite: the hook leaves a print
- *Stage 2*: fibrous chondrite or chondrite with fissures
- *Stage 3*: chondral incisive ulceration 'crab-like coloured' (Fig. 3)
- *Stage 4*: the bone is visible

The soft chondrite is the first cartilaginous reaction. It appears at the edges of the injured intervals 3 or 4 weeks after the trauma. Then, it extends to the convex surfaces (first to the proximal poles of the first row and then to the capitate and lunate poles). It is less visible on the concave surfaces (radial and distal facets of the bones of the first row).

The fibrous chondrite appears as soon as the 4th post-traumatic week on the edges of the injured intervals. It extends to the convex and then to the concave surfaces after the sixth week. Chondral ulceration testifies to a subacute injury which has been lasting for several months.

The exposure of the bone is chronicle. It appears after several years of instability.

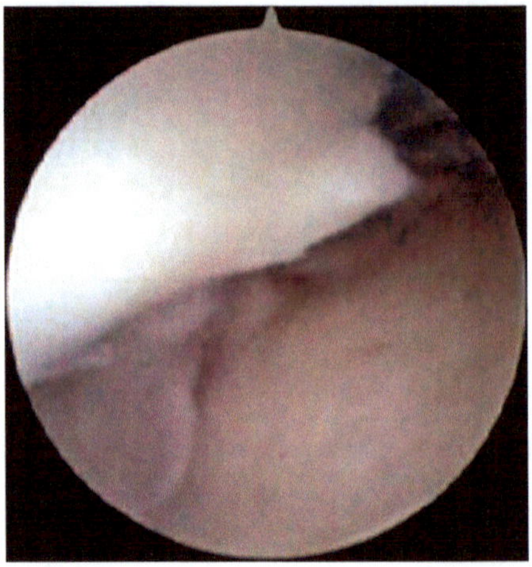

Fig. 3 Incisive ulceration: proximal pole of the triquetrum, C3

4 Scoring Proposal

The author proposes the following scoring:

- T for 'turbidity' followed by a number from 0 to 4
  T0: perfectly transparent fluid
  T4: 1/2 dilution of the arterial blood
- S for 'hematic synovitis' followed by a number from 0 to 2
  S0: absence of hematic synovitis
  S2: hematic synovitis on the whole ligament
- C for 'chondrite' followed by a number from 0 to 4
  C0: absence of chondrites
  C1: soft chondrites
  C2: fibrous chondrites
  C3: incisive chondral ulceration
  C4: exposure of the dome

5 Chart Summing Up the Possible Clinical Aspects

The correlation between each criteria and the post-traumatic delay is the result of a statistical analysis [2].

T0S0C0: normal wrist
T3S2C1: recent trauma dating back from less than 2 weeks
T1S1C2: recent trauma from 2 to 6 weeks
T0S0C2: trauma from 2 to 6 months
T0S0C3: chronicle trauma of more than 1 year

These statistically significant criteria have the merit to objectively evaluate wrist sprains and possible guide treatment.

References

1. Outerbridge RE (1961) The etiology of chondromalacia patellae. J Bone Joint Surg Br 43B: 752–757
2. Overstraeten L, Camus EJ (2012) Arthroscopic criteria for dating wrist sprains. Chir Main 31: 171–175

Part II
Treatment of Ligament Lesions

Management of Wrist Sprain by the General Practitioner

E. Camus

1 Introduction

In case of emergency, wrist sprain diagnosis is often mentioned after a wrist trauma, without fracture or visible luxation on radios. It corresponds to the definition of a sprain for the public at large. A non-pathologic radio sometimes reassures the patient, more often the doctor, and the trauma is usually functionally treated by an elastic or rigid light contention, and even a mere antalgic. It is however necessary to remember that a real sprain corresponds to a trauma of wrist ligaments. Even if a benign sprain will heal without any sequela, the severity of this sprain can be sly. The emergency room doctor has the difficult task to avoid these traps.

2 Clinical Case

This is the case of a 15-year-old girl, victim of a 'benign' wrist trauma. The clinical report at the emergency department mentioned, 'pain at wrist motion, oedema on the wrist, no hematoma, no sensory disorder, no motor disorder'. The initial radio showed a cunean non-displaced fracture of the radius (Fig. 1). The treatment at the emergency department consisted in the application of plaster cast and a prescription of paracetamol.

Four weeks later, when the fracture healed (Fig. 2), the cast was removed, but the patient mentioned a persisting trouble at wrist motion.

One week later, she consulted again as the disorders persisted. The clinical exam mentioned pseudo-blockings with wrist snap, a peri-lunate sensitiveness

E. Camus
Hand Surgery Unit, SELARL Chirurgie de la Main, Polyclinique du Val de Sambre,
162, route de Mons, 59600 Maubeuge, France
e-mail: ejcamus@wanadoo.fr, emmanuel.camus@wanadoo.fr

E. Camus, L. Van Overstraeten (eds.), *Carpal Ligament Surgery*,
DOI 10.1007/978-2-8178-0379-1_12, © Springer-Verlag France 2013

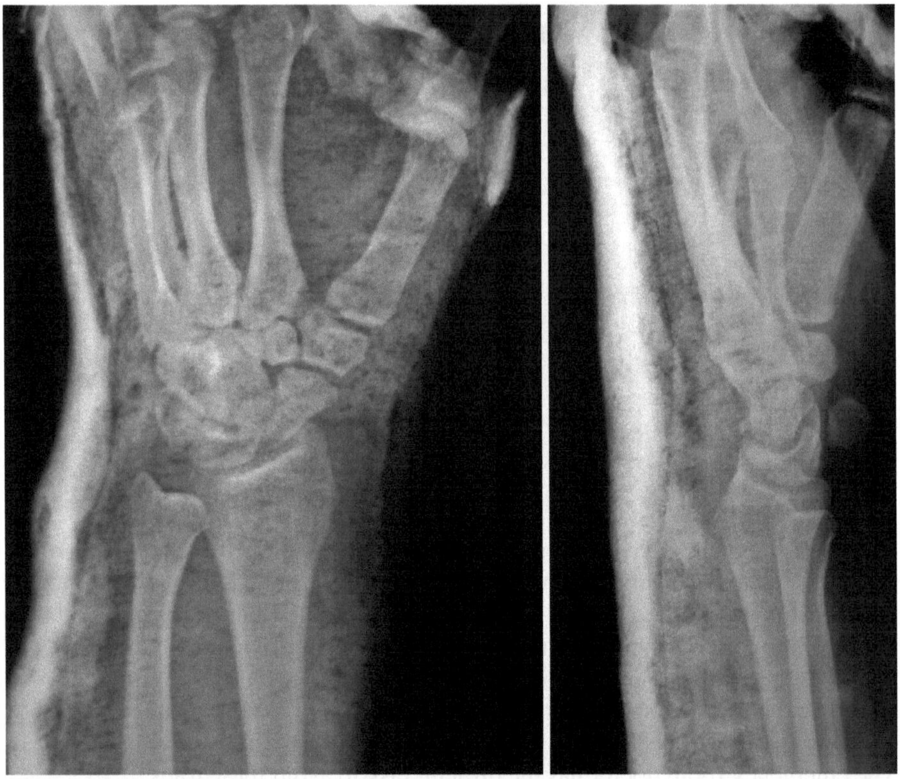

Fig. 1 Initial radiography with the cast

and a doubtful aspect of extension of the lunate on the profile radiography, evoking a possible intracarpal ligament injury. On the one hand, the arthroscanner pointed out an injury of the triangular fibro cartilage complex (TFCC) with a passageway of the contrast fluid into the distal radioulnar joint and on the other hand, an important widening of the scapholunate space, without passage of the contrast fluid (Fig. 3).

Arthroscopy confirmed a rupture of the TFCC (Fig. 4), sutured in the same time (Fig. 5), but also an important scapholunate laxity (Fig. 6) which was immediately pinned with K wires (Fig. 7).

There was a positive evolution after wires had been removed 6 weeks later and after reeducation which had lasted 1 month.

3 Discussion

If the patient had not mentioned her trouble or if her family had not taken her seriously, the trauma would have been diagnosed at a chronic stage. A fracture proves that energy has been delivered by the trauma, which energy could drive to other

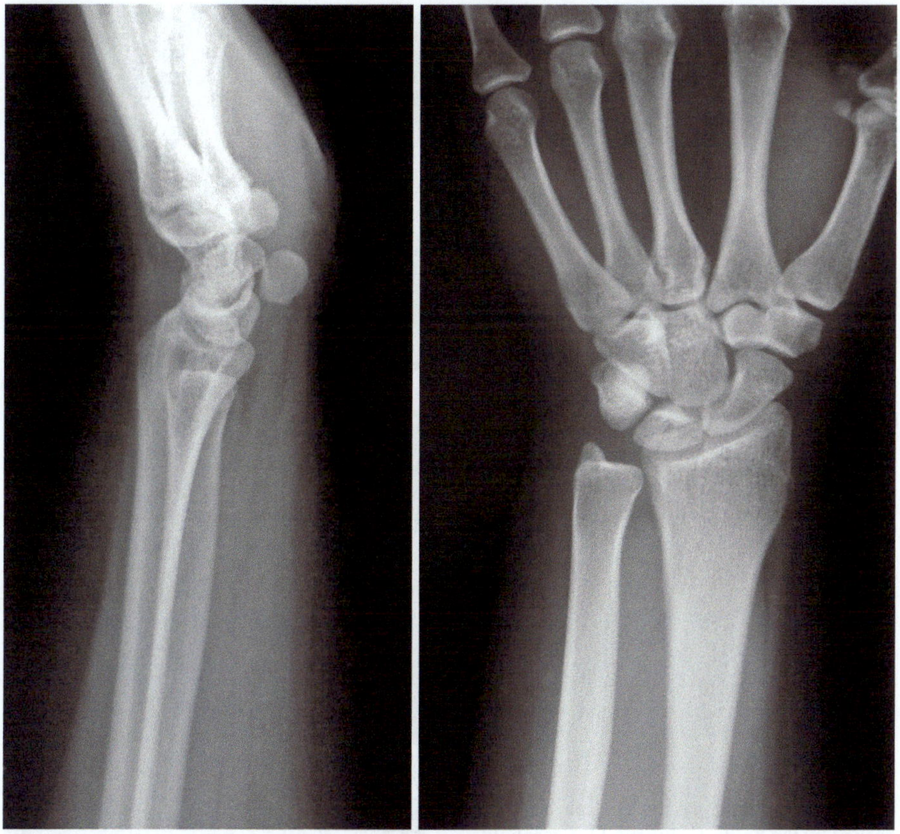

Fig. 2 Radiography once the bone was consolidated

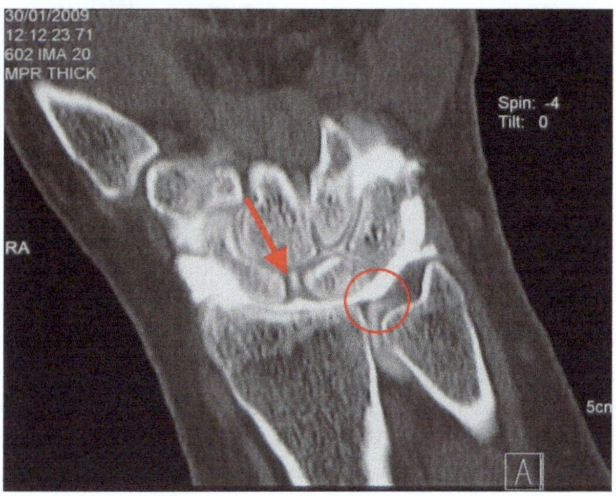

Fig. 3 Arthroscanner. Rupture of the TFCC with passage of the contrast fluid (*circle*). Widening of the scapholunate space (*arrow*)

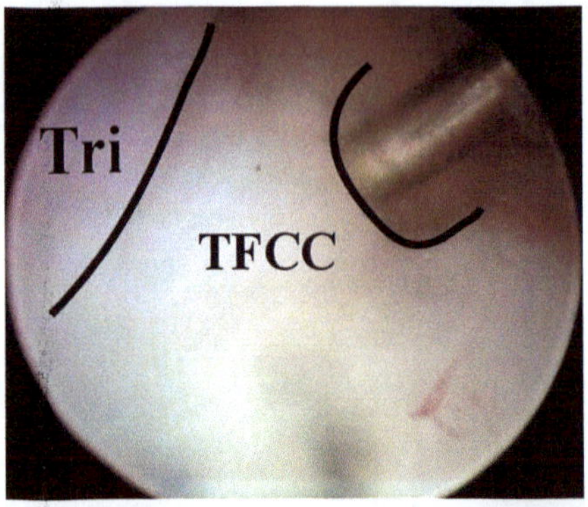

Fig. 4 Arthroscopic image of the perforation of the triangular fibro cartilage complex (TFCC). *Tri* triquetrum

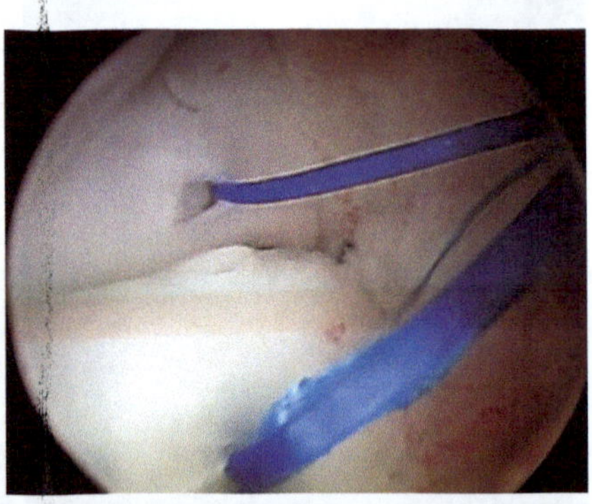

Fig. 5 Arthroscopic suture of the TFCC

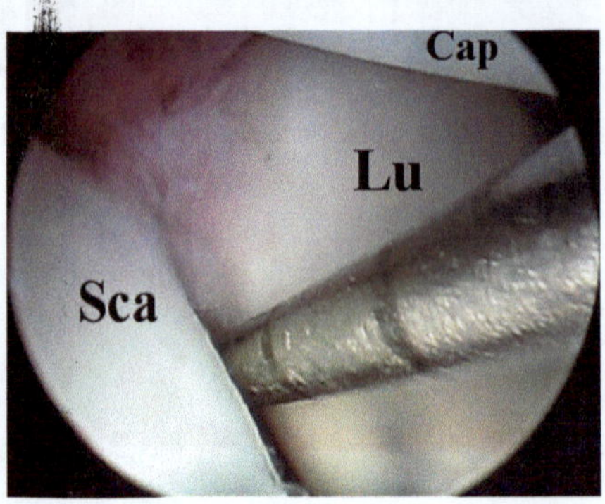

Fig. 6 Scapholunate laxity. The space is easily opened by the hook. *Lu* lunate, *SCA* scaphoid, *Cap* capitate

lesions as ligament tears. Anyway, the absence of fracture does not imply the absence of energy absorbed by the wrist. The history of the trauma, an oedema, snaps or joint blockings, pain at grasp, a bascule of the lunate on the profile radiography, a rupture of Gilula's arcs or a widening scapholunate gap are signs which tend to demonstrate a ligamentous injury. Any wrist trauma has to be followed by a complete clinical exam (Chap. 3). If there is a fracture, it can be difficult to do the exam immediately, but in that case, it must be done at the latest when the plaster cast is removed.

At the slightest doubt, dynamic x-rays can reveal a latent instability, but even at that stage, there can be false negatives. The most important is thus to quickly direct

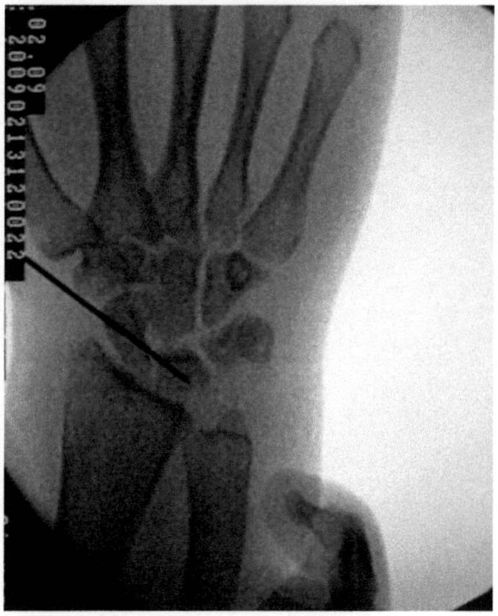

Fig. 7 Scapholunate pinning

the patient towards a surgeon who knows how to deal with carpal pathology when the evolution of the trauma is problematic. Even the arthroscanner can be deficient, and in that case, arthroscopy is the only means to make a report of all the injuries and to test the different wrist ligaments (Chaps. 8 and 9). But it also allows the management of the trauma during the acute phase. The ideal moment to treat the trauma is during the 6 weeks which follow, namely, the period of potential healing of the ligaments. Indeed, after that period, the results of repair are not as good [1]. Non-diagnosed carpal instability, and thus not treated, often leads to advanced arthrosis within a few years [1]. The diagnosis of a sprain and the scoring of severity must be established before a long-lasting immobilization.

4 Conclusion

After a few days or a few weeks, it is paramount to re-examine the injured wrist. During each consultation, the best means to avoid an insidious but invalidating arthrosis is to look for a precursory and clinical sign, which can sometimes be radiological and late. The management of the trauma within the six first weeks allows an ideal treatment often associated with arthroscopy. There is a period of pseudo-silence before chronic instability declares itself, but it can be detected if the signs are well read.

Reference

1. Kuo CE, Wolfe SW (2008) Scapholunate instability: current concepts in diagnosis and management. J Hand Surg 33A:998–1013

Role of the Specialist to Sensitize First-Line Therapists

L. Van Overstraeten

The important impact of wrist traumas among traumatologic emergencies has been known for a long time.

Indeed, the Industrial Accident Fund (IAF) reports statistic datum which are updated every year [1–6].

We also know the important impact of wrist sprains among wrist traumas.

We have been aware of the apparent benign aspect of radiocarpal or intracarpal sprains for a long time. As a matter of fact, pains almost always disappear whatever the sprains (stable or unstable).

Wrist sprains seem to be less seriously taken into account than other traumas of the superior limb. Sprains are often considered as benign, because of ignorance of the clinical and radiological gravity signs.

Yet, once unstable sprains are stabilized within a delay of 6 post-traumatic weeks, there is an anatomic healing of the injuries, and the secondary destabilization and arthrosic adaptation is slowed down or avoided (Chap. 17) [7–9].

During the out-patient clinic activities, we are too often faced to patients who fell on their wrist from 3 to 6 months earlier, and which late diagnosis puts forward an unstable scapho- or triquetrolunate injury while the patient had been examined by a doctor in emergency.

So, there is a public health responsibility in the sensitization of first-line therapeutic actors.

Public powers do not seem to be sensitized to this problem. This is the reason why this responsibility to sensitize first-line therapists should rest on the specialist.

We have to make everything possible to explain emergency room doctors and GPs in each of our health departments:

- That a painful post-traumatic wrist without osseous abnormality can have an unstable ligamentous injury
- That this wrist can be more easily examined after 4 or 5 days of immobilization

L. Van Overstraeten
Hand and Foot Surgery Unit SPRL, Rue Pierre Caille N° 9, B-7500 Tournai, Belgium
e-mail: l.v.o@skynet.be

E. Camus, L. Van Overstraeten (eds.), *Carpal Ligament Surgery*,
DOI 10.1007/978-2-8178-0379-1_13, © Springer-Verlag France 2013

- How to accurately examine a ligamentous wrist
- What the seven stages to examine the wrist are and how to make the round of the joint
- What a manoeuvre of Watson, a triquetrolunate ballottement and a Reagan test is
- That an unstable wrist, even just after the trauma, can remain normal and have a normal mobility and a normal strength
- That if a ligamentous injury is suspected, the patient has to be directed to a hand surgeon and an arthroscanner be quickly made
- That if there is a perilunate ligamentous leak, an appointment must be taken with a surgeon specialized in arthroscopy
- That a period of 6 weeks is a maximum before stabilizing an unstable ligamentous injury
- That if the injury is stable in arthroscopy, a removable orthosis should have a rapid soothing effect and the patient should rapidly go back to work and lead a normal life
- That, on the contrary, if the injury is unstable in arthroscopy, it could be surgically operated within the delay of 6 weeks after the trauma and stabilized with broaches during 6 weeks
- That it is a team work

We have to persuade our colleagues that it is a race against time.

These wrist traumas without osseous injury and these referenced cases by our first-line colleagues have to be our priority in our agendas.

Indeed, if we take into account 15 post-traumatic days before the first consultation and 15 days before a possible arthroscanner, there will be only 15 days remaining to plan a surgical intervention!

A written feedback to our colleagues has to be established to give information on the operating protocol, on the short- and long-term follow-up of the patient and on the efficiency of their action.

It is the easiest way, if not the only one, to reduce the consequence of SLAC-type adaptive decompensations without increasing the consequence of capsulofibrodeses or ligamentoplasties.

References

1. Theme 7 (2007) Private sector: aspects of the injuries engendered by industrial accidents in 2007 at work, Industrial Accident Fund – Fonds voor Arbeisongevallen. www.faofat.fgov.be
2. Theme 19 (2007) Private sector: aspects of the injuries engendered by industrial accidents in 2007 on the way to work, Industrial Accident Fund – Fonds voor Arbeisongevallen. www.faofat.fgov.be
3. Theme 7 (2006) Private sector: aspects of the injuries engendered by industrial accidents in 2007 on the way to work, Industrial Accident Fund – Fonds voor Arbeisongevallen. www.faofat.fgov.be

4. Theme 19 (2006) Private sector: aspects of the injuries engendered by industrial accidents in 2007 on the way to work, Industrial Accident Fund – Fonds voor Arbeisongevallen. www.faofat.fgov.be
5. Theme 6 (2005) Private sector: aspects of the injuries engendered by industrial accidents in 2007 on the way to work, Industrial Accident Fund – Fonds voor Arbeisongevallen. www.faofat.fgov.be
6. Theme 17 (2006) Private sector: aspects of the injuries engendered by industrial accidents in 2007 on the way to work, Industrial Accident Fund – Fonds voor Arbeisongevallen. www.faofat.fgov.be
7. Chloros GD, Wiesler ER, Poehling GG (2008) Current concepts in wrist arthroscopy. Arthroscopy 24(3):343–354, Epub 2008 Jan 7
8. Geissler WB (2006) Arthroscopic management of scapholunate instability. Chir Main 25(Suppl 1):S187–S196
9. Ruch DS, Siegel D, Chabon SJ, Koman LA, Poehling GG (1993) Arthroscopic categorization of intercarpal ligamentous injuries of the wrist. Orthopedics 16(9):1051–1056

Management of Painful Constitutional Laxities

L. Van Overstraeten

1 Introduction

Painful constitutional midcarpal laxities are particular and sometimes block our surgical consultations [1–3, 6, 7].

In 1984, Louis described a capitolunate instability pattern as a distinct form of instability [5]. In 1986, Johnson and Carrera reported chronic capitolunate instability of traumatic origin [8, 9]. In 1984, White and Coll. proved that all the patients who have a CLIP ('capitolunate instability pattern' or capitolunate trigger during Watson manoeuvre) were receptive to a plastered immobilization [14]. In 1996, Ono, Gilula and Coll. disagreed with them [10, 14]. They described the DCT and the VCT ('dorsal and volar capitate displacement test'). In 1996, Schernberg showed on stress views that the dorsal displacement of the capitate was more prominent on lax wrists than on normal wrists [12, 13]. In 2002, out of 100 normal wrists, Park defined the displacement index of the capitate and three types of capitolunate laxity following the direction in dorsal stress of the lunate [11] (Fig. 1). Laxity was definitely more important when the patients were women and young adults (20–29 years old). Neither was there difference between dominant and nondominant wrists nor between dorsal or volar displacements.

In 2002, Kuhlman established that the discomforting SNAP-type trigger was due to a rupture or a loosening of the dorsal radiocarpal ligament [4]. He did not refer to a non-pathologic state.

L. Van Overstraeten
Hand and Foot Surgery Unit SPRL,
Rue Pierre Caille N° 9, B-7500 Tournai, Belgium
e-mail: l.v.o@skynet.be

E. Camus, L. Van Overstraeten (eds.), *Carpal Ligament Surgery*,
DOI 10.1007/978-2-8178-0379-1_14, © Springer-Verlag France 2013

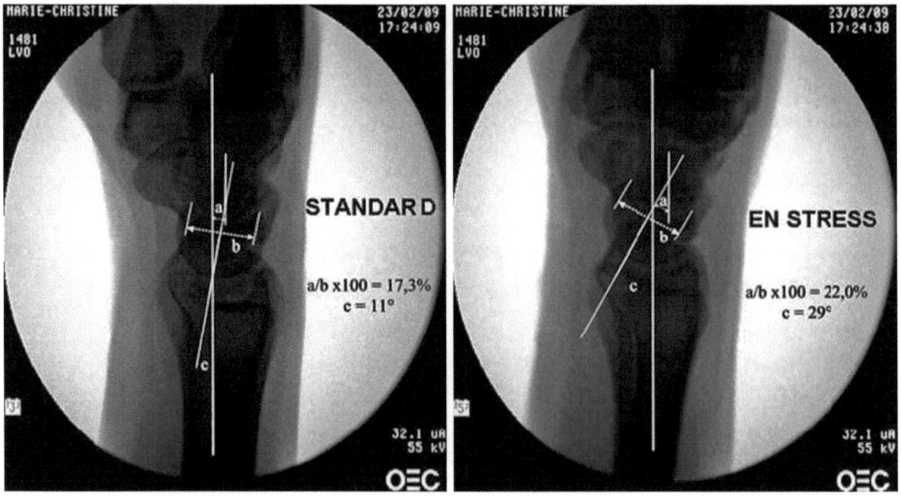

Fig. 1 Park's type II pattern of midcarpal laxity: standard and anteroposterior radiological views. Extension and dorsal displacement stress of the lunate

2 Casuistics

The patients are often young adults from 12 to 20 years old who have no trauma but sometimes suffer from a dorsal wrist pain in the median long fingers as they practise manual activities (gymnastics, gardening, move, athletics). This pain is often associated with the extension of the wrist when we lean on the heel of the hand, by writing, and by ball sports [1]. A dorsal wrist pain spreads to the median long fingers. It can happen at rest and be latent but scarcely engender cramps.

There was no mention of swelling or abnormality. There is no dysesthesia, but cracks or snaps are reported. A shoot up sometimes precedes the painful episode.

The clinical exam usually points out a hypermobility, particularly in the sagittal plane with ranges which come close to or exceed 90°.

The ligamentous testing underlines a sensitive triquetro-lunate ballottement and a midcarpal trigger, sometimes with a CLIP. This trigger is the consequence of the fixing of the dorsal horn of the lunate with the dome of the capitate.

The standard radiographic report is normal.

The differential diagnosis can be established with:

- Hidden arthrosynovitis cysts
- Dorsal synovial pinching
- Early aseptic necrosis of the lunate (Kienböck)
- RUD instability
- Extensor carpi ulnaris instability
- Radiocarpal instability with a deficiency of the extrinsic ligaments

It is a diagnosis of exclusion for which it can sometimes be relevant to resort to scan or NMR.

3 Medical Management

This is a medical, easy and often rapid treatment. Night immobilization in a small antebrachio-palmar orthosis and strengthening of the extrinsic muscles participate in lessening the pain within 2 or 3 weeks. Kapandji proposed to 'reinforce the tendinous cage' [15].

This 'sheath' effect is maintained by daily and long-term exercises of isotonic strengthening of the common flexors of the fingers and the extensor carpi ulnaris. After a few weeks, the orthosis is removed but can be put back whenever necessary.

There is no surgical necessity except in exceptional cases. A fibrosis around the dorsal intercarpal ligament artificially stiffens these hyperlax wrists.

4 Particular Cases: Minor Intracarpal Joint Upsets

Minor joint upsets are rare. The patients who suffer from these upsets are usually hyperlax and the pain, sharp and brutal, spontaneously arises without any initial trauma. The pain can be compared to that of a blade.

The pain is often dorsal and transfixing.

The medical exam of a painful wrist is particularly difficult considering the intensity of the pain.

The aspect of the wrist and the fingers is normal. The wrist is maintained in an 'antalgic' position. On the contrary, the exam of the contralateral wrist generally shows a hypermobile wrist, a small midcarpal trigger. The elbows show a recurvatum and the sub-astragalian are hyperlax.

Usually, there is no significant abnormality on the radiographic report.

Exceptionally, the parallelism between two ossicles is modified (Figs. 2 and 3): capitohamate or triquetro-lunate.

The differential diagnosis is that of a classic midcarpal hyperlaxity.

The paraclinic report is strictly normal:

- 99-m technetium scintigraphy does not reveal any hyper-fixing.
- There is no ligamentous injury or articular foreign body on the arthroscanner; it can confirm the loss of articular parallelism.

The result is strangely similar to that of the minor vertebral articular upsets like lumbagos.

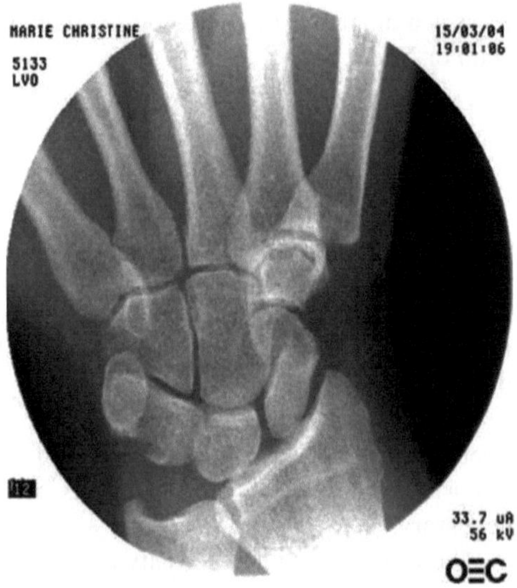

Fig. 2 Minor articular upset: radiological view showing a capitate-hamate interval which is perfectly visible but a superimposed lunate-triquetral interval

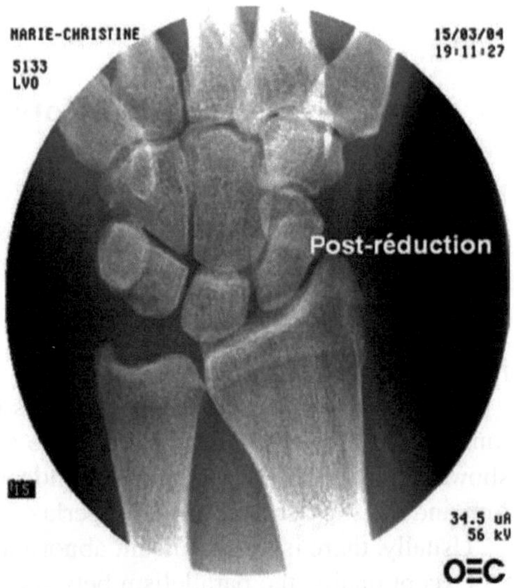

Fig. 3 Post-reduction minor articular upset: radiological view after manipulations. It shows the triquetro-lunate and capitohamate intervals whose bones are not superimposed

The diagnosis is confirmed by axial traction manipulations and anteroposterior joint ballottement. A small trigger almost immediately engenders a disappearance of the pains.

A radiographic report of control shows parallelism has been re-established.

As for wrists with a hyperlax and painful mediocarpus, the strengthening of the extrinsic muscles stays enabled to avoid or decrease the frequency of these 'joint accidents'.

References

1. Apergis EP (1996) The unstable capitolunate and radiolunate joints as a source of wrist pain in young women. J Hand Surg Br 21–13:501–506
2. Berger RA (1997) The ligaments of the wrist: a current overview of anatomy with considerations of their potential functions. Hand Clin 13:63–82
3. Garth WP Jr, Hofammann DY, Rooks MD (1985) Volar intercalated segment instability secondary to medial carpal ligamental laxity. Clin Orthop 201:94–105
4. Kuhlman JN (2002) La stabilité et les instabilités radio et médio-carpienne. Sauramps Médical, Montpellier
5. Louis DS, Hankin FM, Green TL, Braunstein EM, White SJ (1984) Central carpal instability-capitate lunate instability pattern: diagnosis by dynamic displacement. Orthopedics 7:1693–1696
6. Lichtman DM, Schneider JR, Swafford AR, Mack GR (1981) Ulnar midcarpal instability-clinical and laboratory analyses. J Hand Surg Am 6-A:515–523
7. Linscheid RL, Dobyns JH, Beabout JW, Brvan RS (1972) Traumatic instability of the wrist: diagnosis, classification and pathomechanics. J Bone Joint Surg Am 54-A:1612–1632
8. Johnson RP (1980) The acutely injured wrist and its residuals. Clin Orthop Relat Res 149:33–44
9. Johnson RP, Carrera GE (1986) Chronic capitolunate instability. J Bone Joint Surg Am 68-A:1164–1176
10. Ono H, Gilula LA, Evanoff BA, Grand D (1996) Midcarpal instability: is capitolunate instability pattern a clinical condition? J Hand Surg Br 21-B:197–201
11. Park MJ (2002) Normal anteroposterior laxity of the radiocarpal and midcarpal joints. J Bone Joint Surg Br 84-B:73–76
12. Schernberg F (1996) Roentgenographic examination of the wrist: part 1: the standard and positional views. J Hand Surg Br 15B:210–219
13. Schernberg F (1996) Roentgenographic examination of the wrist: part 2: stress views. J Hand Surg Br 15B:220–228
14. White SJ, Louis DS, Braunstein EM, Hankin FM, Greene TL (1984) Capitate-lunate instability: recognition by manipulation under fluoroscopy. AJR Am J Roentgenol 143:361–364
15. Kapandji AI, Martin-Bouyer Y, Verdeille S (1991) Etude du carpe au scanner à trois dimensions sous contraintes de prono-supination. Ann Chir Main 10:36–47

Rotatory Radiocarpal Instability

J.-L. Roux

1 Introduction

Radiocarpal rotatory instability is defined as the increase in longitudinal rotation between the forearm bones and the carpal condyle.

This rotational laxity in the transverse plane constantly provoked by pronosupination is frequently forgotten in clinical and biomechanical studies of carpal stability.

Longitudinal rotation between forearm bones and carpal condyle has nevertheless been described by several authors.

The first was Cyriax [1] in 1917, who showed that an important passive rotation existed between forearm bones and carpal condyle. He emphasized that this rotation cannot be produced actively. He evaluated it clinically at 45°, whereas in a cadaver it was only at 19°.

In 1980, Gagey [2] evaluated intracarpal and radiocarpal rotation at 50° in completely relaxed patients under general anaesthesia in theatre.

In 1991, Kapandji [3] defined 'rotational drift' between the radius and the base of the metacarpals. He measured it in his own wrist under tomodensitometry at 45° in free pronosupination.

In 1992 [4, 5], we clinically measured radiometacarpal rotation RMR, which is the rotation that occurs between the forearm bones fixed in midpronation and the base of the metacarpals. We used a special device that measures simultaneously the RMR, the grip force and the pronosupinator moment arm exerted distally to show that this passive rotation varied for the same moment arm force according to the grip strength. A first measurement was recorded with the wrist relaxed (force less than 5 N), exerting a distal rotation moment arm of 2 Nm in supination and 0.5 Nm in pronation. In these conditions, the RMR was 42°. A second measurement was taken

J.-L. Roux
Hand Surgery Unit, Institut Montpelliérain de la Main,
25, rue Clémentville, 34070 Montpellier, France
e-mail: jlroux.imm@wanadoo.fr

E. Camus, L. Van Overstraeten (eds.), *Carpal Ligament Surgery*,
DOI 10.1007/978-2-8178-0379-1_15, © Springer-Verlag France 2013

with closed wrist (grip force between 80 and 100 N) with distal moment arm of rotation of 1 Nm in pronation and in supination. The RMR was 33°. This decrease in RMR with a distal moment arm almost tripled defines the wrist locking. We used this test to assess 100 healthy wrists.

2 Radiocarpal Rotatory Stability

We have shown in a cadaveric anatomic study that there are radiocarpal and intracarpal ligament structures limiting the passive longitudinal rotation in pronation as well as in supination. We described a 'double ligamentary pronosupinator helix' (Fig. 1) [5, 6].

The pronator helix is activated by active pronation against resistance or passive carpal supination. It originates on the posterior border of the radius and joins the posterior border of the triquetrum ulnarly and is composed mainly of the dorsal radiotriquetral ligament. It is prolonged palmarly by the triquetrocapitate ligament then by the thick capitotrapeziotrapezoidal complex. The supinator helix is activated by active supination against resistance or passive carpal pronation. It originates on the anterolateral border of the radius with the radioscaphocapitate ligament, prolonged by the palmar capitotriquetral ligament. On the dorsal aspect of the carpus, it is continuous with the transverse dorsal carpal ligament by a ligament band

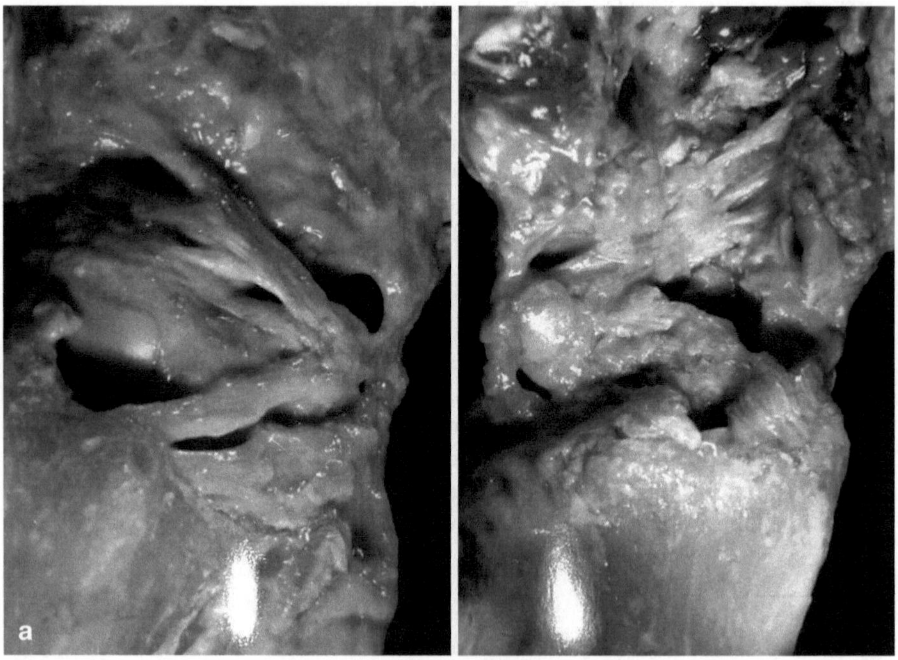

Fig. 1 (**a, b**) Extrinsic ligaments form a double pronosupinator helix. This helix is particularly apparent on pronosupination against resistance

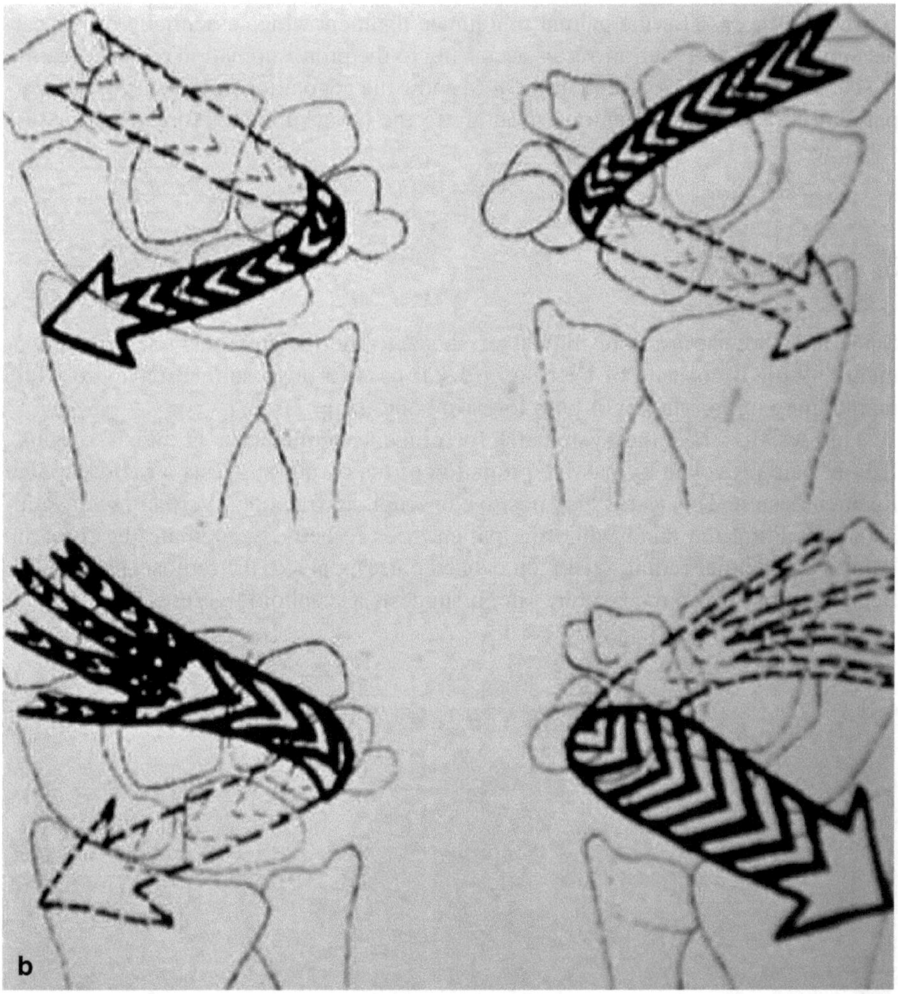

Fig. 1 (continued)

that joins the triquetrum to the trapezoid. This band is more apparent on active supination against resistance.

In a 1995 cadaveric study, Ritt et al. [7] resumed the previous work to study the rotational carpal stability with respect to the radius. He released the anatomic structures activated by a rotational radiocarpal moment arm. When a pronatory moment arm is exerted at the carpal condyle, the radioscaphocapitate ligament is the first to be solicited.

The long and short radiolunate ligaments play a secondary role.

The dorsal radiocarpal ligament is the principal ligament to oppose carpal supination.

Ritt emphasizes that the action of these ligaments depends on the position of the forearm in pronosupination. The ligaments originating from the ulna can be activated by radiocarpal rotation depending on the position of the forearm in pronosupination.

Such is the case for the palmar ulnolunate ligament which essentially resists carpal supination but its action varies according to the pronosupination of the forearm.

The work of Ritt [7, 8] and ours [4–6] show the adaptation of the entire radiocarpal and intracarpal ligamentous structure to the pronosupinator forces the wrist is subjected to.

3 Clinical Test

Since 1992, we use a simple clinical test that activates the previously described ligaments [4–6]. It consists of exerting a distal passive pronosupination force while maintaining midpronation of both forearm bones (Fig. 2).

This test has become systematic for clinical examination of wrist 'sprains'. Palmar pain provoked by passive pronation of the carpus suggests a radioscaphoid ligament lesion. This test is also positive in scaphoid fractures. Verdan used a similar test holding the hand while the patient tries to actively supinate the forearm. Palmar and palmar radial wrist pain evoked corresponds to the radioscaphocapitate ligament pressing on the fracture site. It suggests a scaphoid fracture.

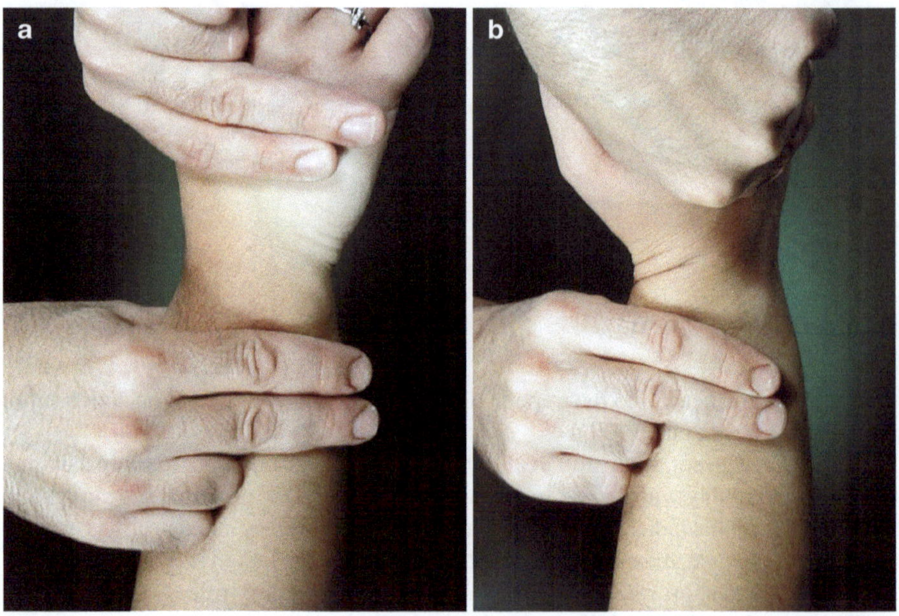

Fig. 2 The test for evaluation of radiometacarpal rotation is a systematic part of our clinical wrist examination, particularly useful if an extrinsic capsular ligament sprain is suspected. (**a**) The forearm is held in midpronation with one hand while the other hand is used to rotate the carpal condyle longitudinally into pronation. (**b**) In supination

The passive carpal supination activates dorsal radiotriquetral ligament and is positive in case of radiotriquetral sprain.

Clinical experience led us to consider results of this test during wrist immobilization [9]. In function of results of this test, we suggest immobilization in slight carpal supination or pronation. This position is independent of the pronosupination of the forearm. We have used this principle for the orthopaedic/closed treatment of dorsal flake triquetral fractures. These fractures are the equivalent of sprain of the dorsal radiotriquetral ligament when this test is positive – this is almost always the case in our experience. For scaphoid fractures and palmar sprains painful in carpal pronation, we place the wrist in mild supination.

4 Radiocarpal Rotatory Instability in Supination

Radiocarpal rotatory instability in supination is defined by increased rotation of the carpal condyle over the distal radius compared to the other side. The clinical test is done symmetrically with one hand holding the forearm in midpronation while the other hand exerts longitudinal rotation in supination at the carpal condyle. In certain cases, simple observation of the wrist shows carpal supination on the distal radius (Fig. 3).

5 Anatomical Reminder

The dorsal radiotriquetral ligament inserts onto the dorsal distal surface of the radius (Fig. 4). Exactly at the dorsal border of the articular surface of the radius, extending from the tubercle of Lister to the sigmoid fossa. It has an oblique pathway passing ulnarly over the posterior horn of the lunate where its deep fibres are attached. These fibres are the reason why the name dorsal radiocarpal ligament is preferred to radiotriquetral. They strengthen the dorsal portion of the lunotriquetral ligament and insert distally on the dorsum of the triquetrum where the ligament merges with the insertion of the dorsal intercarpal ligament. Viegas et al. [10] described the anatomic variations of this ligament but the radiotriquetral fibres are constant.

6 Clinical Experience

Since 1998, we have operated four patients for rotatory radiocarpal instability in supination. To us, this is synonymous with dorsal radiotriquetral ligament insufficiency. We have treated this instability by reconstructing this ligament using extensor retinaculum.

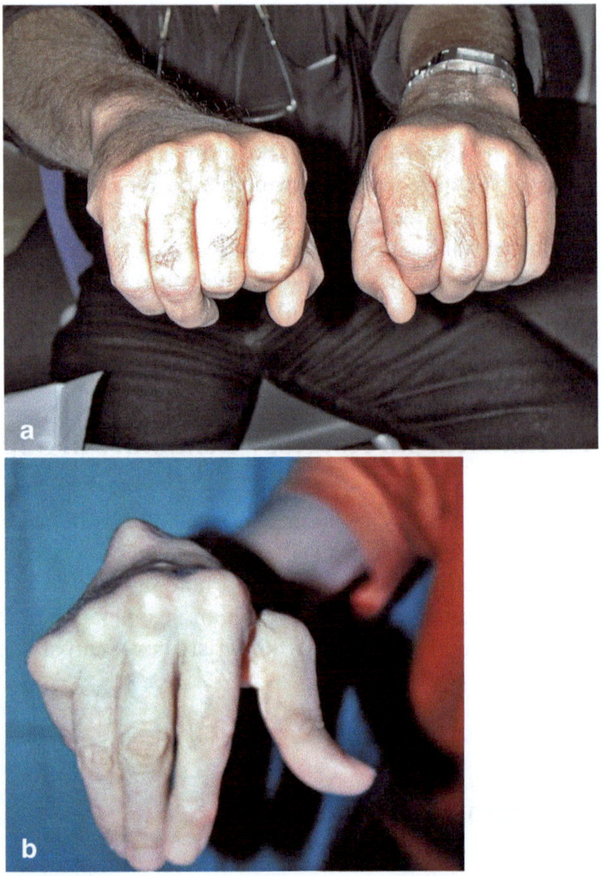

Fig. 3 (**a**) Carpal supination is difficult to observe in case of isolated rupture of the dorsal radiotriquetral ligament. This patient presents with a mild carpal supination of the right wrist following radiotriquetral ligament rupture. (**b**) The carpal supination deformity is apparent in rheumatoid affection or when rupture of ulnocarpal ligaments is associated. Palmar dislocation of the radius with respect to the ulna exacerbates the supination deformity of the carpus

The series includes four men with wrist trauma after a fall. In three cases, the fall was backwards with torsion and supination of the carpus in one case. All cases had posttraumatic oedema. Three patients had radiograms and immobilization, two in a plaster for 3 weeks and one in resin for 1 month. One patient had ignored his initial trauma.

The four patients presented with ulnar wrist pain and acute tenderness on the posterior triquetrum. The radiometacarpal rotation test was positive with pain which increased on carpal supination. In three cases, there was increased radiocarpal rotation in supination compared to the contralateral side. In one case the test was equivocal but the pain sharp. There was no lunotriquetral instability clinically. The radiolunate joint was free with complete pronosupination of the wrist, and normal ROM in other planes with tenderness at extremes of range of motion being the reason for consultation. Patients also complained of a loss of grip strength, measured at 65 % of the contralateral side.

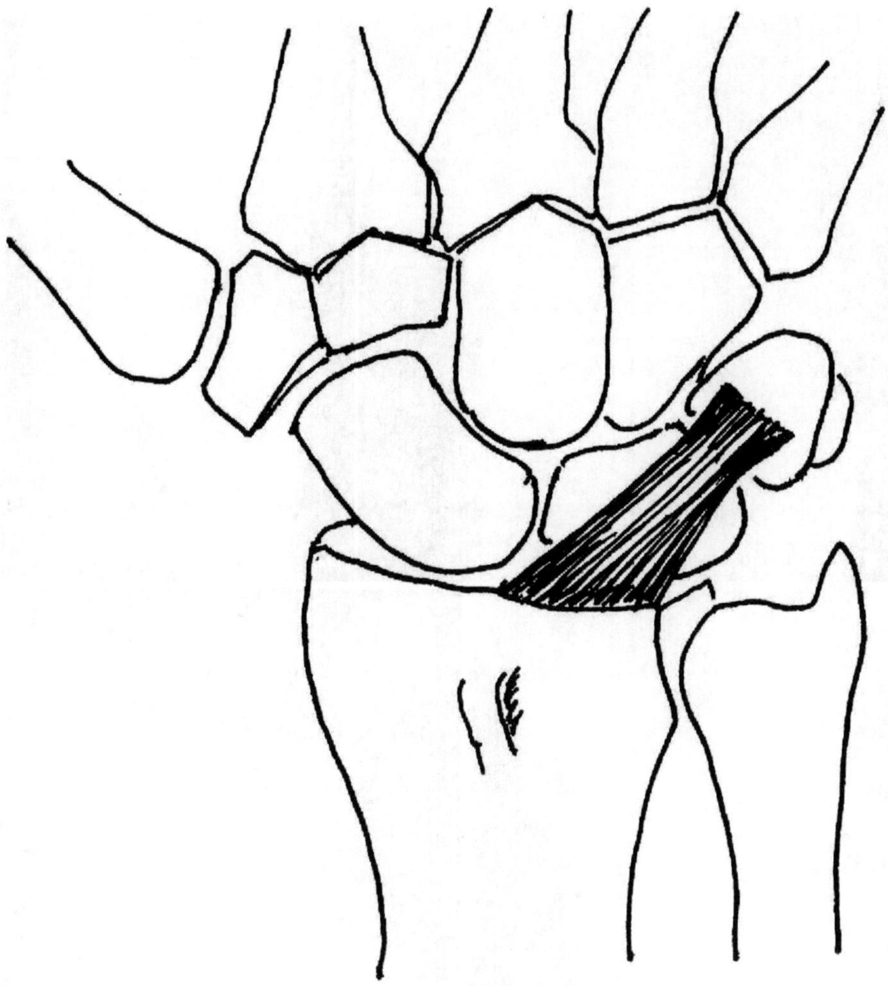

Fig. 4 Dorsal radiotriquetral ligament resists carpal supination. According to Viegas, the radiotriquetral fibres are constant, and in 99 % of cases some fibres terminate on the lunate

In three cases, x-rays showed dorsal avulsion of the ligament off the triquetrum (Fig. 5). There was no ulnar drift of the carpus. The dynamic views showed no disruption of the Gilula lines.

Arthrogram was done in all cases; in two cases there was lunotriquetral incompetence, TFCC was intact in all cases. In one case, a scapholunate ligament lesion without diastasis was found.

Scintigraphy was done in two cases showing isolated ulnar fixation.

Patients were operated at 12–30 months from the initial trauma.

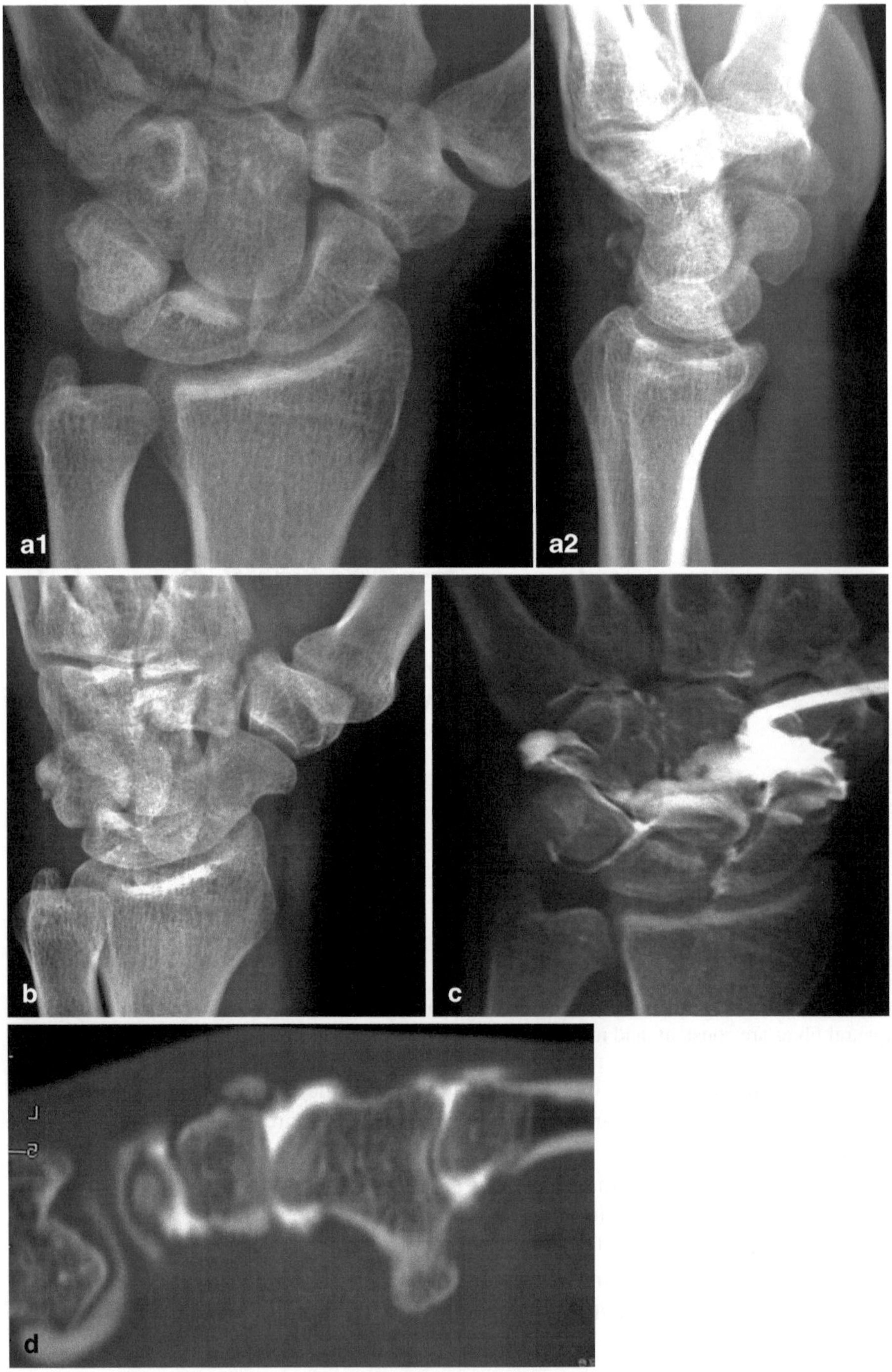

Fig. 5 (**a1, a2**) A 32-year-old patient presents with dorsal avulsion of the triquetrum on x-ray where the fragment is seen on the lateral view. (**b**) The oblique view shows the dorsal surface of the triquetrum. (**c**) Arthrogram shows a leak through the lunotriquetral ligament. (**d**) Sagittal cut through the triquetrum of the arthrogram shows the avulsed dorsal fragment

7 Operative Technique

7.1 Reconstruction of the Radiotriquetral Ligament

The operation is performed under general anaesthesia with a tourniquet at the upper arm through a dorsal longitudinal incision in the axis of the third ray medial to the tubercle of Lister. The dorsal extensor retinaculum is identified and the tubercle located. A flap of retinaculum is drawn 6–8 mm wide parallel to its fibres (Fig. 6a). This flap needs to be long enough to reach the dorsal surface of the triquetrum. The retinaculum is incised parallel to its fibres taking care of the extensor tendons beneath (Fig. 6b). Once the flap is harvested, the retinaculum is then opened longitudinally and distally. We identify the dorsal radiocarpal interval and identify the radiotriquetral ligament. In four cases, we found substantial fibrosis and the ligament was difficult to isolate. In three cases, a bony fragment was found on the dorsal

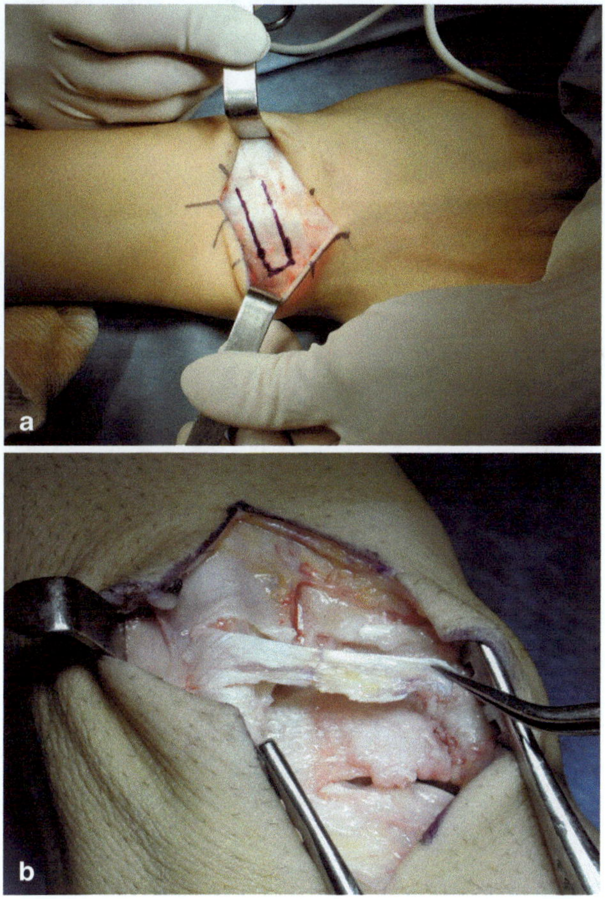

Fig. 6 Operative technique for radiotriquetral ligament reconstruction: (**a**) Right wrist: plane of the extensor retinaculum after longitudinal incision in the axis of the third ray. (**b**) Left wrist: harvesting the retinacular flap; its insertion on the tubercle of Lister is preserved. (**c**) Left wrist: removal of a fragment of the avulsed triquetrum and reaming the radiotriquetral ligament insertion zone. (**d**) Left wrist: fixation of the ligamentoplasty, the carpus is placed in pronation over the radius. (**e**) Left wrist: the extensors resume their position onto the ligamentoplasty. (**f**) Postoperative immobilization using a malleable splint holding the carpus in pronation to the radius

Fig. 6 (continued)

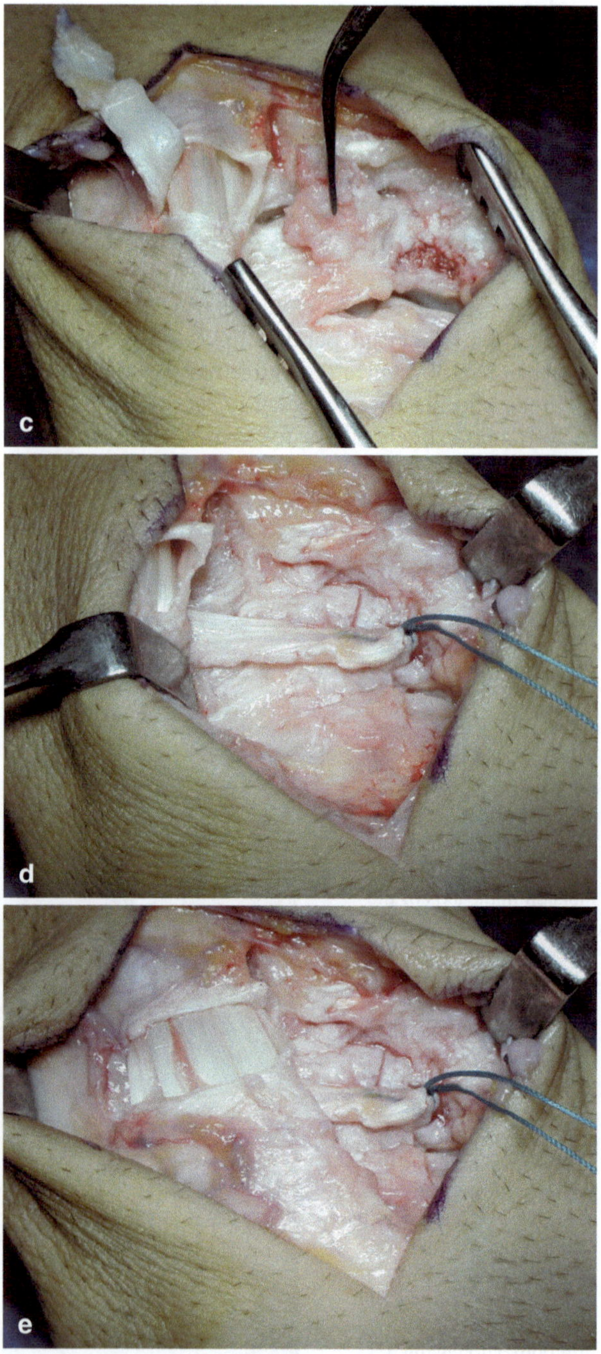

Fig. 6 (continued)

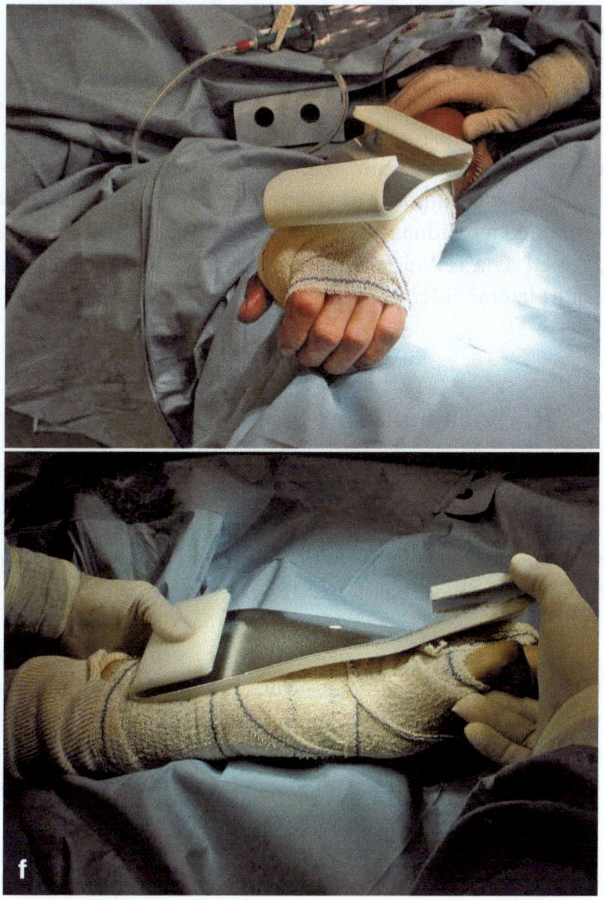

aspect of the triquetrum in the midst of fibrous tissue with difficulty to identify the ligament fibres (Fig. 6c). The ulnocarpal interval was explored and partial minute insignificant lesions of the lunotriquetral ligament were found in three cases without instability. Nothing was done for the lunotriquetral. In one case we sutured the scapholunate ligament which was partially ruptured.

The dorsal aspect of the triquetrum is reamed at the ligament insertion. The retinacular flap is passed under the extensor tendons; its tension is adjusted and fixed onto the dorsal triquetrum using an anchor with the carpus held in maximum pronation to the forearm (Fig. 6d, e). The dorsal retinaculum is resutured so as to re-establish the extensor gliding plane and the continuity of the ligament curtain that resists the carpal supination. A drain is inserted. The hand and forearm are immobilized on a malleable splint maintaining the carpus pronated with respect to the radius (Fig. 6f). At 48 h postoperative, the drain is removed and a resin splint is used to keep the carpal pronation. This splint is renewed at suture removal at 15–20 days and is kept for a total of 45 days.

8 Results

The four patients were reviewed with a final follow-up of at least 1 year. Pain was improved in all four patients. One patient suffered from pain on strength grip, the other three had no pain.

Pronosupination was complete, and extension recovered. In all cases there remained a residual flexion deficit of about 20 % compared to the contralateral side as well as a radial inclination. An increase of force was recorded at 90 % of the contralateral side.

9 Radiocarpal Rotatory Instability in Pronation

The radiocarpal rotatory instability in pronation is defined as the increase in carpal rotation on the distal radius in pronation compared to the contralateral side. Testing is done symmetrically, with one hand maintaining the forearm in midpronation while the other hand exerts a longitudinal rotation at the carpal condyle in pronation.

This clinical test is systematic for us in traumatic wrist examination. We did not find a frank asymmetry of rotation as in the test in supination. This test is positive if painful. Pain is felt on the palmar and radial aspects of the wrist; direct pressure on the wrist between flexor carpi radialis and abductor pollicis longus reproduces this pain. We attribute this pain to a radioscaphocapitate sprain or a scaphoid fracture.

We exclude scaphoid rotatory instability in the setting of scapholunate dissociation. In case of scapholunate dissociation, scaphoid instability occurs in pronation but it involves the scaphoid and not the carpal condyle. This is associated with dissociative intracarpal instability: scapholunate instability.

Radioscaphoid ligamentoplasty as described by Blatt aims to correct the rotator instability between the radius and the scaphoid. Some clinical results are good despite an absent scapholunate ligament. These observations related to our analysis of radiocarpal instability lead us to question: Can dissociative scapholunate instability be secondary to a primary lesion of the radioscaphocapitate ligament?

10 Discussion

Radiocarpal rotatory stability is necessary to transmit pronosupination from the forearm to the hand [6]. The role of the wrist ligaments in the transverse plane is seldom studied. It is in this plane that pronosupination is exerted.

For over a century, radiography has led us to analyse the stability of the carpus in the frontal and sagittal planes while masking the transverse plane.

The advent of CT and MRI that offered a view of the transverse plane in multiple cuts was very conducive to the study of instability, and the 3-D reconstructions facilitate the interpretation of the relative position of the bones.

For the study of instability of ligamentous origin, the available imaging today remains inadequate. The visualization of the interosseous ligaments is good but that of the capsular ligaments is still mediocre. Arthroscopy shows the wrist ligaments directly, and visualization of the radiocarpal capsular ligaments that can be put under tension by pronosupination emphasizes the importance of the transverse plane in carpal stabilization.

Slutsky [11, 12] studied the dorsal radiotriquetral ligament arthroscopically using a palmar radiocarpal portal. This work showed the frequency of lesions of this ligament. Unfortunately, the test of passive carpal supination to detect radiotriquetral ligament lesions did not correlate with the findings of Slutsky. This work showed the frequent association of this lesion with other ligament lesions: scapholunate, lunotriquetral or TFCC. No association of triquetral fracture seems to have been found.

Three of the four patients operated presented with avulsion of the dorsal fragment of the triquetrum. Arthroscopy was not done for these patients. It would have shown the bony fragments found on operation on the distal part of the ligament. We think the lesions we describe are different from those intraligamentous ones reported by Slutsky. Ours were primary lesions of the radiotriquetral ligament; isolated or associated with nonsignificant lesions of the interosseous ligaments. In one case we sutured the scapholunate interosseous ligament.

On the other hand, lesions identified by Slutsky are frequently associated with interosseous ligament lesions. They could be secondary ligament lesions as their diagnosis was very remote from the initial trauma. They could be microtraumatic due to excessive use in case of rupture of the interosseous ligaments. These findings lead us to think that capsular ligament lesions activated by the rotatory pronosupination force are often the site of 'adaptative' secondary lesions. This is what we define as secondary or 'adaptative' rotatory instability. With this instability, the fine radiotriquetral ligament is vulnerable, which may explain the frequent lesions found by Slutsky.

This secondary rotatory instability is probably the cause of the difficulties encountered in the treatment of interosseous ligament injuries – a theory that correlates well with the known evolution pattern of the scapholunate ligament injury. In an initially isolated SL ligament injury, the so-called secondary stabilizers will progressively be affected [13]. At surgery, all the ligaments should be repaired if possible [14].

We think that most primary ligament lesions are acute result of trauma in extension mainly, less frequently in flexion, and the secondary chronic ligament lesions are the result of repeated pronosupination against resistance.

When the wrist is relaxed, pronosupination force induces radiocarpal rotation which places the radiocarpal ligaments under tension. If the force increases, rupture will occur which will, in turn, increase the radiocarpal rotation [15].

Rarely, torsion can induce carpal rotation on the radius and cause acute lesions such as the avulsion of the triquetral insertion of the dorsal radiotriquetral ligament.

The exact mechanism of these fractures is debated between the advocates of avulsion and those of triquetrum impaction against the ulnar styloid [16]. Practically, both mechanisms are probably involved. The four radiotriquetral avulsion patients treated were asked about the trauma. Only one reported torsion with carpal supination, while the other three reported a fall backwards with impaction of the hypothenar eminence in extension. In this case the forearm is pushed behind and the carpal supination may be secondary to forearm pronation; ulnar styloid impaction onto the triquetrum is also possible.

Carpal supination is marked in rheumatoid deformity and palmar ulnocarpal lesions are most probably associated with a radiotriquetral ligament lesion [7].

This idea is reinforced by the distal radioulnar instability and palmar subluxation of the radius. In rheumatoid polyarthritis, rotatory instability in rotation is associated with ulnar drift of the carpus. This drift was never found in our patients. In rheumatoid, the deformity is often treated by tendon transfers of ECRL on to ECU which reproduces the course of the radiotriquetral ligament. In more advanced affection, partial arthrodesis (radiolunate or radioscapholunate) is done for stabilization, to correct supination and ulnar shift of the carpus.

11 Conclusion

Radiocarpal rotatory instability has to draw our attention on the transverse plane, plane of pronosupination, plane where imaging is still deficient.

Only an accurate account of the ligament lesions can provide basis for efficient ligament reconstruction. We thus think that acute posttraumatic ligament lesions are complicated by secondary 'adaptative' lesions that need to be diagnosed and treated.

References

1. Cyriax EF (1917) On the rotatory movements of the wrist. J Anat 51:396–399
2. Gagey O (1980) Contribution à l'étude de la biomécanique du carpe: mécanique statique des tendons moteurs du carpe. Thesis, Montpellier
3. Kapandji IA (1991) Etude du carpe au scanner à trois dimensions sous contraintes de pronosupination. Ann Chir Main 10:36–47
4. Roux JL (1992) La rotation longitudinale radio-métacarpienne. Thesis, Montpellier
5. Roux JL, Micallef JP, Rabischong P, Allieu Y (1997) La rotation Longitudinale Radio-Métacarpienne. La Main 2:169–179
6. Roux JL, Micallef JP, Rabischong P, Allieu Y (1996) Etude de la transmission des mouvements de pronosupination au niveau du poignet. Ann Chir Main 15(3):167–180
7. Ritt MJPF, Stuart PR, Berglund LJ, Linscheid RL, Cooney WP, An KN (1995) Rotational stability of the carpus relative to the forearm. J Hand Surg 20A:305–311
8. Ritt MJPF, Stuart PR, Berglund LJ, Linscheid RL, Cooney WP, An KN (1996) Rotational laxity and stiffness of the radiocarpal joint. Clin Biomech 11(4):227–232

9. Roux JL, Allieu Y (1996) Immobilisation du poignet: un positionnement vicieux insoupçonné. J Trauma Sport 13:50–62
10. Viegas SF, Yamaguchi S, Boyd NL, Patterson RM (1999) The dorsal ligaments of the wrist: anatomy, mechanical properties and function. J Hand Surg 24A:456–468
11. Slutsky DJ (2005) Arthroscopic dorsal radiocarpal ligament repair. Arthroscopy 21:1486
12. Slutsky DJ (2008) Incidence of dorsal radiocarpal ligament tears in the presence of other intercarpal derangements. Arthroscopy 24:526–533
13. Short WH, Werner FW, Green JK, Sutton LG, Brutus JP (2007) Biomechanical evaluation of the ligamentous stabilizers of the scaphoid and lunate: part III. J Hand Surg 32A:297–309
14. Garcia Elias M, Lluch AL, Stanley JK (2006) Three-ligament tenodesis for the treatment of scapholunate dissociation: indications and surgical technique. J Hand Surg 31A:125–134
15. Roux JL, Micallef JP, Allieu Y (2000) Biomechanical considerations for wrist arthroplasty. In: Simmen BR, Allieu Y, Lluch A, Stanley J (eds) Hand arthroplasties. Martin Dunitz, London, pp 183–191
16. Garcia Elias M (1987) Dorsal fractures of the triquetrum: avulsion or compression fractures. J Hand Surg 12A:266–268

Vertical Instability of the Carpus – Axial Dislocation and Fracture-Dislocation: Review of the Literature

J. Vogels, A.-P. Uzel, and O. Delattre

1 Definition, Epidemiology, Classification

Carpal axial dislocation with preservation of the radio-luno-capitate axis on a lateral view is extremely rare.

According to Herzberg [1], it is a combination of dislocation of the second carpal row and the second carpometacarpal joint (the intermetacarpal space).

Since Oberst [2] in 1901, about 70 cases have been reported in the literature. The largest series was reported by Garcia-Elias et al. [3] from the Mayo clinic and was conducted over 16 years as a retrospective analysis of nearing on 1,140 carpal trauma and fracture cases, among which 16 cases (1.4 %) were diagnosed as axial dislocation (Fig. 1).

Garcia-Elias et al. [3] describes three types of axial dislocation according to the affected column:

- Radial axial (RA) (Fig. 2) with instability and proximal radial displacement of the radial column (first and second metacarpals, trapezium, trapezoid, scaphoid), while the ulnar column maintains stable relations with radius and ulna.
- Ulnar axial (UA) (Fig. 3) where the ulnar column (fourth and fifth metacarpals, hamate, triquetrum) is displaced proximal and ulnar, while the radial column maintains stable relations with the radius and ulna.

J. Vogels (✉) • O. Delattre
Hand Surgery Unit and Hands Emergency Care Unit,
CHU et SOS mains de Fort-de-France,
BP 632, Fort-de-France Martinique 97200, France
e-mail: jerome.vogels@gmail.com; olivier.delattre@chu-fortdefrance.fr

A.-P. Uzel
MCU-PH Chirurgie, Orthopédique, CHU,
Guadeloupe, France

E. Camus, L. Van Overstraeten (eds.), *Carpal Ligament Surgery*,
DOI 10.1007/978-2-8178-0379-1_16, © Springer-Verlag France 2013

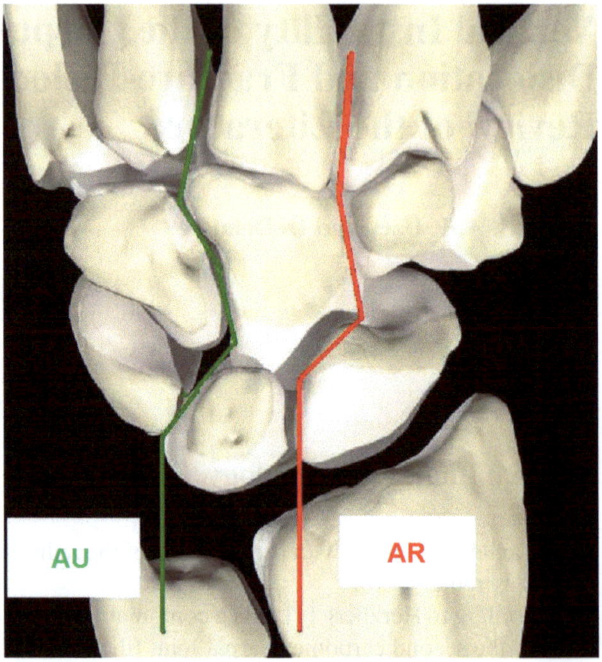

Fig. 1 Radial and ulnar columns with axial dislocation lines. *AU* axial ulnar, *AR* axial radial

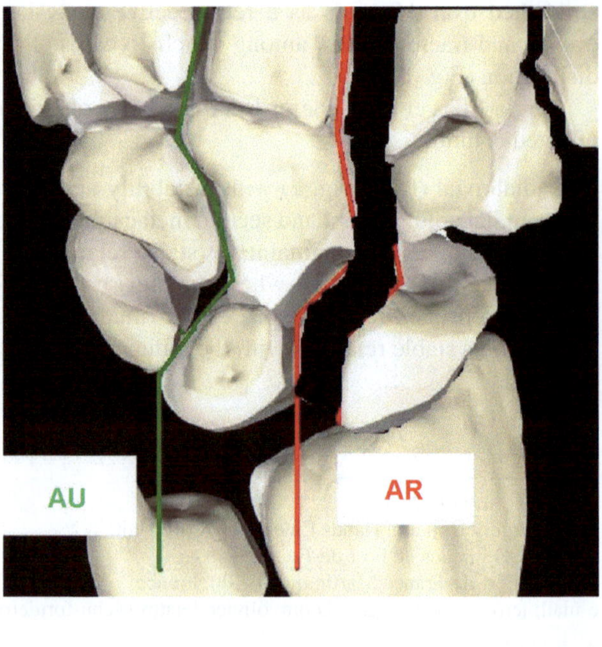

Fig. 2 Radial axial dissociation: *AU* axial ulnar, *AR* axial radial

Fig. 3 Ulnar axial dissociation. *AU* axial ulnar, *AR* axial radial

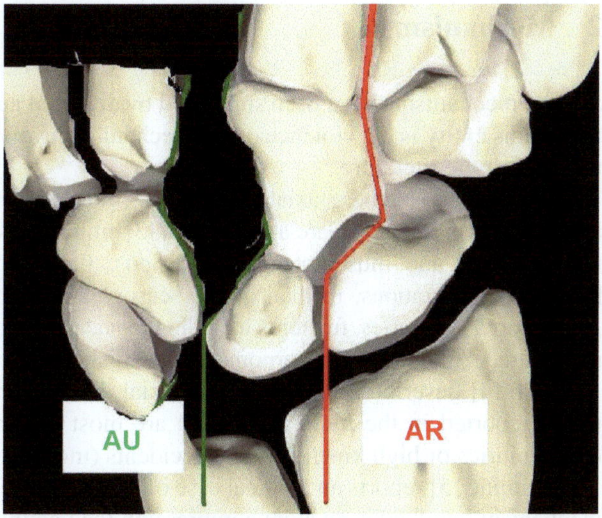

Fig. 4 Radioulnar axial dissociation. *AU* axial ulnar, *AR* axial radial

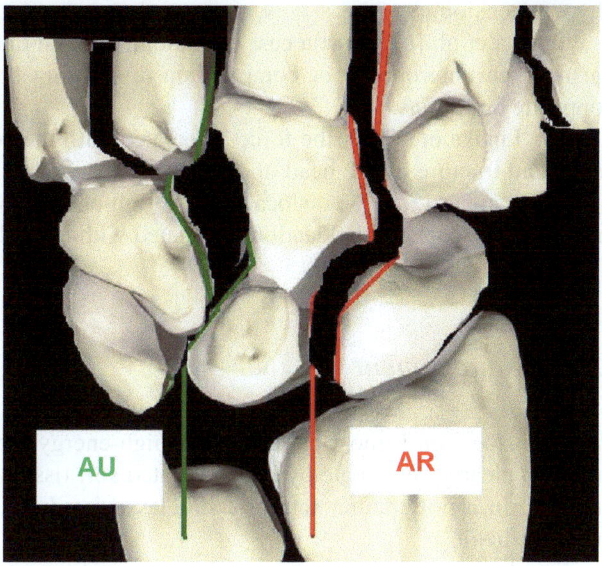

- Radioulnar axial (Fig. 4) with instability and displacement of both columns parting in opposite directions. Here, the third column (third metacarpal, lunate, capitate) is stable onto the radius and ulna, while the two other columns are displaced.

Garcia-Elias describes subgroups for the forms RA and UA:

- For RA, three subgroups: peritrapezial/peritrapezoid, peritrapezial, transtrapezial
- For UA, three subgroups: trans-hamatal/peri-pisiform, peri-hamatal/peri-pisiform, peri-hamatal/trans-triquetral

2 Mechanism

Several mechanisms have been suggested by different authors, but the common factor for this entity is the violence of the mechanism involved which has been reported throughout the literature.

According to Herzberg, axial dislocation is most often associated with blast injuries and open crush injuries. Garcia-Elias et al. [3] emphasizes the frequency of associated neurovascular and musculotendinous lesions: flexor/extensor injuries, thenar and hypothenar lacerations, median nerve, sensory and motor branches of ulnar nerve lesions, arterial injuries, fractures including metacarpal, hook of hamate, fracture avulsion of trapezium, pisiform, carpometacarpal dislocations and digital amputations.

Tabib [4] describes a case of radial axial dislocation and describes the mechanisms reported in the literature. These are most commonly manual work-related crush injuries or high kinetic energy accidents (motorcycle).

Yammine [5] reports an atypical case of scapholunate axial dislocation where the mechanism involved is an axial compression load acting as a major vector surpassing other associated forces in a longitudinal axis of the wrist associated with hyperextension.

Tanaka et al. [6] report a case of radioulnar axial dislocation where the mechanism is an anteroposterior compression dislocating both columns which part in opposite directions.

For Tanaka et al. [6], the force associated with the compression may result in a scaphoid fracture by the head of capitate.

The scaphoid may be dislocated by a high-energy force; Horton [7] describes a rare case of scaphoid dislocation associated with axial disjunction.

2.1 Management

Axial dislocation is most often due to a high-energy mechanism. When isolated, it is often clearly detectable by the associated soft tissue damage and clinical deformation. In a polytrauma setting and/or associated lesions, the diagnosis may be more difficult.

Standard x-rays remain key to diagnosis. The posteroanterior view shows the radial, ulnar ulnoradial inclination of the displacement, while the lateral view shows the radio-lunato-capito-3rd metacarpal axis and indicates the palmar or dorsal displacement of the affected columns.

Management is in emergency; however, an immediate diagnosis may be difficult due to the complexity of interpretation of PA and lateral views, and certain authors propose further investigations.

In a series of eight patients, Inoue and Miura [8] reports eight delayed diagnoses: 2 weeks in five patients and over 1 month in three patients. The worst outcomes are correlated with delayed diagnosis. In radiological abnormality associated with clinical functional deficit or oedema, the diagnosis may require a CT scan which should not – nevertheless – delay management.

MRI may be useful but unavailable. It is of special interest in the diagnosis of ligament lesions and incomplete fractures. Horton [7] describes the use of MRI away from the trauma to diagnose ligamentous palmar, dorsal, intrinsic and extrinsic lesions. These lesions are confirmed by radiocarpal and midcarpal arthroscopy and unravel scapholunate and capitohamatal instability.

2.2 *Treatment and Results*

The mechanism is often high-energy trauma, with skin laceration and severely displaced fractures. The associated ligamentous lesions are usually severe, causing great instability. Management is often surgical by closed reduction and fixation. A palmar or dorsal approach is recommended with reduction and pinning or screw fixation [9]. Some authors [3, 10] report closed reduction and immobilization in a cast. There is no evidence in the literature to favour surgical approach and fixation over closed fixation.

The mean immobilization is 4–6 weeks.

Functional prognosis is correlated to the severity of the initial trauma as well as associated neurovascular and other lesions. Good results reported in the literature are only around 60 %.

References

1. Herzberg G (2008) Perilunate and axial carpal dislocations and fracture – dislocations. J Hand Surg 33A:1659–1668
2. Oberst M (1901) Fracturen und luxationen der finger und des carpus, die fracturen des metacarpus und der vorderarmknochen. Forstchr Geb Roentg 5(suppl):1–21
3. Garcia-Elias M, Dobyns JH, Cooney WP, Linscheid RL (1989) Traumatic axial dislocations of the carpus. J Hand Surg 14A:446–457
4. Tabib W, Banallec L, Banallec Y, Lamelin JC (2001) Traumatic axial separation of the radial midcarpal joint. Case report and review of the literature. Chir Main 20(5):391–396
5. Yammine K (2000) Luxation axiale du carpe interscapholunaire. Rev Chir Orthop 86:193–196
6. Tanaka Y, Ohshige T, Hanakawa S (2002) Traumatic axial dislocation of the carpus: a case report of transscaphoid pericapitate transhamate axial dislocation. J Orthop Sci 7:414–416
7. Horton T (2004) Isolated scaphoid dislocation associated with axial carpal dissociation: an unusual injury report. J Hand Surg 29A:1102–1108
8. Inoue G, Miura T (1991) Traumatic axial-ulnar disruption of the carpus. Orthop Rev 20:867–872
9. Freeland AE, Rojas SL (2001) Traumatic combined radial and ulnar axial wrist dislocation. Orthopedics 24:1161–1163
10. Irwin LR, Paul R, Kumaren R, Bagga TK (1995) Complex carpal dislocation. J Hand Surg 20B(6):746–749

Arthroscopic Debridement Pinning: Management of Recent and Unstable Perilunate Injuries

L. Van Overstraeten

1 Introduction

When a scapholunate or triquetrolunate injury is stabilized within 6 weeks from the date of the trauma, its midterm or long-term outcome is usually favourable. Indeed, the use of wires to stabilize the joint in anatomic reduction for a period from 6 to 8 weeks slows down or prevents adaptive collapse [1, 3, 4, 5].

In 1980, Green and O'Brien were the first to insist on rapid treatment of these traumas, which they described as being acute scapholunate instability without perilunate dislocation [2].

As already mentioned, the establishment of a diagnosis of interosseous instability is a 'race against time'.

2 Surgical Indications

For medicolegal reasons, it is our practice that an arthroscopy will always be indicated by an arthro-CT abnormality. This means there will be a small group of false negatives that will be neither identified nor stabilized—those presenting a ligamentary instability but without any arthro-CT abnormality.

Even if the number of patients with an unknown unstable wrist is significant, we are determined not to advise arthroscopy on clinical signs only [6]. Indeed, sooner or later, a 'borderline' stabilization (for instance, in stage 0 of scapholunate injury [9], associated with a type 2 laxity of the radio-scapho-capitate (Chap. 9)) risks

L. Van Overstraeten
Hand and Foot Surgery Unit SPRL,
Rue Pierre Caille N° 9, Tournai B-7500, Belgium
e-mail: l.v.o@skynet.be

E. Camus, L. Van Overstraeten (eds.), *Carpal Ligament Surgery*,
DOI 10.1007/978-2-8178-0379-1_17, © Springer-Verlag France 2013

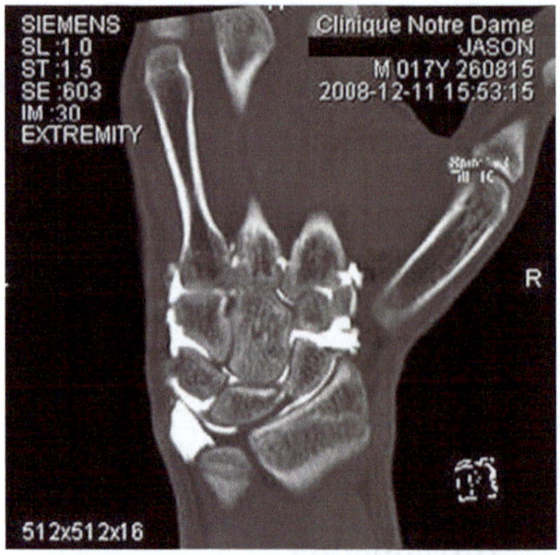

Fig. 1 Arthroscanner at the 15th post-traumatic day: triquetrolunate leak

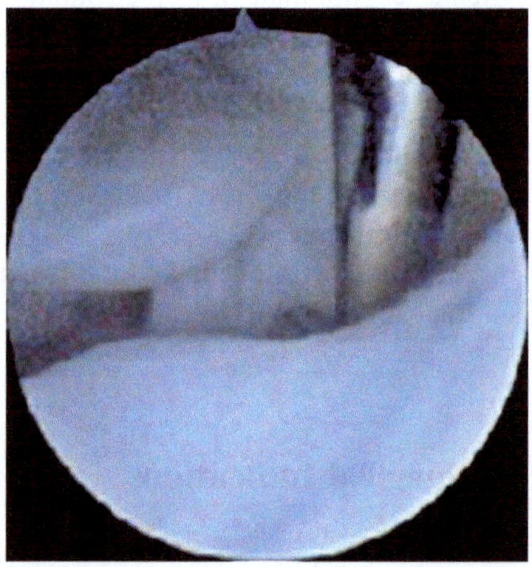

Fig. 2 Arthroscopy at the 20th post-traumatic day: midcarpal compartment—spontaneously opened interval, easy widening with the hook, hypermobility of the triquetrum (Dautel 2)

being criticized or rejected by the insurer (NIHDI—National Institute for Health and Disability Insurance, insurance law, third-party insurance).

For the author, arthroscopic stabilization rests on the following conditions:

- Anamnesis: <6 post-traumatic weeks
- Doubtful clinical examination (SL or TL pain; Watson or TL ballottement; painful Reagan or [+])
- X-ray examinations (–) or (+): RL angle, SL angle, SL diastasis, arcs of Gilula
- Arthroscan (+) (Fig. 1–3)
- Criteria to date the trauma [7]
- Interosseous instability by Dautel (2–3) [9] (Fig. 2)
- Little or no interosseous instability according to Dautel (0–1) but laxity on one of the three extrinsic bolts (Chap. 9) [9]

3 Surgical Technique

This is a simple technique. The patient is under plexus anaesthesia and in dorsal decubitus with the upper limb in an abducted position, with traction from 8 to 10 kg and upper arm support. There is a pneumatic tourniquet at the extremity of the limb.

Arthroscopy is standard, 5–6 portals (1–2, 3–4, 4–5, (6U), RMC, UMC). The following information can be obtained:

- Turbidity of the synovial fluid (T0–T4) [7]
- Haematic synovitis (S0–S2) [7]
- Aspect of the cartilage (C0–C4)
- Laxity of the extrinsic ligaments (E0–E3) and analysis of the extrinsic bolts (Chap. 9)
- In radiocarpal: RSC, RL(T)L, RL(T)S, UTL, RCDorsal
- In midcarpal: distal scapho-capitate, STT, DIC
- SL and TL interosseous testing according to Dautel (0–3) (parallelism)

If the following conditions are completed, stabilization is made:

>T0 –>S0 –<C3
D123 (+E0) or D0123 (+>E0)

An optional shaving is made on the reinserted osseous edge. A small fissure can be ploughed with a burr. Stabilization is realized by Kirchner wire 12/10° under arthroscopic and fluoroscopic control. A correction of the DISI by joystick is possible.

Scapholunate instabilities are pinned in scapholunate and scaphocapitate.

Triquetrolunate instabilities are stabilized in triquetrolunate and triquetrohamate (Fig. 3).

The ends of the wires remain on the outside and are folded and fixed one to the other by Steri-Strips. This sterile fixing is very simple. It increases the stability of the mount as it turns it into a real osteotaxis. It significantly diminishes the risk of fracture and secondary infection of the K-wires. At first, there is no antibiotic prescription. An antebrachial plastered splint is made. Three days later, the state of the wrist is checked. The dressing is renewed after a disinfection by alcohol of the wires. Wrist swelling linked to arthroscopic drainage is always resorbed. A circular plaster cast is placed for a period of 6–8 weeks if there is no sign of an exceptional and local inflammation. A little cell is prepared using the base of a plastic cup to avoid any contact between the plaster cast and the K-wires. A radioclinical control is made 1 month later.

When the wires are removed during consultation, perilunate and midcarpal joints will be stiff. From 20 to 30 physiotherapy sessions are necessary. Manual workers can go back to work 4 months after the operation. The wrist gets a below normal suppleness back between the 12th and 18th month after operation.

Stabilizations which are made on only one lunate side have a quicker recovery time. (Triquetrolunate stabilizations are significantly faster.) It is possible to go back to work about 10 weeks after the operation. Physiotherapy is necessary 50 % of the time. The wrist is supple 6 months later.

These results confirm those reported in literature.

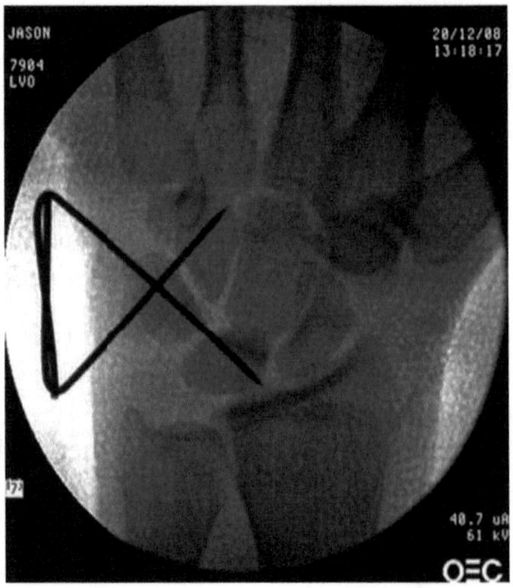

Fig. 3 Stabilization of a triquetrolunate instability by triquetrolunate and triquetrohamate pinning (Kirschner wire 12/10 exteriorized and fixed)

4 Conclusion

Pinning debridement is dedicated to acute or subacute scapholunate or triquetrolunate instabilities which are less than 6 weeks old and which come within the frame of Garcia-Elias stage 1 or 2 [8].

References

1. Chloros GD, Wiesler ER, Poehling GG (2008) Current concepts in wrist arthroscopy. Arthroscopy 24(3):343–354
2. Green DP, O'Brien ET (1980) Classification and management of carpal dislocations. Clin Orthop Relat Res (149):55–72
3. Geissler WB (2006) Arthroscopic management of scapholunate instability. Chir Main 25(Suppl 1):S187–S196
4. Kuo CE, Wolfe SW (2008) Scapholunate instability: current concepts in diagnosis and management. J Hand Surg Am 33(6):998–1013
5. Ruch DS, Siegel D, Chabon SJ, Koman LA, Poehling GG (1993) Arthroscopic categorization of intercarpal ligamentous injuries of the wrist. Orthopedics 16(9):1051–1056
6. Slutsky DJ, Nagle DJ (2008) Wrist arthroscopy: current concepts. J Hand Surg Am 33(7):1228–1244
7. Van Overtsraeten L, Camus EJ (2012) Arthroscopic criteria for dating wrist sprains. Chir Main 31:171–175
8. Garcia-Elias M, Liuch AL, Stanley JK (2006) Tree-ligament tenodesis for the treatment of scapholunate dissociation: indications and surgical technique. J Hand Surg 31A:125–134
9. Dreant N, Dautel G (2003) Development of a arthroscopic severity score for scapholunate instability. Chir Main 22(2):90–94

Technique of Open Scapholunate Ligament Repair

J. Garret

This technique is ideally used for recent scapholunate ligament rupture associated with arthroscopically irreducible malalignment (Figs. 1 and 2).

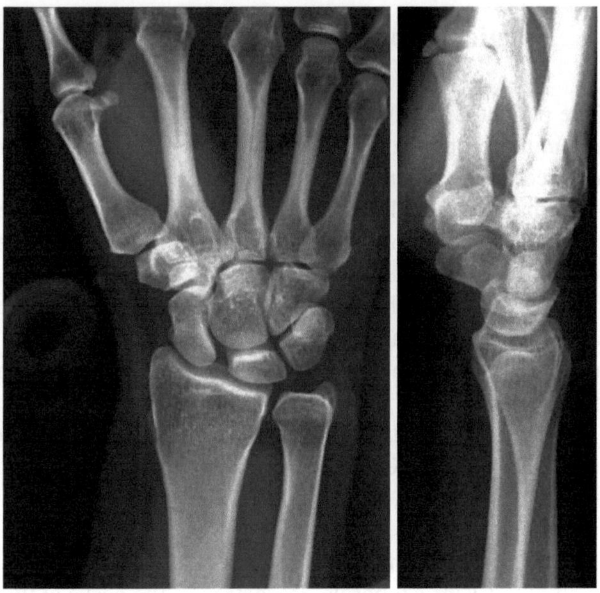

Fig. 1 Recent scapholunate ligament rupture with static malalignment, widened scapholunate gap, DISI of the lunate and palmar tilt of the scaphoid

J. Garret
Hand Surgery Unit, Clinique du Parc, 155 ter, bd de Stalingrad, Lyon 69006, France
e-mail: j.garret@cliniqueduparclyon.com

E. Camus, L. Van Overstraeten (eds.), *Carpal Ligament Surgery*, DOI 10.1007/978-2-8178-0379-1_18, © Springer-Verlag France 2013

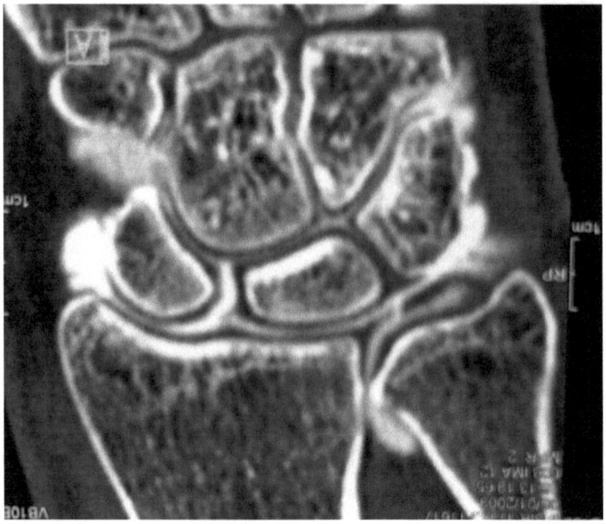

Fig. 2 Scapholunate ligament rupture with wide SL gap. Note the asymptomatic central degenerative TFCC lesion

1 Surgical Approach

The patient is supine with the upper limb on an arm table and an upper arm pneumatic tourniquet in place. The wrist is flexed and a dorsal longitudinal incision is centred on the tubercle of Lister (Photo 1).

Skin is dissected medially and laterally to expose the extensor retinaculum. The articular branches of the radial nerve are divided, thus performing a partial denervation of the carpus (Photo 2).

A ‘free’ flap is harvested from the proximal extensor retinaculum transversely along its entire breadth across the wrist – 3 cm × 0.5 cm. This will function as a ligament to strengthen the posterior portion of the scapholunate interval (Photo 3, Fig. 3).

This extensor retinaculum is divided between the third and fourth compartments; the intercompartmental septum between the first and second compartments is released. The EPL, ECRL and ECRB tendons are retracted radially and the EDC medially.

The posterior interosseous neurovascular bundle is identified subperiosteally, medial to Lister’s tubercle. Resection of the nerve at this point completes the carpal denervation. Lister’s tubercle is minimized using a rongeur (Photo 4, Fig. 4).

The posterior capsule and posterior scapholunate ligament are exposed. A posterior capsulotomy in extended Z shape is performed as described by G. Herzberg (Photo 5, Fig. 5).

Photo 1

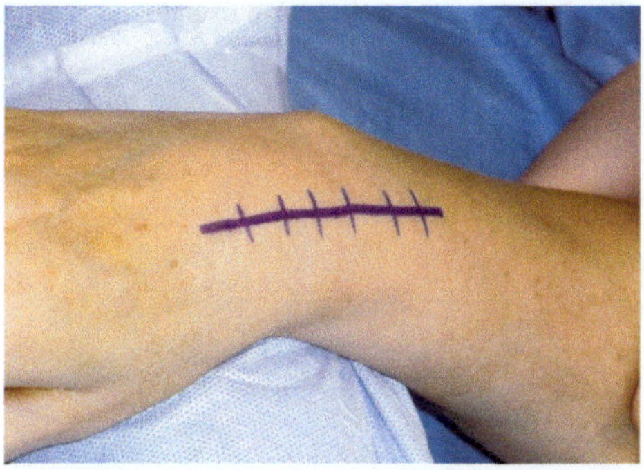

Photo 2

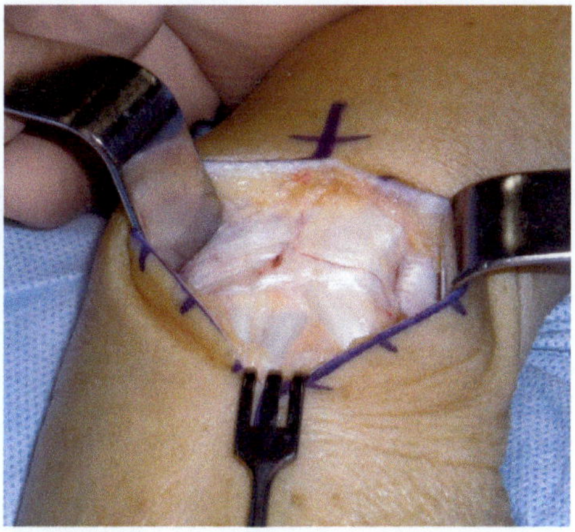

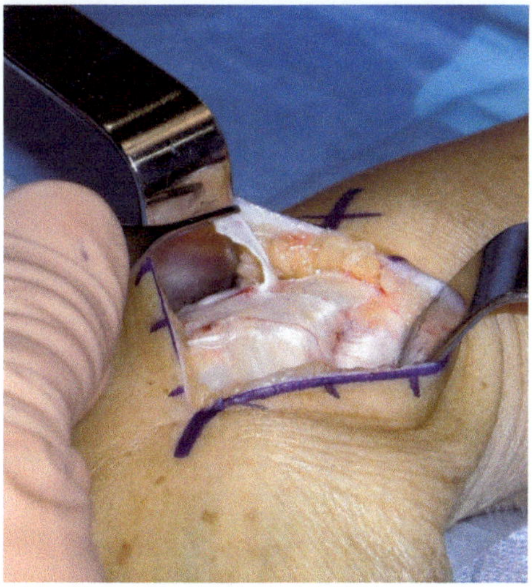

Photo 3

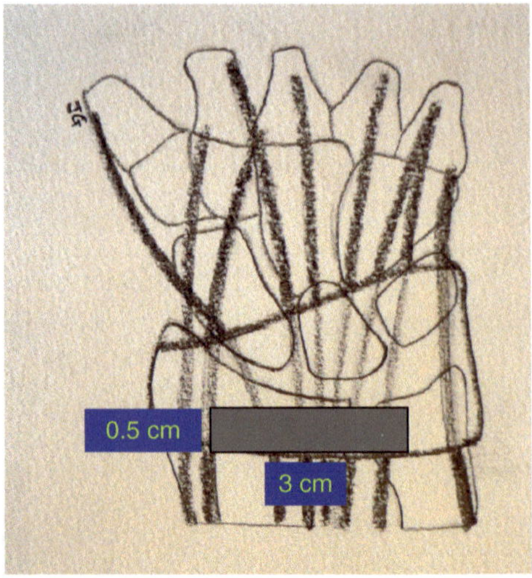

Fig. 3 Harvesting a 'free' flap from the extensor retinaculum

Photo 4

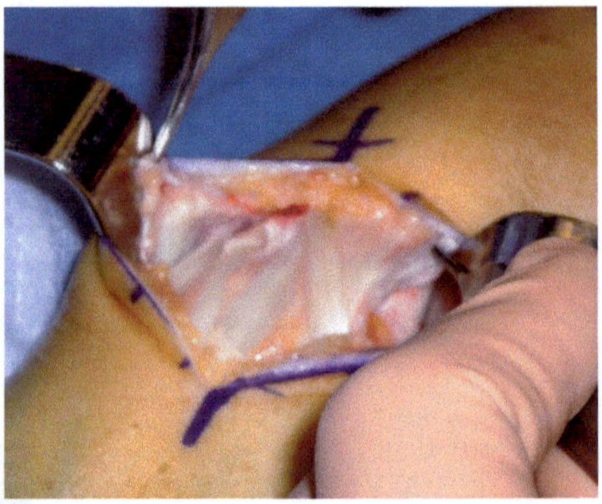

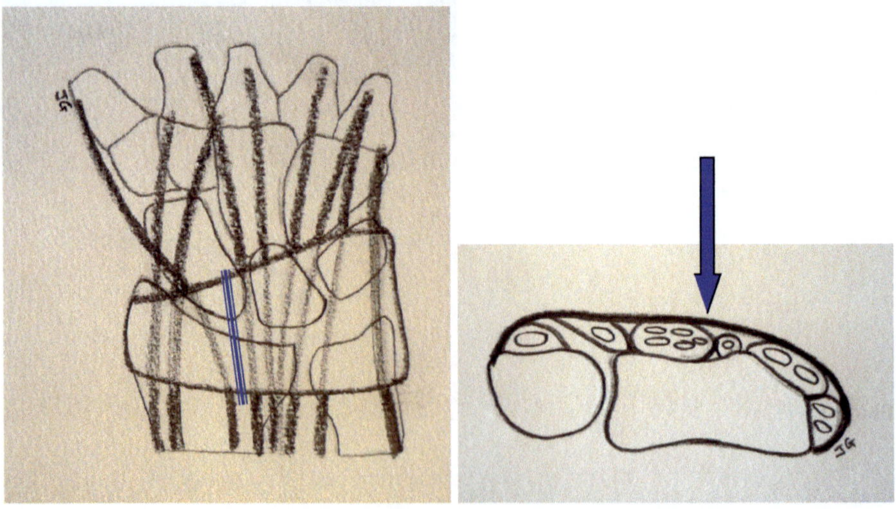

Fig. 4 Incision of the extensor retinaculum between third and fourth compartments (*arrow*)

Photo 5

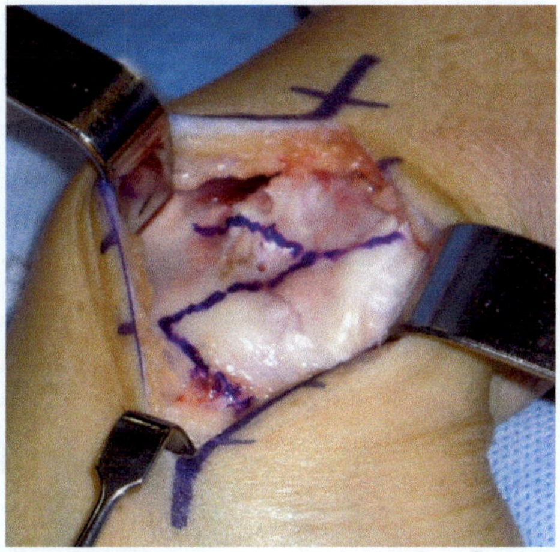

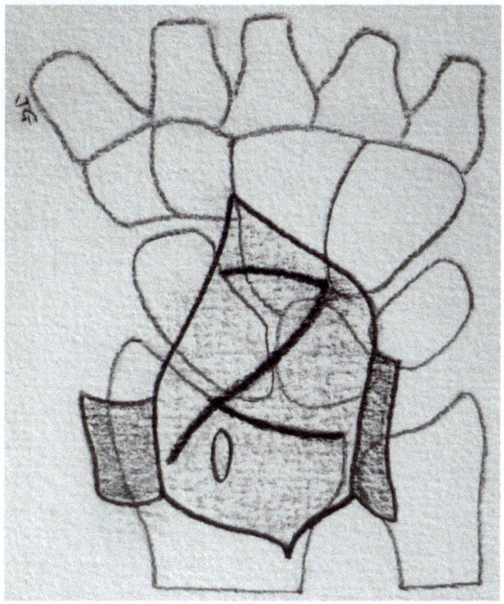

Fig. 5 Posterior capsulotomy in extended 'Z' as described by G. Herzberg

2 Suturing the Scapholunate Ligament

The scapholunate interval is thus exposed revealing scapholunate instability with an abnormal scapholunate gap, a horizontalized scaphoid with a tendency for dorsal subluxation and a dorsally tilted lunate (Photo 6).

A small curette is used to revive the insertion arc of the scapholunate ligament at the proximal scaphoid pole. Three transosseous tunnels are drilled using a 10/10 K-wire between dorsal waist and the freshened area proximally. Two U-shaped 3-0 PDS sutures are passed directly into the transosseous tunnels (Photo 7 and Fig. 6).

Photo 6

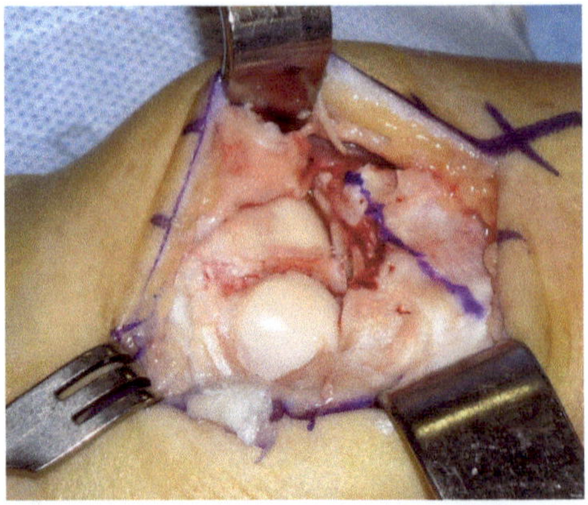

Photo 7

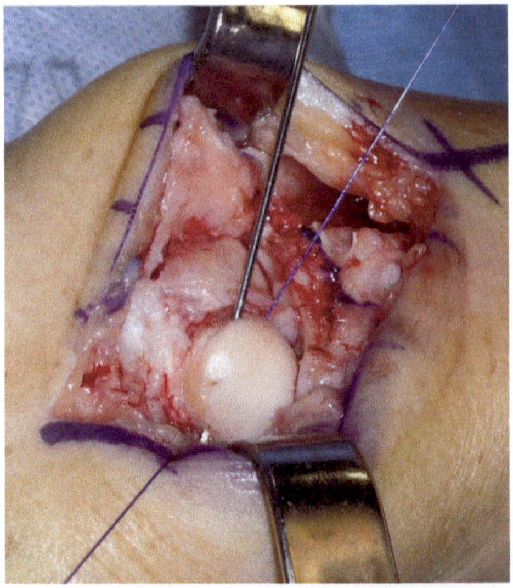

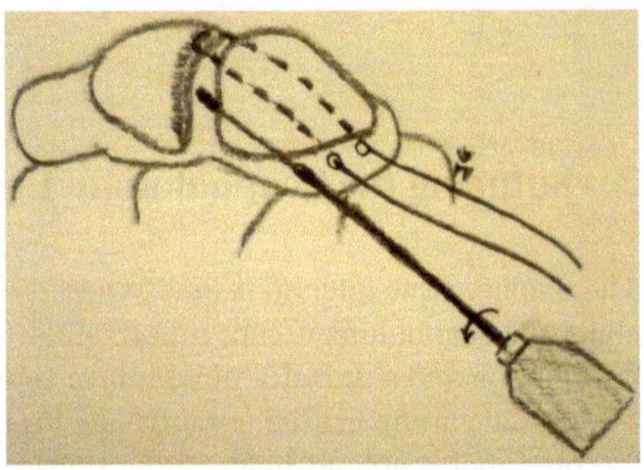

Fig. 6 The creation of three intraosseous tunnels through the scaphoid using 10/10 pins to pass the two 'U' sutures for scapholunate ligament reinsertion

The stage of realignment of the scapholunate complex then follows and is the most difficult part of the operation. The lunate tilt in dorsiflexion must be reduced; the scaphoid flexion must be corrected as well as the posterior subluxation of its proximal pole and reduction of the scapholunate gap. Once reduction is achieved, fixation is performed using two 12/10 scapholunate K-wires and two 12/10 scaphocapitate wires. These temporary intracarpal pins are removed at 6 weeks to allow for ligament healing.

The following tips may be useful to obtain a perfect scapholunate reduction:

- The use of 'joystick' K-wires to manipulate the scaphoid and the lunate.
- Reduction of the lunate dorsiflexion is performed in wrist flexion followed by scapholunate pinning (Linscheid manoeuvre).
- Use a towel clip style fracture holder (Backhauss).
- Pin position is verified by fluoroscan.

We bury our pins and use a cap on the sharp tip to minimize subcutaneous irritation postoperative. Care must be taken to avoid conflict with the EPL and the sensory branch of the radial nerve (Photo 8 and Figs. 6 and 7).

The two 'U' sutures for scapholunate ligament reinsertion may now be tied (Photo 9).

The retinacular flap is used to reconstruct posterior scapholunate ligament reinforcement. A small anchor is placed in the posterior horn of the lunate and another in the dorsal part of the proximal pole of the scaphoid. The transplant is fixed between these two anchors (Photos 10 and 11).

The direct repair of the scapholunate ligament can be complemented by a capsulodesis using a mini anchor on the posterior aspect of the scaphoid waist which is fixed to a radial capsular radiocarpal flap (Fig. 8).

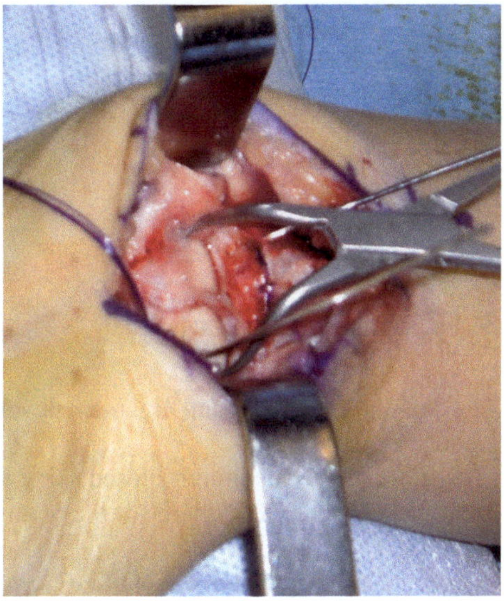

Photo 8

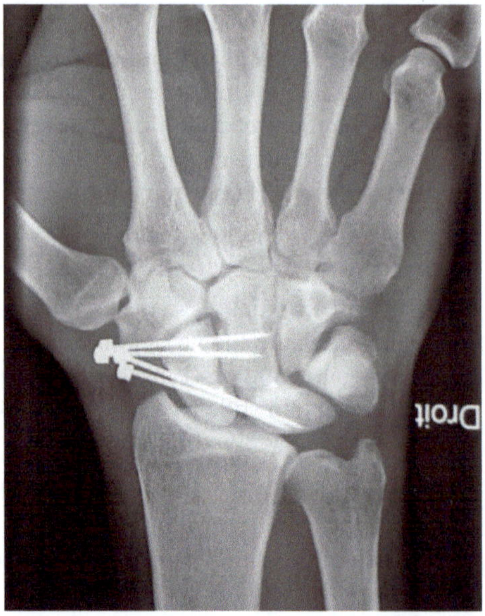

Fig. 7 K-wire fixation for temporarily scapho-lunar and scapho-capitate arthrodesis

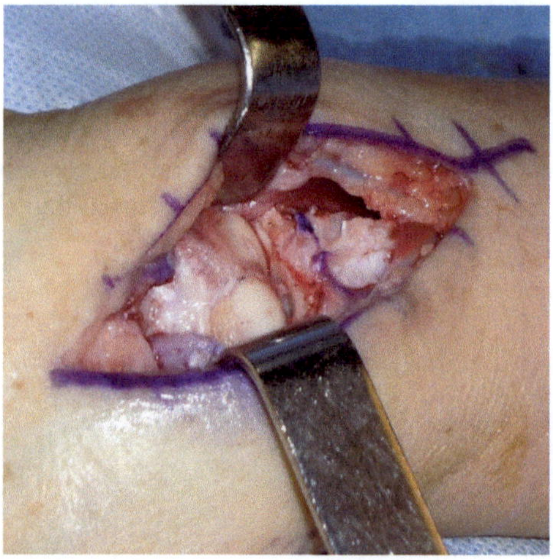

Photo 9

3 Closure in Layers

The posterior capsule and ligament layer are closed using interrupted PDS 4/0 sutures.

The dorsal retinaculum is closed using a double row 'to and fro' continuous PDS 4/0 as described by L. Erhard for the repair of pronator teres (Photos 12 and 13 and Fig. 9).

A hand-forearm volar slab is used for postoperative immobilization for 45 days.

Photo 10

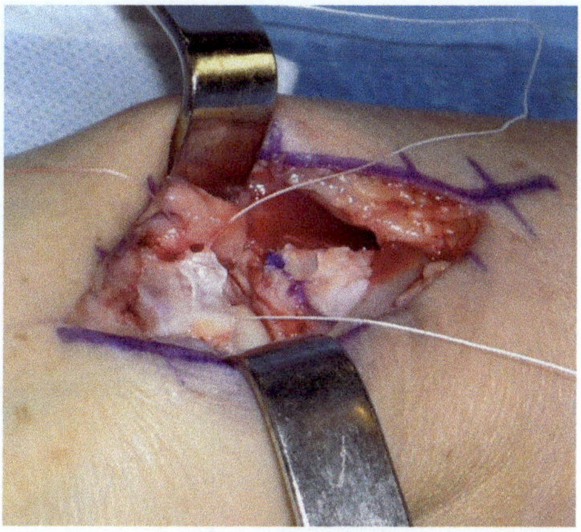

Photo 11

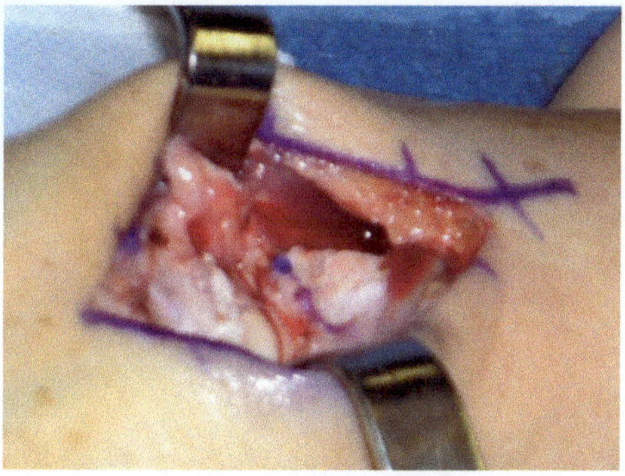

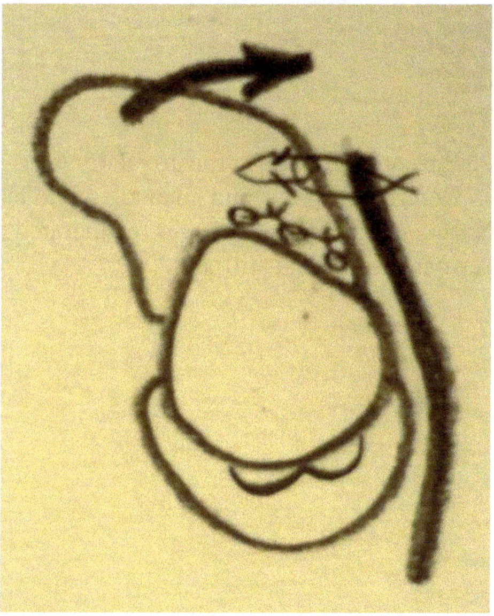

Fig. 8 Posterior capsulodesis

Photo 12

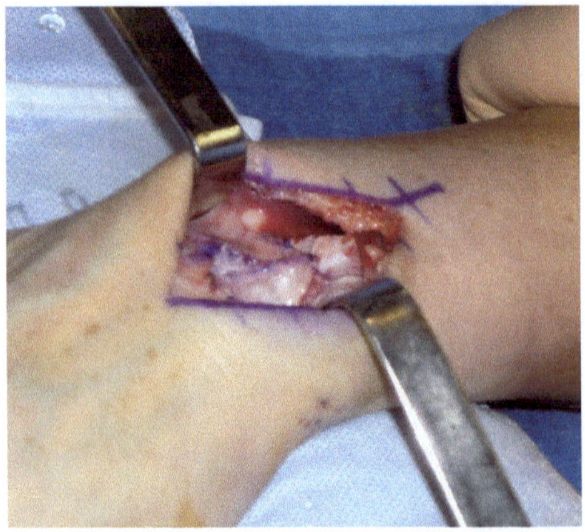

Photo 13

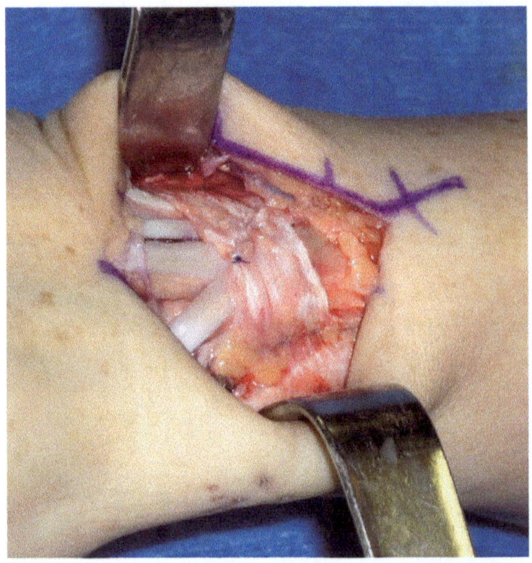

Pins are removed in theatre at 45 days.

Return to sports and manual work is authorized at 3 months postoperative. Normal range of movement is recuperated at 3–6 months with a considerable risk of permanent residual stiffness.

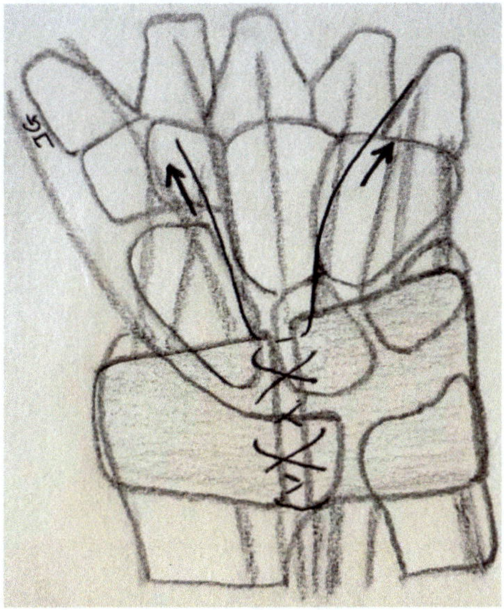

Fig. 9 Closure of the dorsal retinaculum using a double row continuous PDS 4/0

Management of Scapholunate Instabilities Resorting to Blatt's Capsulodesis

L. Van Overstraeten

1 Introduction

Blatt's capsulodesis, which uses a dorsal capsular flap with a proximal hinge, was described in 1987 to treat rotative dissociations of the scaphoid and to stabilize a distal ulna following the excision of its head [1]. Capsulodesis is like a mechanical brake to avoid the volar flexion of the scaphoid.

At that time, this capsulodesis was an alternative to Taleisnik's treatment of the scapholunate ligament.

For about 10 years, surgeons resorted to it as an isolated treatment or, more often, together with a suture of the interosseous ligament [2, 3].

Nowadays, this technique is still widely used. In 2004, a Canadian study questioned North American hand surgeons and reported that, among the 468 surgeons who answered the questionnaire, most of them preferably resorted to a repair of the scapholunate ligament together with capsulodesis when the injury was acute. In their opinion, the best means of treating chronic instabilities is Blatt's capsulodesis, capsulodesis combined with scapholunate repair or scaphotrapeziotrapezoid (STT) arthrodesis [4].

2 Surgical Technique

The incision is dorsoradial and longitudinal and goes to the ulnar side of the long flexor of the thumb, between the third and fourth compartments of the extensors. It goes from Lister's tubercle to the scaphotrapezial joint. The thumb

L. Van Overstraeten
Hand and Foot Surgery Unit,
Rue Pierre Caille N° 9, B-7500 Tournai, Belgium
e-mail: l.v.o@skynet.be

E. Camus, L. Van Overstraeten (eds.), *Carpal Ligament Surgery*,
DOI 10.1007/978-2-8178-0379-1_19, © Springer-Verlag France 2013

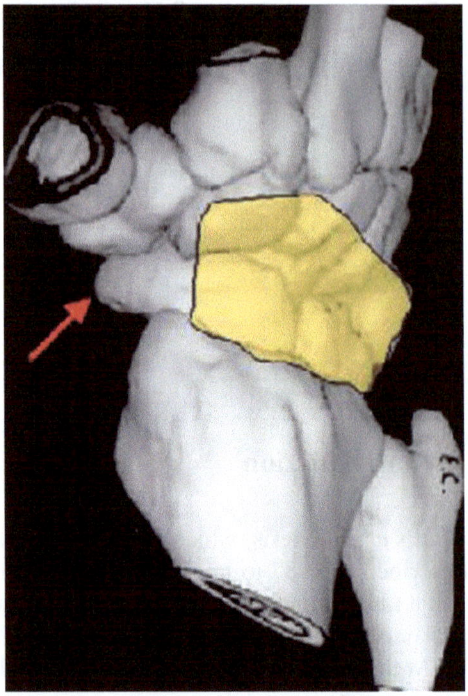

Fig. 1 The dorsal capsule. The *arrow* shows the scaphoid: it is flexed before the capsulodesis

long extensor and the radial long extensor of the carpus are lowered to the radial side; the radial short extensor of the carpus is lowered either in ulnar or in radial. A 1 cm wide dorsal capsular flap with a proximal hinge is cut from the distal extremity of the radius to the distal side of the scaphoid (Figs. 1 and 2). The scaphoid may be reduced by volar pressure as the wrist rests in ulnar deviation. Reduction is maintained by scaphocapitate or scapholunate Kirchner wire. The dorsal bridge of the scaphoid, which separates the radiocarpal and midcarpal articular surfaces, is exposed. The capsular flap is reintroduced under tension in a fissure which is ploughed on the dorsal side of the distal scaphoid (this bridge is used as a reference point), as distally as possible. Fixing is either made by a clamp or by one or two mini anchors [2, 5], with a Ticron 2/0 suture. The repair tension is adjusted so as to reach the minimum flexion or, at least, the neutral position.

The capsular repair and then the skin are fastened. The column of the thumb is maintained by a plaster cast during 6½ weeks. At that stage, the plaster cast and the wires are removed and the patient starts physiotherapy.

It would seem that American surgeons prefer to resort to a scapholunate and scaphocapitate pinning [4].

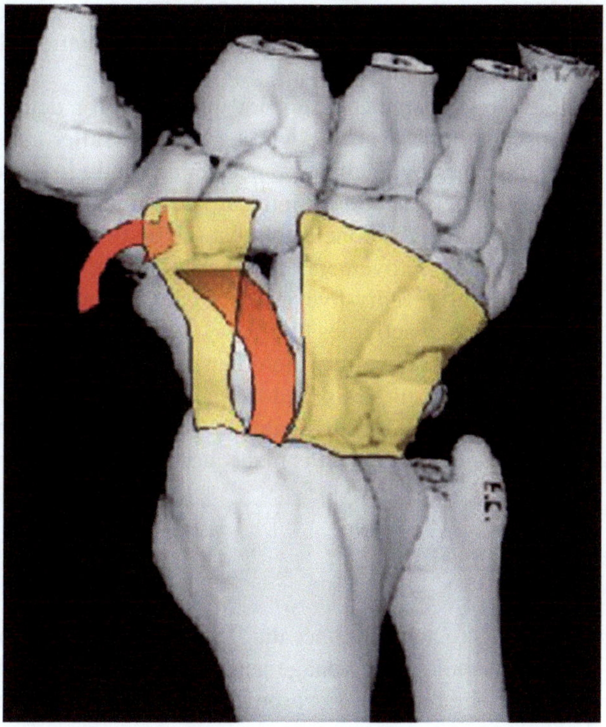

Fig. 2 Blatt's capsulodesis. This procedure allows a verticalization of this scaphoid (*arrows*)

3 Results

Results depend on how long patients have been followed up. Short-term results (1–2 years) are usually favourable [6]. However, they deteriorate at midterm (5 years), especially when important daily constraints are applied to the wrists [6].

In Blatt's original survey, which concerned twelve indications, most scapholunate instabilities are static and chronic. Long-term results were very satisfactory as extension was completely recovered and flexion loss was only 20°. Average grip strength was recovered to 80 %. Most patients returned to their pre-operatory level of daily activities [1].

The series studied are short. Some of them mostly deal with indications of pre-radiologic or dynamic instability [2, 7], others with indications of chronic static instability [1, 8]. The most important series contains 44 patients [9]. Pain, normally studied by subjective analogical scale, often improves (except in Pommerance's scale on which it is estimated at 3/10 before and after capsulodesis [1, 10]). However, it seldom disappears [11].

Clinical improvement is constant, with a decrease of the pain in all cases, at the expense of a loss of mobility. The deficiency of post-operatory flexion reaches

11–32° depending on the series [2, 7, 9]. The deficiency of extension reaches 11–22° [2, 9]. Grip strength is not improved by the operation [11] and reaches 66 % of the contralateral strength [9].

Radiologic parameters do not modify [9] or deteriorate [6, 11] with surgery. Scapholunate diastasis is about 1 mm wider after capsulodesis, the scapholunate angle increases by 5°. In a biomechanical study in a cadaver model, Slater made a comparison between dorsal intercarpal ligament capsulodesis and Blatt's capsulodesis. He came to the conclusion that the first method reduces the scapholunate diastasis and the improvement of the scapholunate angle is better than Blatt's [10].

Sixty-six to seventy-five percent of the patients can return to the same job and/or to heavy manual activities [7, 9].

According to Lavernia, there is no significant difference between the results of an isolated capsulodesis and a capsulodesis combined with the repair of the interosseous scapholunate ligament. There is no difference either when the repair of the scapholunate ligament is made alone [8].

4 Conclusion

Authors agree with the fact that Blatt's dorsal capsulodesis remains a useful and efficient technique to manage acute instabilities (together with a repair of the scapholunate ligament), or chronic instabilities, whether they are pre-radiologic, dynamic or static.

Blatt's capsulodesis is used in Garcia-Elias' stages 1, 2 and 3.

References

1. Blatt G (1987) Capsulodesis in reconstructive hand surgery. Dorsal capsulodesis for the unstable scaphoid and volar capsulodesis following excision of the distal ulna. Hand Clin 3(1):81–102
2. Muermans S, de Smet L, van Ransbeeck H (1999) Blatt dorsal capsulodesis for scapholunate instability. Acta Orthop Belg 65(4):434–439
3. Saffar P, Sokolow C, Duclos L (1999) Soft tissue stabilization in the management of chronic scapholunate instability without osteoarthritis. A 15-year series. Acta Orthop Belg 65(4):424–433
4. Zarkadas PC, Gropper PT, White NJ, Perey BH (2004) A survey of the surgical management of acute and chronic scapholunate instability. J Hand Surg Am 29(5):848–857
5. Konduru RS, Scott I, Mehdi R, Dent JA, Abboud R, Wigderowitz C (2006) Dorsal capsulodesis for scapholunate instability. Effect on patient disability and wrist pain. J Hand Surg 31 B(3):311–316
6. Pomerance J (2006) Outcome after repair of the scapholunate interosseous ligament and dorsal capsulodesis for dynamic scapholunate instability due to trauma. J Hand Surg Am 31(8):1380–1386
7. Wintman BI, Gelberman RH, Katz JN (1995) Dynamic scapholunate instability: results of operative treatment with dorsal capsulodesis. J Hand Surg Am 20 A:971–979

8. Lavernia CL, Cohen MS, Taleisnik J (1992) Treatment of scapholunate dissociation by ligamentous repair and capsulodesis. J Hand Surg 17-A:354–359
9. Deshmukh SC, Givissis P, Belloso D, Stanley JK, Trail IA (1999) Blatt's capsulodesis for chronic scapholunate dissociation. J Hand Surg Br 24 B:215–220
10. Slater RR Jr, Szabo RM, Bay BK, Laubach J (1999) Dorsal intercarpal ligament capsulodesis for scapholunate dissociation: biomechanical analysis in a cadaver model. J Hand Surg Am 24(2):232–239
11. Moran SL, Cooney WP, Berger RA, Strickland J (2005) Capsulodesis for the treatment of chronic scapholunate instability. J Hand Surg Am 30(1):16–23

Management of Chronic Scapholunate Ligament Tears Before Arthritis Occurrence or to Prevent Arthritis

Ch. Mathoulin, E. Papadogeorgou, and A. Pagliei

1 Introduction

The scapholunate ligament injury is the most frequent lesion that results from supination and extension trauma of the wrist [1]. It engenders a chronic instability that may turn to arthritis.

This lesion can be associated with a fracture of the radial epiphysis [2]. Acute injuries (less than 2 months old) are difficult to diagnose. Wrist arthroscopy is useful to detect these injuries at an early stage and to treat them by stable fixing, without open surgery of the wrist. The management of chronic injuries of the scapholunate ligament before occurrence of arthritis remains a challenge for the surgeon who often manages to correctly stabilize the instability but may not prevent wrist stiffness. We report a new therapeutic scheme based on the classification proposed by Marc Garcia-Elias et al. [3], using two new methods: an arthroscopic technique and an open surgery with ligamentoplasty. Both techniques enabled us to obtain encouraging results, even if many series showed that the result of the early treatment was superior to any attempt of secondary stabilization [1, 2, 4–11].

2 Anatomic Basis

As a full part of a sophisticated multiarticular system, the scapholunate joint is a critical joint, which is very ductile for man and essential for a 'skilful hand'. The structural integrity of the bone and the stabilization means, static and dynamic, allow the scaphoid to play a key role in the dynamics of the carpal rows which are

Ch. Mathoulin (✉) • E. Papadogeorgou • A. Pagliei
Hand Surgery Unit, Institut de la main, Clinique Jouvenet,
6, square Jouvenet, Paris 75016, France
e-mail: cmathoulin@orange.fr

E. Camus, L. Van Overstraeten (eds.), *Carpal Ligament Surgery*,
DOI 10.1007/978-2-8178-0379-1_20, © Springer-Verlag France 2013

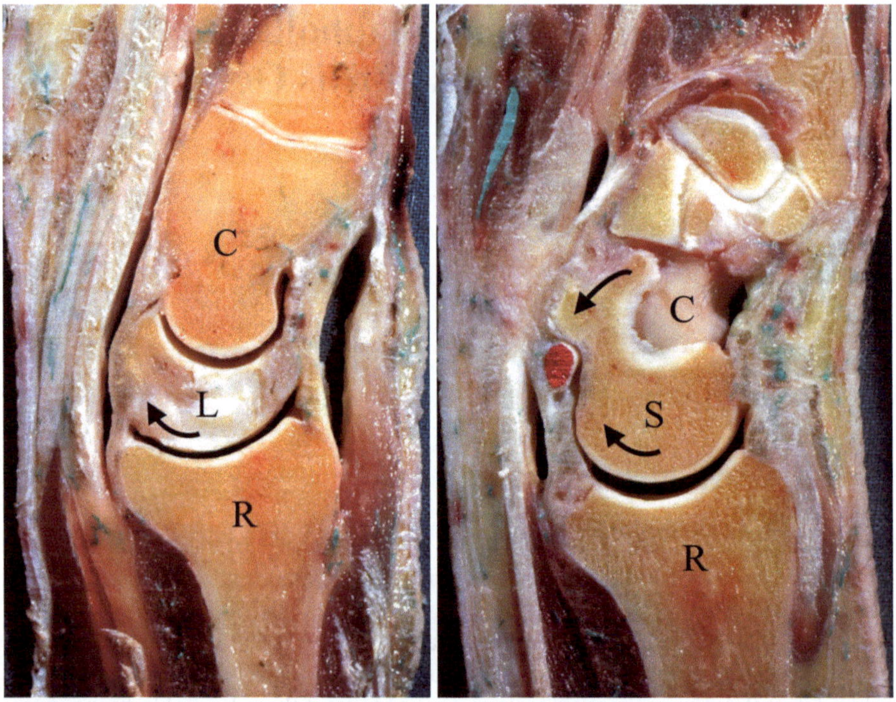

Fig. 1 Fresh cadaver, frozen wrist: lateral section showing the constraints applied on the scapholunate complex. We can notice the thickness of the palmar capsulo-ligamentous structures creating a sort of cushion positioned against the anterior translation of the carpus. *C* capitate, *L* semilunate, *S* scaphoid, *R* radius

in a precarious balance, considering the opposite constraints acting on the proximal and distal poles. The distal pole tends to flex in response to the strengths applied on the first ray, while the proximal pole extends due to its links with the semilunate. This condition, which is peculiar to the scaphoid, follows the acquisition of opposition of the thumb (anteposition of the first ray, scaphoid anteversion), a fundamental progressive event for the man's hand.

As it is related to the progressive flexion of the scaphoid, the trapezium comes on a much volar plane: the structure of the trapezio-metacarpal favours the opening of the first ray of the palm, which gives it the possibility to oppose the four digital other rays. This recent phylogenetic acquisition makes the scaphoid no longer parallel to the other elements of the carpus, with the application of important unbalanced strengths on the opposite poles (Fig. 1).

2.1 Means to Stabilize the Distal Pole of the Scaphoid

Devices meant to stabilize the distal pole of the scaphoid play a quite important part considering the constraints transmitted by the first ray due to its anteposition. The

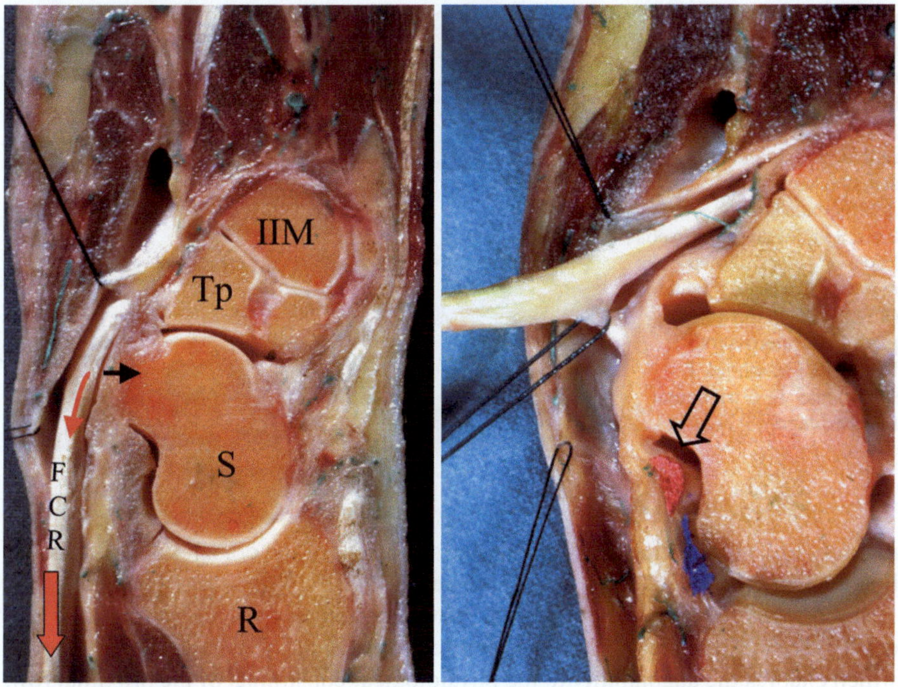

Fig. 2 Fresh cadaver, frozen wrist: lateral section showing the distal ligamentous complex of the scaphoid. The tendon of the flexor carpi radialis (*FCR*) can have accessory insertions on the scaphoid (*S*), on the trapezium (*Tp*) or on the scapho-trapezoid along its course towards the base of the 2nd metacarpal (*IIM*); through the trapezio-trapezoid complex, it exerts constraints in flexion on the scaphoid (*red arrows*). The *black arrow* represents the active stabilizing function of the *FCR*. In fact, this musculotendinous entity is opposed to an excessive volar dislocation of the tubercle of the scaphoid. The radio-scapho-capitate ligament can be clearly seen (*in red*, *empty arrow*) in its function of tense pivot between the radius and the capitate, around which the scaphoid makes movements of flexion and extension. *R* radius

flexor carpi radialis system (FCR) has both an active and a passive part: its osteofibrous canal is a real anterior abutment which is superimposed to the distal ligamentous complex of the scaphoid (scapho-trapezio-trapezoidal and scapho-capitate ligaments) (Fig. 2).

2.2 Interosseous Scapholunate Ligament

The scaphoid is linked to the semilunate by an interosseous ligament which acts like a twisting bar as it creates a system with viscoelastic dampers. It is a nonhomogeneous system composed of three parts: the anterior part is fitted into the long and short radio-lunate ligament and the radioscapholunate ligament. The intermediate proximal part is a real avascularized fibrocartilaginous membrane that corresponds to the depressed zone during arthroscopic palpation. The posterior part is strong and

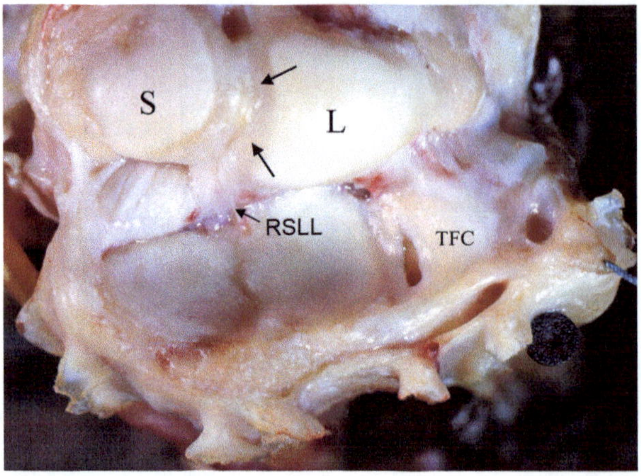

Fig. 3 Fresh cadaver, anatomic preparation of the radiocarpal: the carpus has been placed in exaggerated flexion to show the volar radiocarpal ligaments and the articular section only – intermediate section – of the scapholunate interosseous ligament (*black arrows*). The radioscapholunate ligament (*RSLL*) covers the anterior part of the interosseous ligament. *S* scaphoid, *L* semilunate, *TFC* triangular fibrocartilage

securely linked to the dorsal capsule as it is adjacent to the dorsal scapho-triquetral ligament and the dorsal intracarpal ligament (Fig. 3).

The carpus has also a capsulo-ligamentous system (extrinsic, intracapsular and extra-synovial ligament) organized in different ways at the volar and dorsal level, which enables the adaptability to the physiological constraints of the proximal row, especially that of the scapholunate complex (Fig. 4).

2.3 *Assessment of the Anatomic Aspects*

From a strictly anatomic point of view, the scapholunate joint is characterized by the superimposition of two smooth articular facets, creating an arthrodia in the presence of a syndesmotic element at the level of the proximal pole between two bones. The clinical experiment shows smooth joints, and especially syndesmoses show particular sensitivity to the passage of a metallic synthesis tool as it develops an important secondary fibrosis. Thus, if we want to make an 'arthrofibrosis' as close to the physiological condition as possible, it seems logical to treat an instability resulting from the injury of a syndesmosis by stabilization using trans-articular synthetic means.

Although we noticed an anatomic division of the interosseous scapholunate ligament into three parts, it would be an error to give a major role to particularly ligamentous parts. The mere notion of 'interosseous ligament' should be restricted to the intermediate section, that is to say, the sole fibrocartilaginous, avascularized and thus unrepairable section. On the contrary, the anterior and posterior parts of the scapholunate ligament are perfectly integrated into the volar and dorsal extra-synovial ligamentous system and consequently reminiscent of the system of all extra-articular ligaments with many cells and well-developed vascularization.

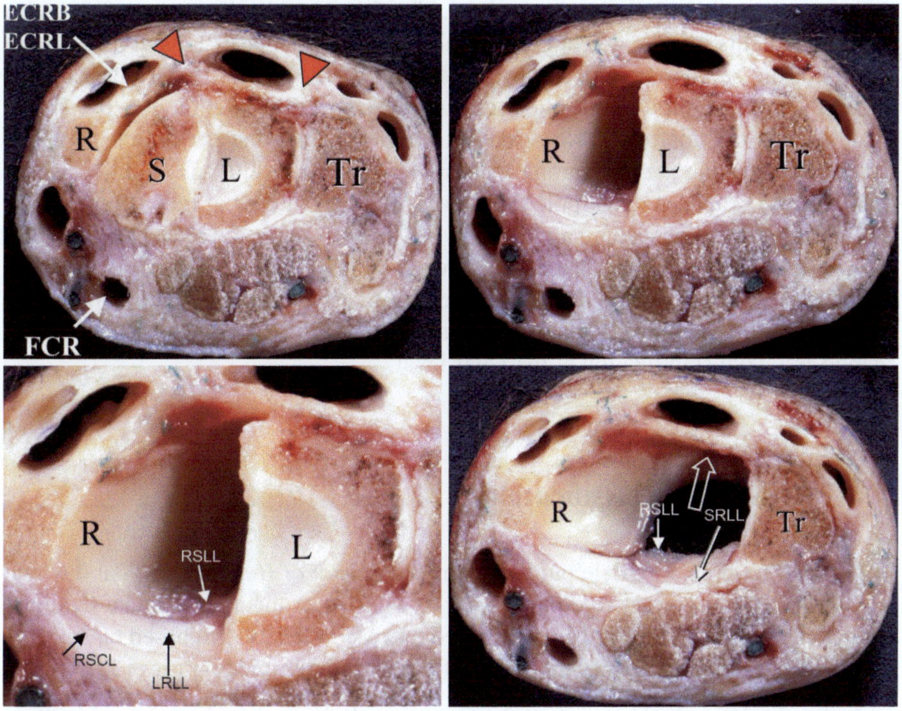

Fig. 4 Fresh cadaver, frozen wrist: coronal section at the level of the midcarpal, after the removal of the proximal pole of the scaphoid (*S*) and the semilunate (*L*). (*R*) radius, (*Tr*) Trapezium. We can notice: The correct osseous covering that the styloid section of the radial socket gives the proximal pole of the scaphoid. The structural differences between the volar and dorsal capsulo-ligamentous complex. We can underline the orientation of the volar radiocarpal ligaments (*RSCL* radio-scapho-capitate ligament, *LRLL* long radio-lunate ligament, *SRLL* short radio-lunate ligament) which have a reversed V-shape with converging arms on the capitate and lunate, making a less elastic and more stable system with 'a central symmetry' and with shorter and stronger ligaments: *RSLL* the radio-scapholunate ligament or the ligament of Testut and Kuentz. On the contrary, the dorsal capsule, which is thinner, seems to be reinforced by the dorsal intercarpal ligament which is tensed between the pyramidal and the *STT* complex (scapho-trapezio-trapedoidal) and linked to the posterior and more dorsal parts of the scapholunate and luno-triquetral interosseous ligaments (*tips of the red arrows*), where the posterior scapho-triquetral ligament originates. The dorsal intercarpal ligament and the dorsal radio-triquetral ligament (or dorsal radiocarpal, which belongs to the carpal ulnar sling of Kuhlmann – *empty white arrow*) form an oblique ligamentous 'V' with the apex centred on the pyramidal: a ligamentous system with an 'eccentric symmetry', longer and thinner but much more elastic oblique ligaments. The carpal tendinous cage created by the extra-articular slings (retinaculum of the flexors and retinaculum of the extensors; the latter is made more visible once the tendons are removed), insures a dynamic control system which elements are set in rays, forms a system with 'radial symmetry' which allows and adjusts wrist motion in all directions: *FCR* flexor carpi radialis, *ECRB* extensor carpi radialis brevis, *ECRL* extensor carpi radialis longus

The proximal row is a complex system that has to present both a twisting elasticity enabling the flexion-extension of the scaphoid and stability enough to resist without bending too much the constraints of compression transmitted by the distal row and more particularly by the capitate. The far more elastic system of the volar carpal ligaments and the dorsal intercarpal ligaments enables the distal parts of the scaphoid, the semilunate and the pyramidal to execute limited movements on the sagittal plane and allows controlled twisting of the scaphoid-semilunate pyramidal chain. The correction of a rotary instability of the scaphoid at a chronicle level has to take into account the execution of a scapholunate 'arthrofibrosis' and the stabilization of the scaphoid distal pole. Surgical techniques aimed at reconstructing the capsulo-ligamentous system and preserving the anatomic characteristics of the physiological stabilization means must be given priority. The reconstruction of a dorsal capsulo-ligamentous system, especially that of the dorsal intercarpal complex, seems to guarantee limited stiffness and can be associated, if necessary, to scapho-trapezial stabilization at the volar level.

3 Garcia-Elias Classification

In January 2006, in an article published in the *Journal of Hand Surgery*, and which has become an important reference as far as injuries of the scapholunate ligament are concerned, Marc Garcia-Elias proposed a new scoring system based on answers to five questions dealing with the status of the wrist in chronic injuries [3]:

1. Is the scapholunate ligament, and more particularly its dorsal section, intact?
2. Is the injury of the scapholunate ligament partial or not?
3. Is the scapholunate ligament repairable?
4. Are osseous connections normal?
5. Is the scaphoid reducible?
6. Are cartilages normal?

This questionnaire results in a six-stage classification distributed as follows:

- *Stage 1*: There is a mere partial injury which is likely to be repaired thanks to a normal line, a reducible scaphoid and healthy cartilages.
- *Stage 2*: The injury is complete but intact repair seems possible.
- *Stage 3*: There is an important injury of the scapholunate ligament but the osseous connections are still normal.
- *Stage 4*: There is a complete tear of the scapholunate ligament with a dislocation of the scaphoid, but reduction appears possible.
- *Stage 5*: Reduction is not spontaneous as the horizontalization of the scaphoid is settled.
- *Stage 6*: Cartilages are affected (SLAC 1–4).

On this basis, Marc Garcia-Elias proposed the following therapeutic chart:

- *Stage 1*: It should be considered scapholunate broaching under arthroscopic control for acute cases and scapholunate broaching associated with dorsal capsulodesis for chronic cases.

- *Stage 2*: Suture of the scapholunate ligament by open surgery.
- *Stage 3:* Reconstruction either by bone-ligament-bone fixing or reconstruction by the three-ligament technique.
- *Stage 4*: Reconstruction by ligamentoplasty.
- *Stage 5*: Scapho-trapezio-trapezoidal arthrodesis is the most logical indication but in some cases after cleaning periosseous fibrosis and eventual reduction, stage 5 could be turn into stage 4 with reconstruction by ligamentoplasty.
- *Stage 6*: Potential surgery depending on the progression of arthrosis with palliative techniques such as resection of the first carpal row and arthrodesis of the 4 internal bones.

4 Arthroscopic Capsuloplasty (Stages 2–4)

In stages 2, 3 and 4 in particular, no matter if the ligament appears repairable or not, when the lines are strictly normal, we suggest a new technique of dorsal capsuloplasty associated with scapholunate and scapho-capitate pinning associated with arthroscopic control and support. The technique is based on a suture between the dorsal capsule and the scapholunate ligament. The arthroscope is introduced between the radiocarpal joint and the midcarpal. An internal knot is made between the scaphoid and the semilunate, and an external knot is made at the level of the capsule so as to create a link between the dorsal capsule and the dorsal part of the scapholunate ligament to reinforce the dorsal section of this ligament (Figs. 5, 6, 7, 8, and 9).

We used this technique to operate on 11 male patients, aged from 19 to 45 years (averaged age: 36 years). Most of them (nine cases) had sport accidents and three cases were high-level sportsmen.

Real effects of the procedure could not be assessed so early since the average period lasts 12 months (from 7 to 17 months). Pain disappeared in all cases except two who still suffer from moderate climatic pains. Mobility is normal in seven cases, as well as muscular strengths.

To date, no surgical failure occurred and these results are really favourable, but more time is necessary to analyse long-term results after the patients returned to sports activities (Figs. 10, 11, 12, 13, 14, and 15).

5 ECRB Ligamentoplasty and Scapholunate Stabilization

In stage 5, in particular when lines are disturbed and with a reducibility of the scaphoid which is easy or not, we systematically suggest by an open portal to perform reconstructive ligamentoplasty using a strip of the extensor carpi radialis brevis (ECRB). This technique aims at making an arthrofibrosis through the scapholunate joint and stabilizing the distal pole of the scaphoid thanks to this ligamentoplasty.

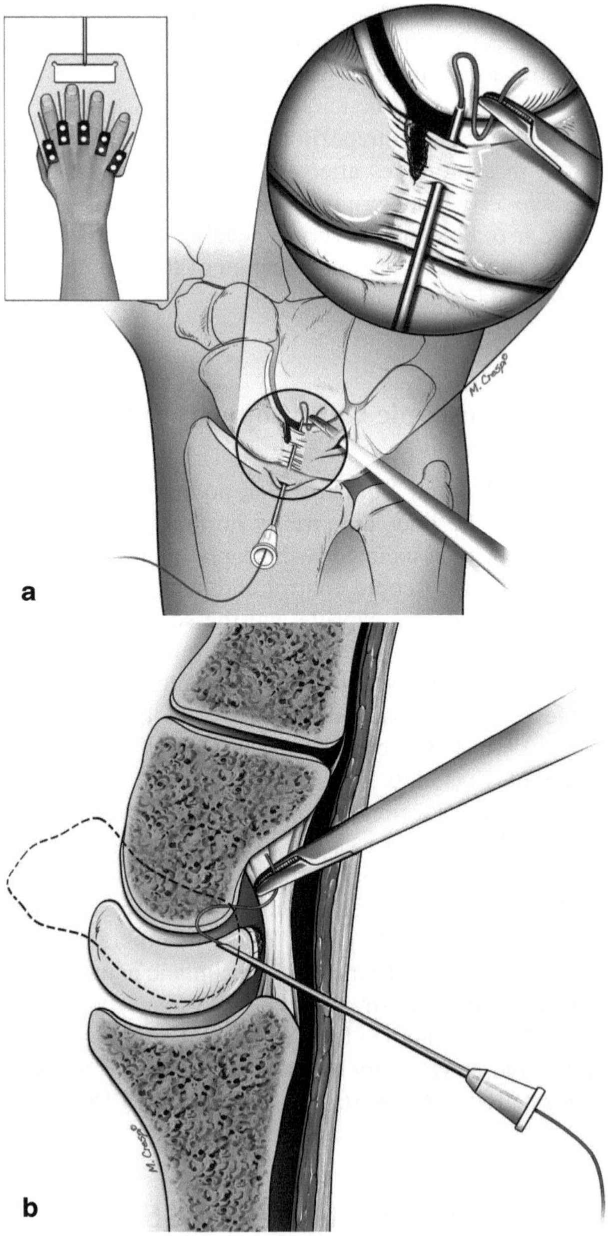

Fig. 5 (**a**, **b**) First introduction of a thread between the dorsal capsule and the scapholunate ligament. Under arthroscopic control, the thread is placed inside a needle and goes from the radiocarpal joint to the midcarpal joint where the thread is got back and removed by the radial midcarpal portal

The therapeutic principle was to fix the scapholunate joint in a reduced position for a long period (6 months). Following our anatomic studies, a new ligamentoplasty using a strip from the extensor carpi radialis brevis (ECRB) stabilized the complex of the carpal first row.

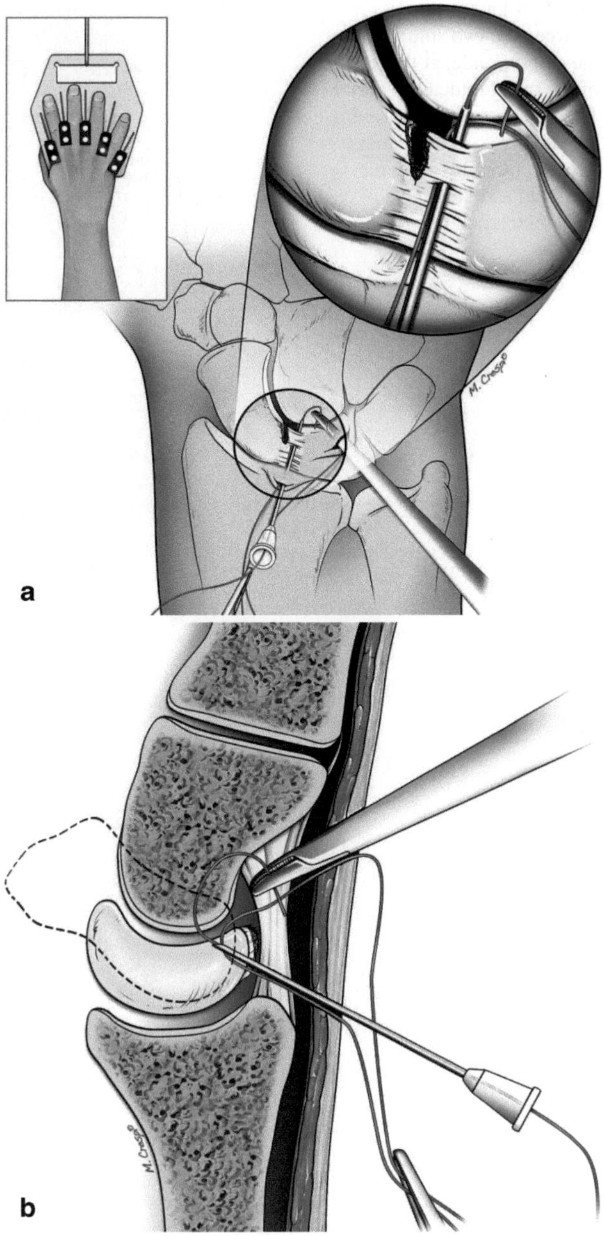

Fig. 6 (**a**, **b**) A second thread, parallel to the first one, is introduced using the same technique

Arthroscopic assessment was always made after surgery, following the same techniques, to check the presence of potential arthrosis and the importance of the dislocation.

The technique is based on an arciform approach. After the strip had been removed from the ECRB and fixed on the distal 2nd metacarpal, we performed dorsal arthrotomy and explored the scapholunate joint (Fig. 16). Reducing the radio-lunate joint

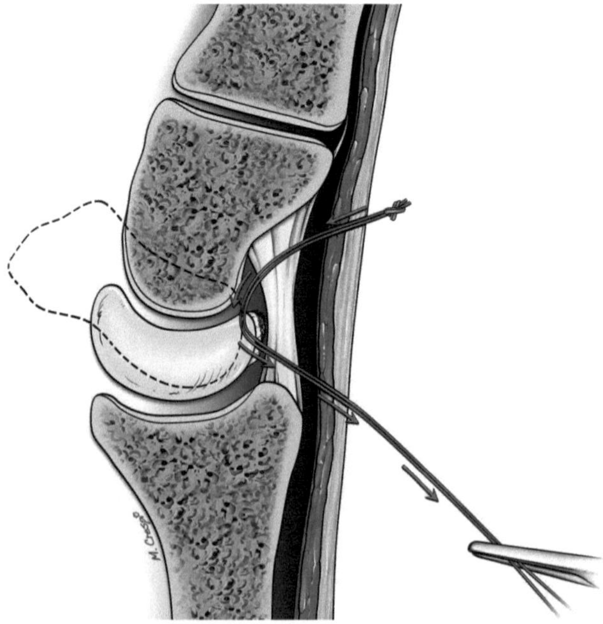

Fig. 7 A knot is done between the two sutures at the external side, at the level of the radial midcarpal portal. Then the thread is removed proximally so that the first knot is placed between the scaphoid and the lunate in intra midcarpal

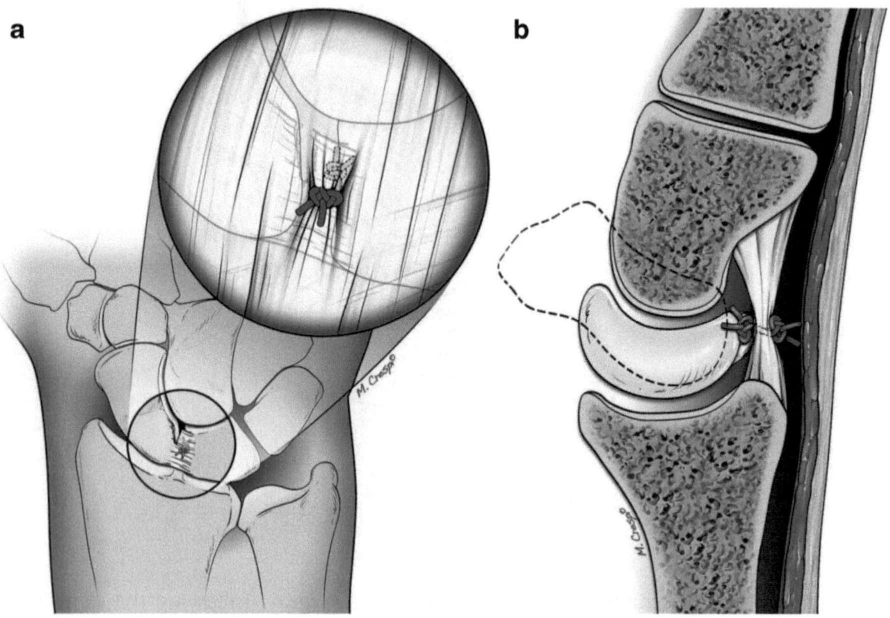

Fig. 8 (**a, b**) A suture is done at the radiocarpal so as to create a capsuloplasty between the dorsal capsule and the dorsal section of the scapholunate ligament

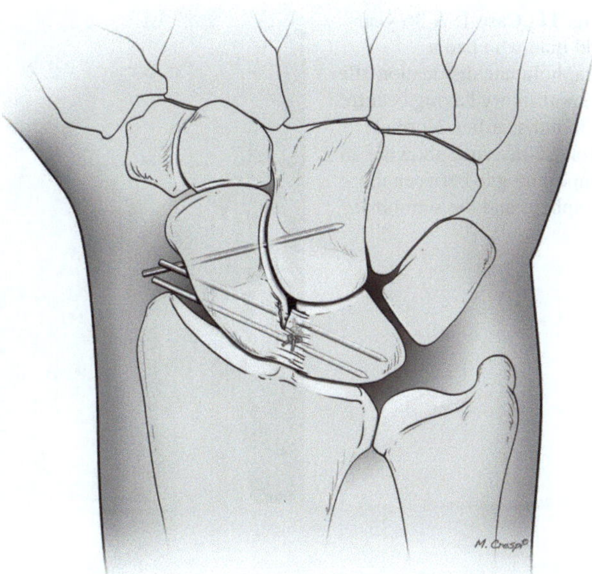

Fig. 9 The reduction of the scapholunate interval is maintained by a crossed scapholunate double pining and sometimes a scapho-capitate K-wire

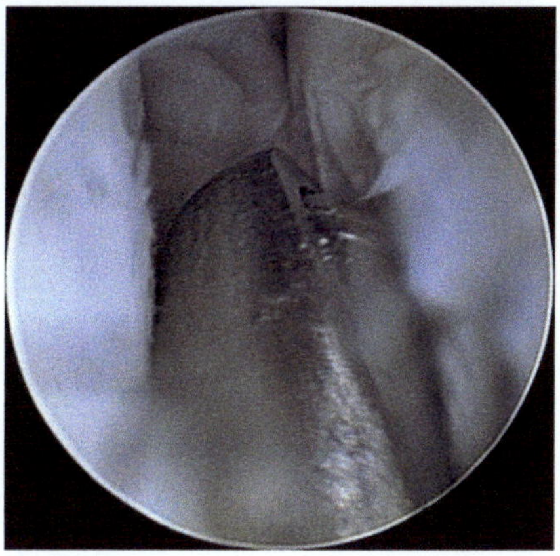

Fig. 10 Case 1: Midcarpal arthroscopic view of a stage four injury showing quite an important gap between the scaphoid and the semilunate with space enough to let a 3-mm shaver being introduced from the radiocarpal to the midcarpal joint

was sometimes difficult (Fig. 17) and scapholunate pinning maintained temporarily this reduction (Fig. 18).

The scapholunate space is then fixed either with staple and K-wires or with a cannulated screw.

The strip from the ECRB was placed from the midcarpal joint to the radiocarpal joint inside the dorsal radio-luno-triquetral ligament (Fig. 19) and then fixed in the neutral position of the wrist in the distal dorsal part of the scaphoid using an intraosseous anchor (Fig. 20). Associated capsulodesis was performed by the introduction of two anchors into the posterior horn of the lunate and the dorsal section of

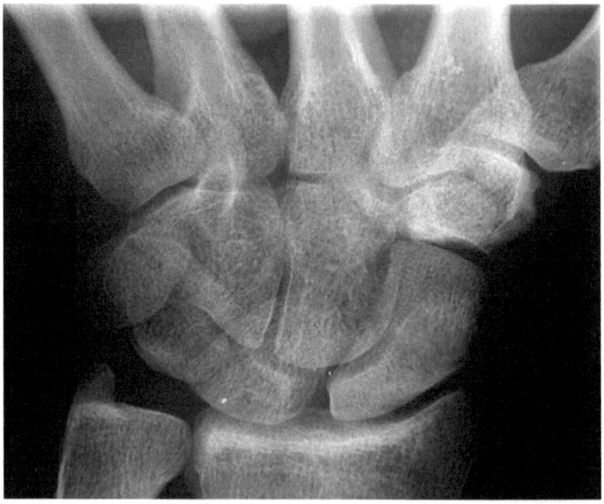

Fig. 11 Case 1: A 36-year-old man who had a scapholunate dislocation after a sport injury having occurred 5 months earlier. Normal front X-ray view showing an important gap between the scaphoid and the semilunate

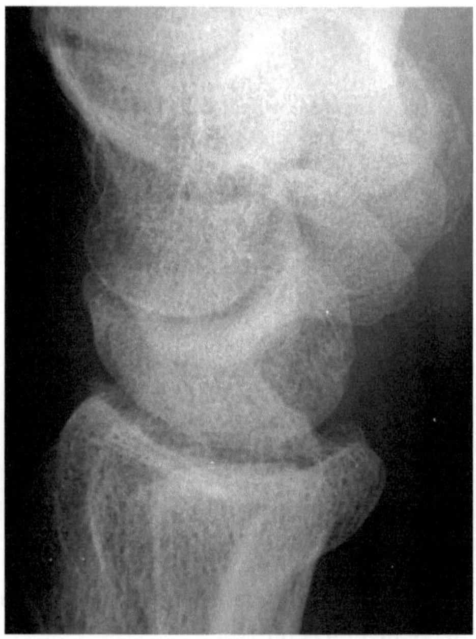

Fig. 12 Case 1: Profile view showing a dorsal drift of the semilunate (*DISI*) and a 80° scapholunate angle

the proximal pole of the scaphoid. The aim of this ligamentoplasty is double: first, the ligamentoplasty, by tenodesis, is expected to fight naturally against the horizontalization of the scaphoid and when the wrist flexes (Fig. 21). Moreover, it should establish a narrowing between the luno-triquetral complex and the scaphoid. Its distal fixing on the dorsal side of the scaphoid distal tubercle achieves easier stabilization of the distal pole of the scaphoid (Fig. 22).

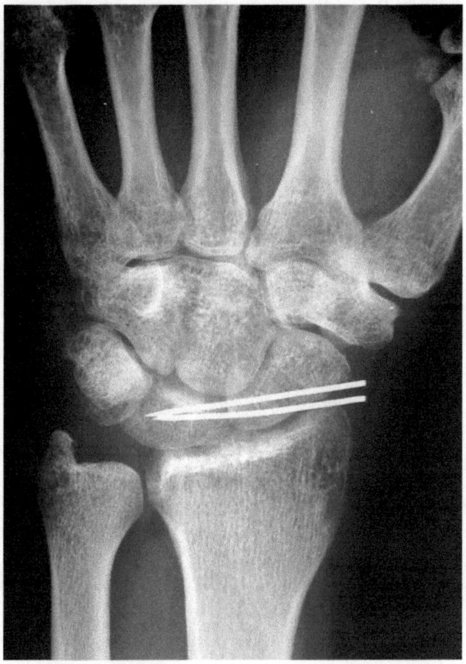

Fig. 13 Case 1: X-ray after capsuloplasty with two pins placed with arthroscopic assistance

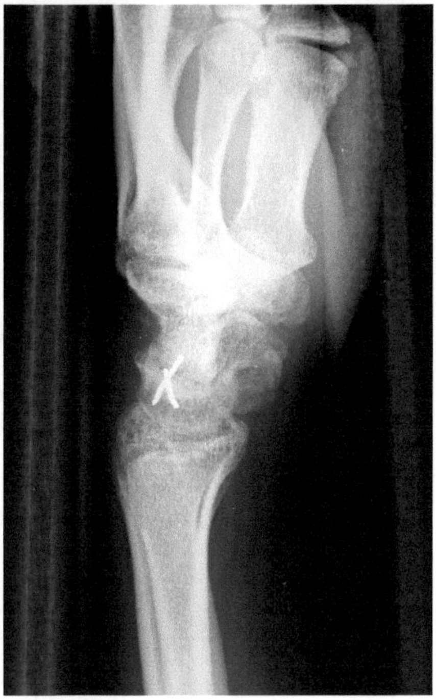

Fig. 14 Case 1: Profile view showing the good position of the K-wires and the correct reduction of the lunate, with disappearance of the DISI and a normal 45° scapholunate angle

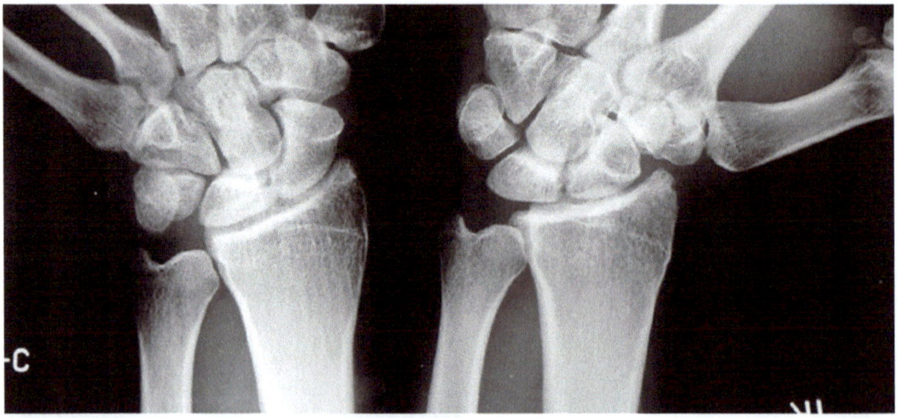

Fig. 15 Case 1: Radial frontal X-ray and ulnar deviation 2 years after the repair, with the recovery of normal anatomy and mobility of the scaphoid

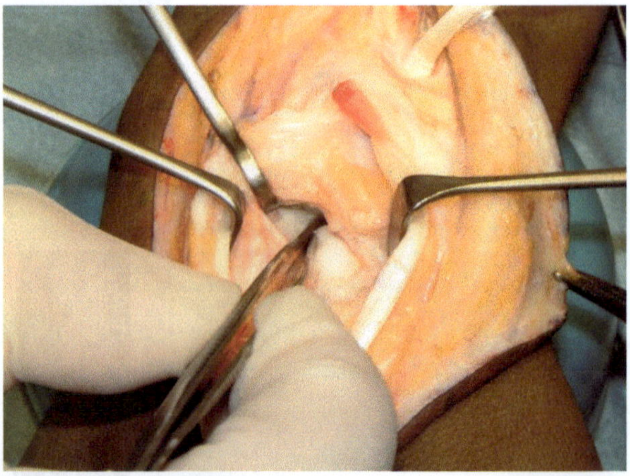

Fig. 16 After arthrotomy, the investigation of the joint shows a rupture of the scapholunate ligament (it is a stage III after arthroscopy)

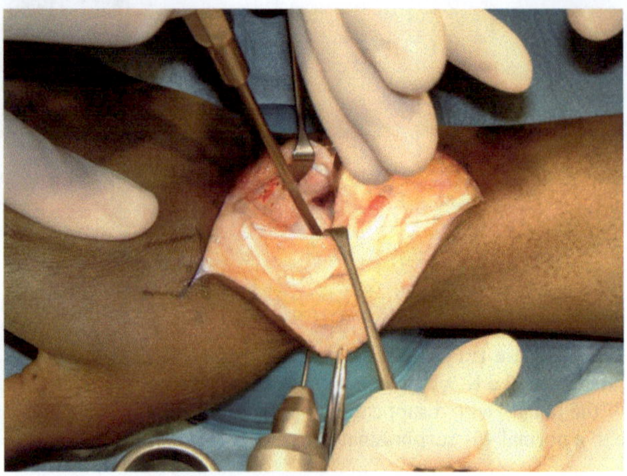

Fig. 17 The reduction of the scaphoid when it is well positioned can be made with a peak bone, the wrist in slight traction, in extension and in ulnar drift. A temporary K-wire maintains the reduction

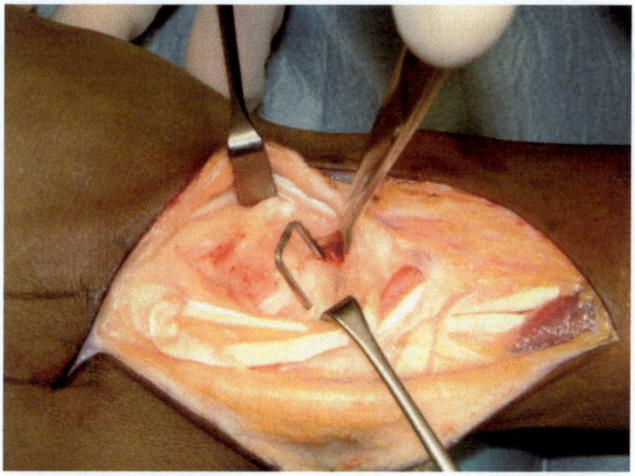

Fig. 18 Dorsal staple is placed over the scapholunate joint and fix the reduction. The oblique position of the staple allows normal mobility in extension

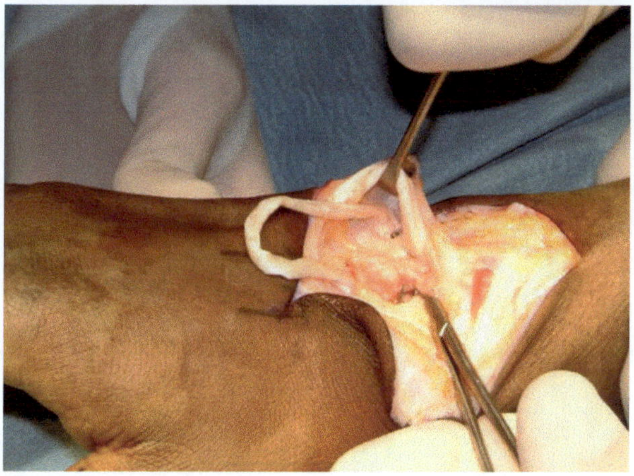

Fig. 19 A strip from the ECRB is distally placed on the 2nd metacarpal and goes from the midcarpal joint to the radiocarpal joint inside the dorsal radio-luno-triquetral ligament

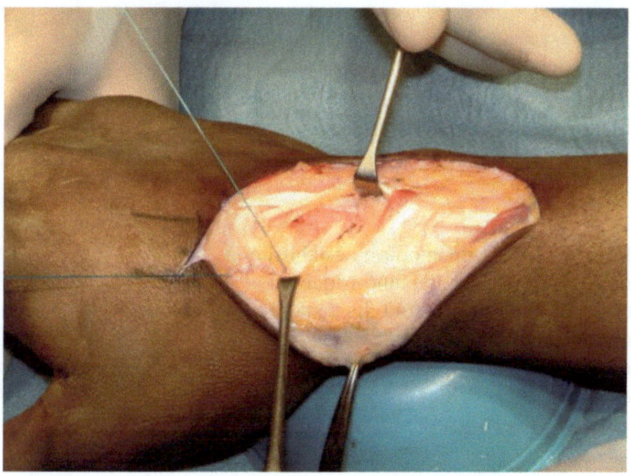

Fig. 20 The ligamentoplasty is fixed in the dorsal section of the distal tubercle by an intraosseous anchor, the wrist in a neutral position

Fig. 21 By tenodesis effect, the ligamentoplasty is going to naturally resist the horizontalization of the scaphoid and when the wrist flexes

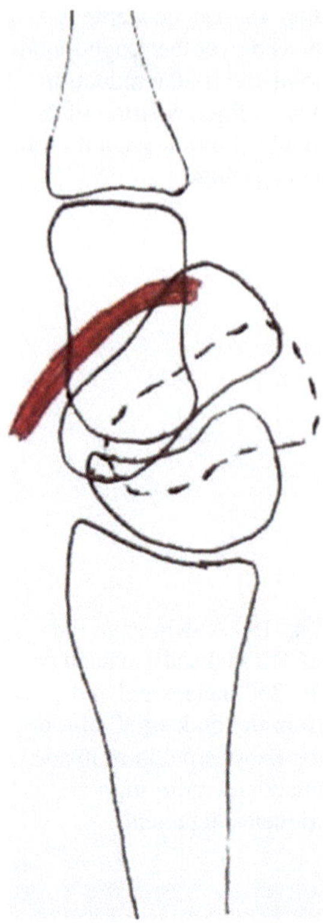

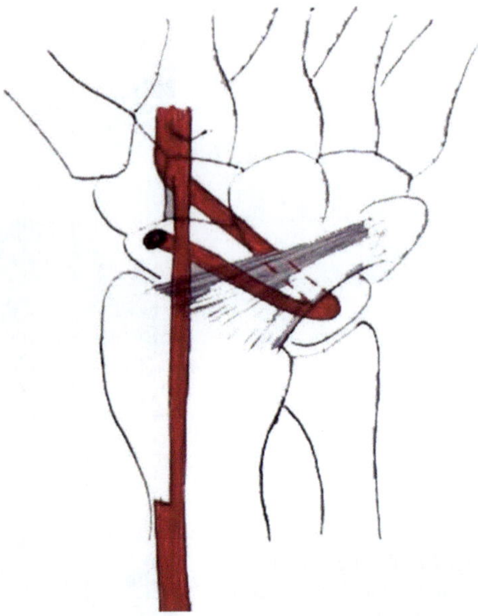

Fig. 22 The ligamentoplasty establishes a narrowing between the luno-triquetral complex and the scaphoid. Its distal fixing on the scaphoid dorsal side of the distal tubercle makes easier the stabilization of the scaphoid distal pole

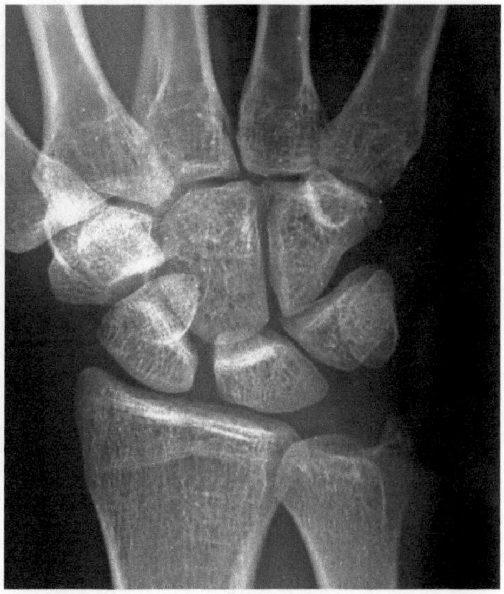

Fig. 23 Case 2: A 25-year-old tennis player (high level). Eight months after a tennis accident (smash), he had wrist pains and cracks at ulnar deviation. X-ray view shows a horizontalization of the scaphoid and a scapholunate gap

Then, a plastered splint was placed for a 2-month period after which patients could use their wrist normally. The fixing equipment was removed 6 months later.

We operated on 32 patients (23 men and 9 women). The average age was 39 (20–55 years of age).

The average follow-up was 50 months (27–67 months). Twelve patients had no pain, 12 patients had climatic pains only. Four patients had moderate pains and four others had permanent moderate pains. No patient experienced invalidating pain. Mobility in extension was about 70° and 42° in flexion, the moderate but real loss of flexion was the price to pay for this type of stabilization. Strength was about 86 % compared to the opposite side (Figs. 23, 24, 25, 26, 27, 28, and 29).

The complications that occurred were four complete losses of flexion, two Südeck's dystrophy which were treated and healed, and a staple which was expelled and necessitated the modification of our system of scapholunate fixing to systematically choose a cannulated screw.

6 Discussion

The analysis of the state of the scapholunate ligament with the help of wrist arthroscopy and the analysis of the peripheral structures allow, as Marc Garcia-Elias pointed out, to refine the classifications of chronic scapholunate injuries.

The use of mere immobilization by pinning in acute injuries of the scapholunate ligament resulted in satisfactory outcome.

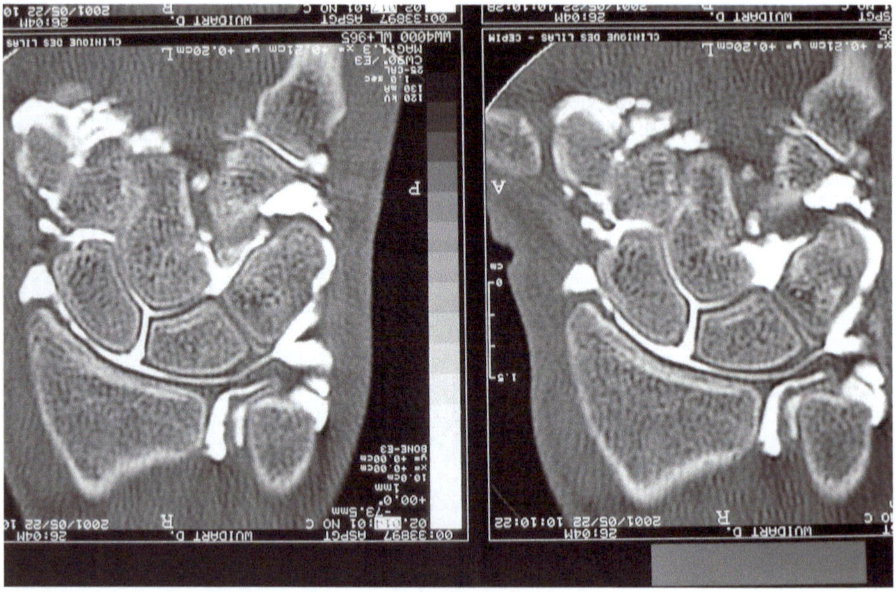

Fig. 24 Case 2: The arthro CT-scan confirms a rupture of the scapholunate ligament. The associated arthroscopy showed a stage IV

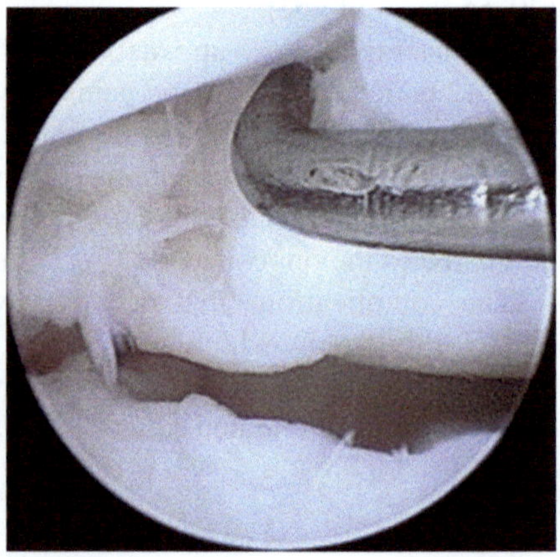

Fig. 25 Case 2: Radiocarpal arthroscopic view of a stage IV injury showing a more important gap with space enough to let a hook being introduced between the scaphoid and the lunate from the radiocarpal to the midcarpal joint

The repair of the intermediate part of the scapholunate ligament is illusory as it is a fibrocartilaginous tissue which structure is close to that of the free section of a meniscus or the central section of the triangular ligament. The correction of the rotary instability of the scaphoid must then be associated with a scapholunate arthrofibrosis and the stabilization of the distal pole of the scaphoid. Therefore, surgical techniques aimed at reconstructing the capsulo-ligamentous system should be preferred as they respect the anatomic characteristics of the physiological stabilization means. The

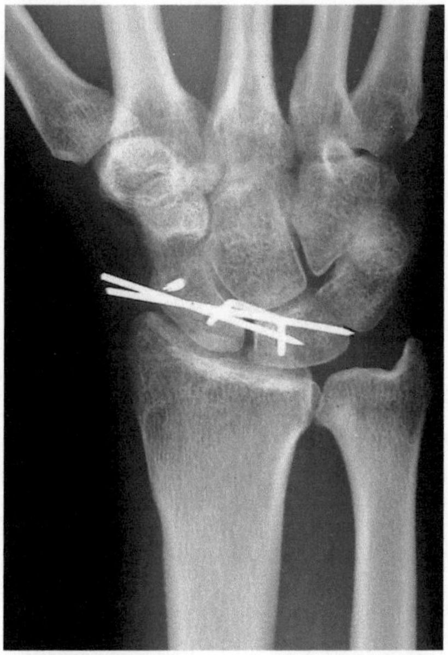

Fig. 26 Case 2: Radiography 6 months after the surgery and before the removal of the staple. We can notice a correct reduction of the scapholunate interval

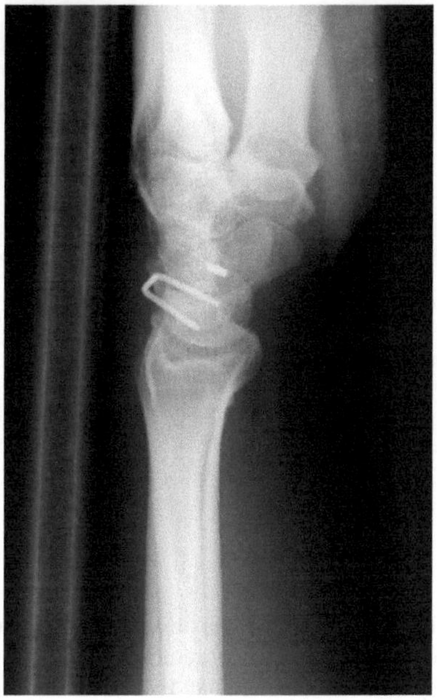

Fig. 27 Case 2: Profile radiography 6 months after the surgery showing a normal scapholunate angle

repair of the dorsal and volar systems of the scapholunate ligament but also the distal volar scapho-trapezial section looks logical. Brunelli suggested a technique with similar ambition, but it was often responsible for a post-operative stiffness that jeopardized the functional result [12]. The three-ligament tenodesis suggested by Garcia-Elias

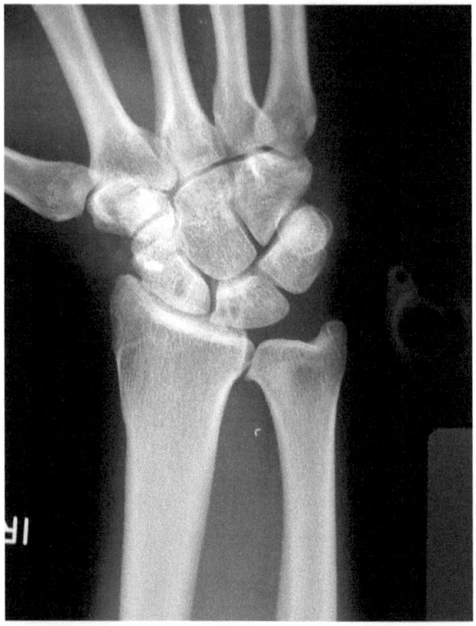

Fig. 28 Case 2: Full front radiography in radial drift 3 years after the surgery. It shows normal mobility with normal osseous connections

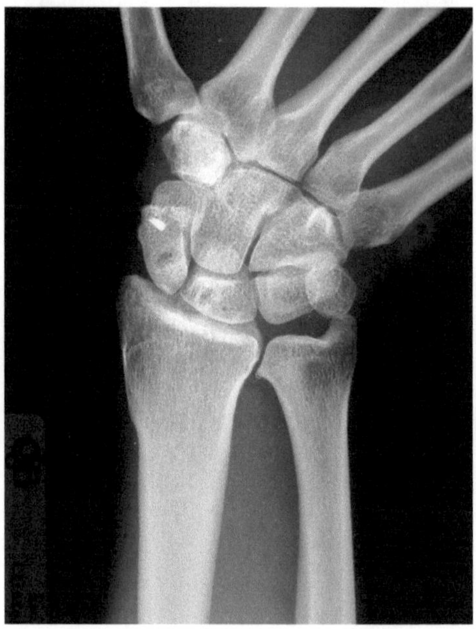

Fig. 29 Case 2: Same observation in ulnar deviation. The patient returned to all his sports activities without discomfort and at the same level

improves this problem, but it remains quite stiffening in extension [3]. Moreover, capsuloplasties fixed on the radius, as mentioned by Blatt, are also stiffening [13].

Posterior arthroscopic capsulodesis prevents these complications at stages which keep normal carpal architecture. At more advanced stages, reconstruction of a capsulo-ligamentous system of the mere dorsal intercarpal complex seems to limit the effects of stiffening. The results of the ligamentoplasty using ECRB associated with temporary fixing of the scapholunate interval result in good long-term stabilization as they maintain correct mobility despite a moderate loss of flexion.

References

1. Kozin SH (1999) The role of arthroscopy in scapholunate instability. Hand Clin 15(3): 435–444, vii
2. Peicha G, Seibert FJ, Fellinger M, Grechening W, Schippinger G (1997) Lesions of the scapholunate ligaments in acute wrist trauma – arthroscopic diagnosis and minimally invasive treatment. Knee Surg Sports Traumatol Arthrosc 5(3):176–183
3. Garcia-Elias M, Lluch A, Stanley J (2006) Three-ligament tenodesis for the treatment of scapholunate dissociation: indications and surgical technique. J Hand Surg 31A(1):125–134
4. Ruch DS, Smith BP (2001) Arthroscopic and open management of dynamic scaphoid instability. Orthop Clin North Am 32(2):233–240
5. Westkaemper JG, Mitsionis G, Giannakopoulos PN, Soteranos DG (1998) Wrist arthroscopy for the treatment of ligament and triangular fibrocartilage complex injuries. Arthroscopy 14(5):479–483
6. Weiss AP, Sachar K, Glowaski KA (1997) Arthroscopic debridement alone for intercarpal ligament tears. J Hand Surg Am 22(2):344–349
7. Rush DS, Poehling GG (1996) Arthroscopic management of partial scapholunate and lunotriquetral injuries of the wrist. J Hand Surg Am 21(3):412–417
8. Whipple TL (1995) The role of arthroscopy in the treatment of scapholunate instability. Hand Clin 11:37–40
9. Wintman BI, Gelberman R, Katz JN (1995) Dynamic scapholunate instability: results of operative treatment. J Hand Surg Am 20:971–979
10. Linscheid RL, Dobyns JH (1991) Treatment for scapholunate dissociation. Hand Clin 8: 645–652
11. Geissler W, Haley T (2001) Arthroscopic management of scapholunate instability. Atlas Hand Clin 6(2):253–274
12. Brunelli GA, Brunelli GR (1995) A new technique to correct carpal instability with scaphoid rotary subluxation: a preliminary report. J Hand Surg 20A:S82–S83
13. Blatt G (1987) Capsulodesis in reconstructive hand surgery. Dorsal capsulodesis for the unstable scaphoid and volar capsulodesis following excision of the distal ulna. Hand Clin 3: 81–102

Berger's Capsulodesis with Dorsal Intercarpal Ligament in Chronic Scapholunate Instability

N. Dréant

When a completely torn scapholunate ligament is associated with a deficiency of the distal joints of the scaphoid base, there is a scapholunate instability. A scapholunate diastasis, a lunate extension (DISI) and a rotary subluxation of the scaphoid appear. When this pathologic flexion of the scaphoid (radio-scaphoidal angle >45°) is still reducible, and before arthrosis appears, preserving treatments aiming at reconstructing good scapholunate congruence are indicated [1]. Among the different capsular techniques, tendinous or ligamentous as proposed in literature, one of them, as described by R. Berger [2] particularly called our attention and is to be explained.

1 Wrist Arthroscopy

Before ligamentoplasty as such is made, arthroscopy is systematically made on an unstable and painful wrist. It aims at seeing the stump of the scapholunate ligament and making sure it cannot heal anymore. Arthroscopy is useful to test the good reducibility of flexion of the scaphoid, which must be easy, as it slightly presses on the capital facet of the scaphoid thanks to the hook palpator which is introduced in midcarpal. Finally, it enables to examine all the cartilages, especially the proximal pole of the scaphoid, the scaphoidal facet of the radius and the radial styloid, since they are the first to be affected by arthrosis [3]. If arthroscopic data confirm the resort to a scapholunate ligamentoplasty, the technique consisting in using the intercarpal ligament is thus proposed.

N. Dréant
Pole Urgence Main Nice,
10 Bd Pasteur, Nice 06000, France
e-mail: ndreant@sfr.fr

E. Camus, L. Van Overstraeten (eds.), *Carpal Ligament Surgery*,
DOI 10.1007/978-2-8178-0379-1_21, © Springer-Verlag France 2013

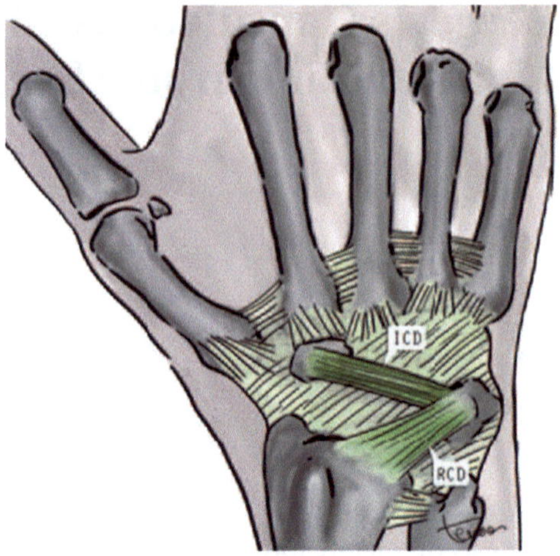

Fig. 1 The dorsal radio-carpal (DRC) and dorsal inter-carpal (DIC) ligaments

2 Surgical Technique

Under locoregional anaesthesia and tourniquet placed at the base of the arm, the portal is dorsal and transversal as it joins the radiocarpal entry points of the arthroscopy (3–4 and 4–5 portals). This is a variant of the original technique which sole interest is to be more aesthetic since it is in the bend of extension of the wrist, especially when the patient is a young woman. The retinaculum of the extensors is split lengthwise in its distal half, between the third and fourth compartment. There is a systematic avulsion of the posterior interosseous nerve.

R. Berger [4] insisted on the importance of the osseous landmarks before beginning the capsulotomy, and we follow these indications. The idea is to make a portal respecting the dorsal radiocarpal (DRC) and dorsal intercarpal (DIC) ligaments (Fig. 1).

These landmarks are (Fig. 2):

1. The middle of the section between Lister's tubercle and the radioulnar joint, which gives the centre of the radial joint of the DRC ligament
2. The top of the dorsal tubercle of the triquetrum, towards which the DRC and the DIC ligaments converge
3. The scapho-trapezial joint, which gives the distal insertion zone of the DIC ligament

Thus, the capsule is lifted as if it were a flange with a distal joint. The proximal half of the DIC ligament is also lifted on its scaphoidal joint (Fig. 3).

Two 1.2 mm diameter Joystick pins are placed in the scaphoid and the lunate (Fig. 4) and used to reduce the scapholunate diastasis, the flexion of the scaphoid and the extension of the lunate (Fig. 5). Two parallel pins maintain the reducing of the scapholunate couple, and a scaphocapitate pin cancels out the strengths which create the flexion of the scaphoid (Fig. 6). The DIC ligament is thus introduced on the posterior horn of the lunate thanks to an intraosseous anchor (Fig. 7).

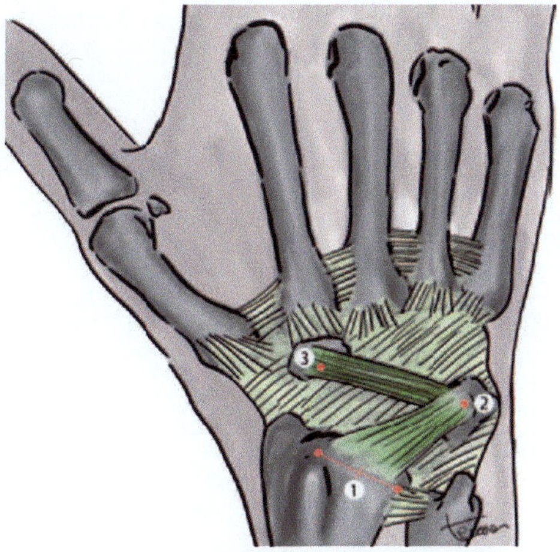

Fig. 2 The landmarks of the capsulotomy

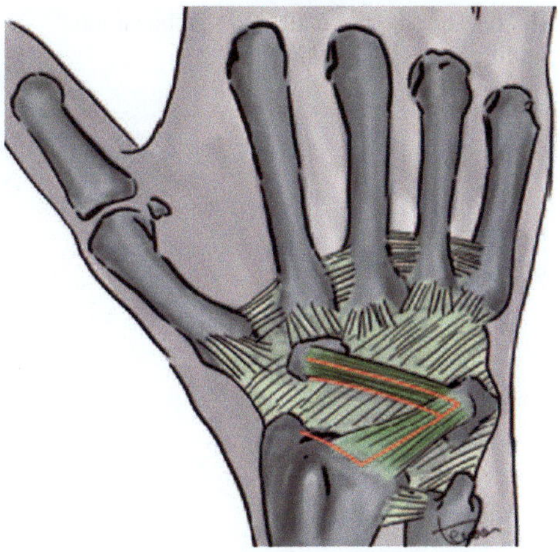

Fig. 3 The drawing of the capsular flaps

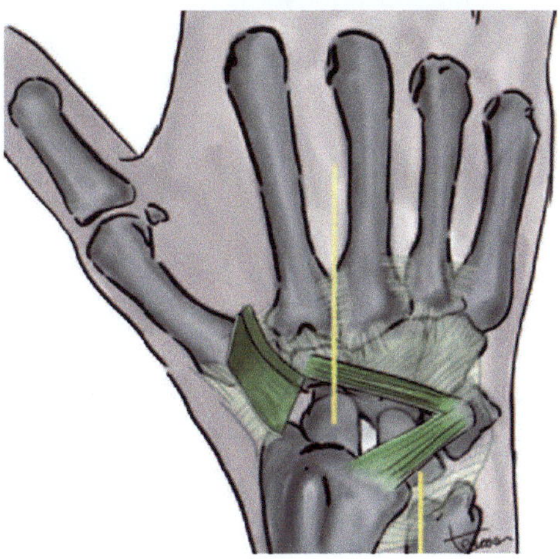

Fig. 4 The two joystick pins placed in the scaphoid and the lunat

Fig. 5 The reduction maneuver

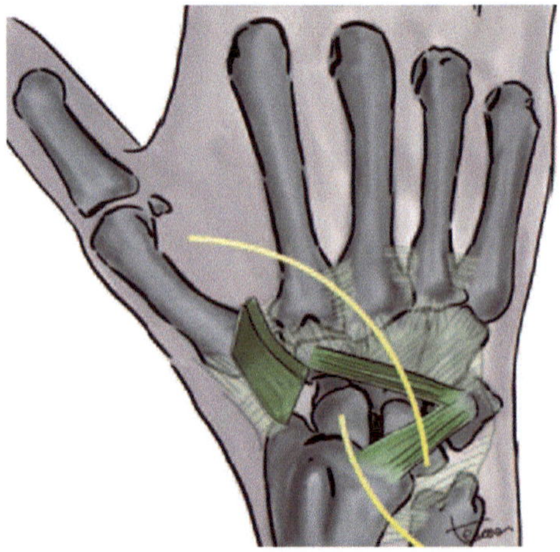

Fig. 6 The scapholunate and scaphocapitate pinning

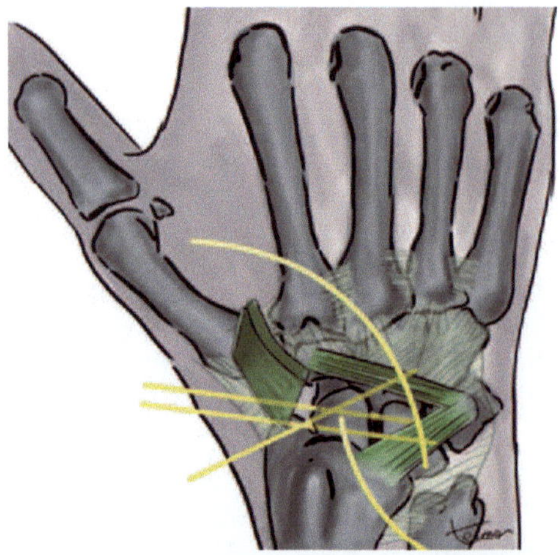

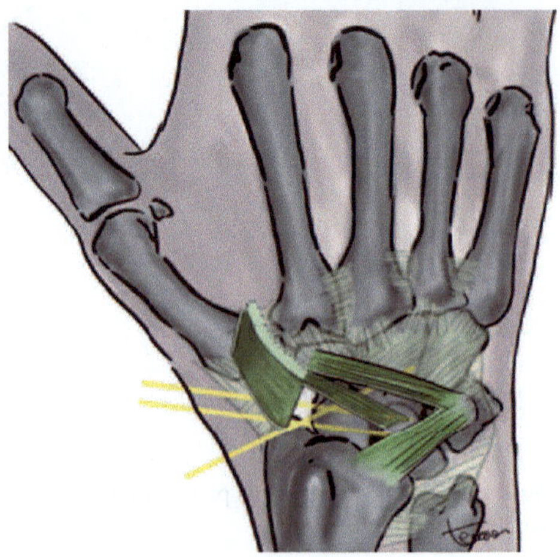

Fig. 7 The anchoring of the DIC ligament

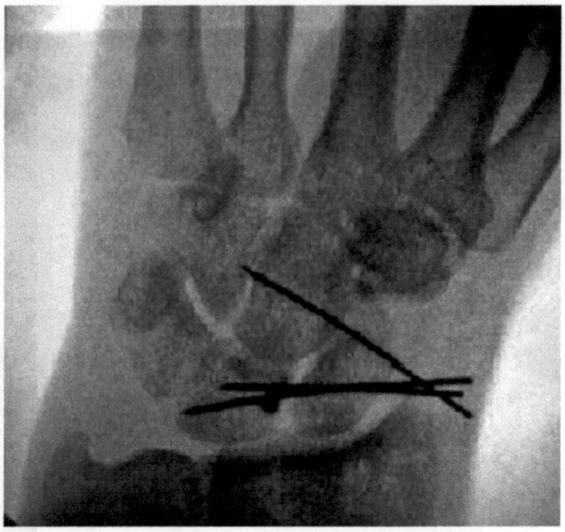

Fig. 8 The pins are cut under the skin

The triquetral's tip of the capsular flap is sutured thanks to a resorbing thread. It seems to us that this anatomic capsular suture *a minima* minimizes the loss of flexion of the wrist.

The retinaculum of the extensors is closed in the proximal half of its open section. The pins are cut under the skin so that they hamper the patient as less as possible (Fig. 8) and are removed 6 weeks later. An antebrachia-palmar splint in neutral position of the wrist which completely frees the metacarpophalangeal joints of the long fingers and the thumb is carried during 6 weeks.

When the pins are removed, a soft and progressive physiotherapy of the wrist begins.

3 Clinical Series

3.1 Material and Method

Our experience of this surgery rests on 40 patients among which 25 have been examined again about 41 months later. They were operated by the same surgeon between January 2002 and January 2007. They all suffered from a chronic scapholunate instability with a traumatic origin dating back to more than 3 months. The average age was 28. The delay between the trauma and the surgery was about 10 months (3 months to 5 years). Each patient was clinically evaluated in preoperative and 3, 6, 12 and 24 months after the surgery by a same independent observer who uses the computer system EVAL.

The ranges in flexion-extension and in radial and ulnar inclination of the painful wrist and the healthy wrist were reported, as well as grip strength thanks to Jamar's dynamometer.

The comparative static and dynamic radiographic report was systematically established at the same periods. The dynamic report was composed of a view in

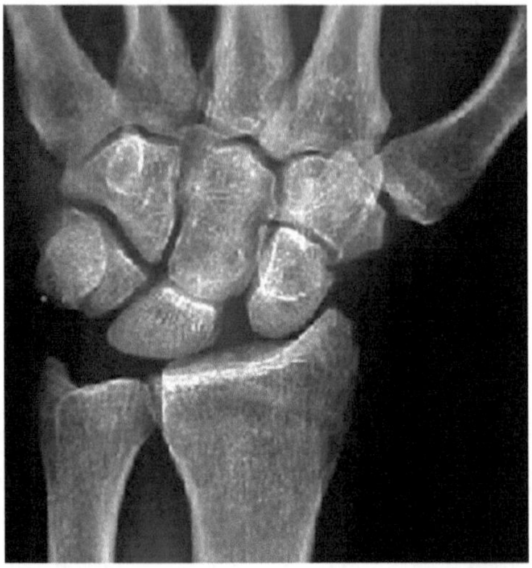

Fig. 9 Radiographic static instability

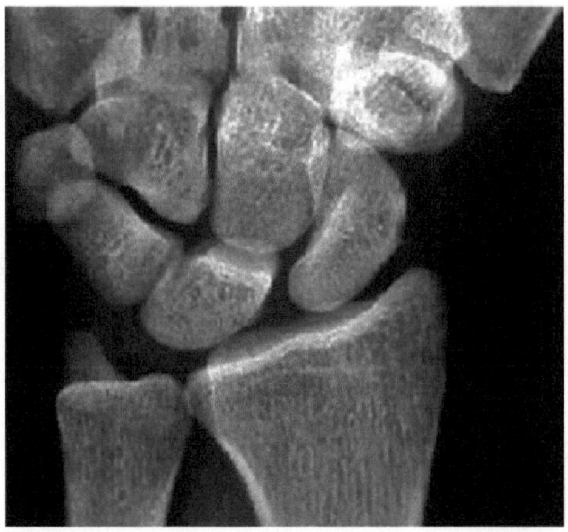

Fig. 10 Radiographic dynamic instability

radial inclination, a view in ulnar inclination and a view in supination with clenched fist. Twelve patients had a static instability (Fig. 9) and 13 had a dynamic instability (Fig. 10). The radio-lunate and scapholunate angles as well as the scapholunate interval were measured for each series of views at the different periods.

Each patient benefited from wrist arthroscopy to quantify the degree of instability following Dautel's classification [5] and to check the absence of arthrosis, the correct reducibility of flexion of the scaphoid and the absence of associated ligamentous injury.

Eighteen instabilities were stage 3 and 7 were stage 2. The surgical technique which was used was the one described above.

Three complications should be reported in this series: 2 superficial sepses on the pins which did not imply the early removal of the material. One patient had to be reoperated 2 years later for a curettage and to fill a cyst of the lunate which appeared around a resorbing anchor, but without consequence on the efficiency on the capsulodesis.

Table 1 Compared results with other series

	Moran (Brunelli)	Moran (Berger)	Garcia-Elias (tenodesis 3LT)	Talwalkar (tenodesis 3LT)	Chabas (modified Brunelli)	Dreant (Berger)
Moderate pain 0–3	27 %	43 %	73 %	62 %	80 %	58 %
Extension	43°	49°	52°	55°	50°	56°
Flexion	40°	44°	51°	45°	41°	48°
Radial inclination	16°	19°	16°	18°	24°	22°
Ulnar inclination	26°	26°	29°	29°	29°	30°
Grip strength	87 %	91 %	65 %	80 %	78 %	88 %
Scapholunate interval	2–6 mm	4 mm			2–4 mm	3 mm
Scapholunate angle	54°	66°			62°	64°

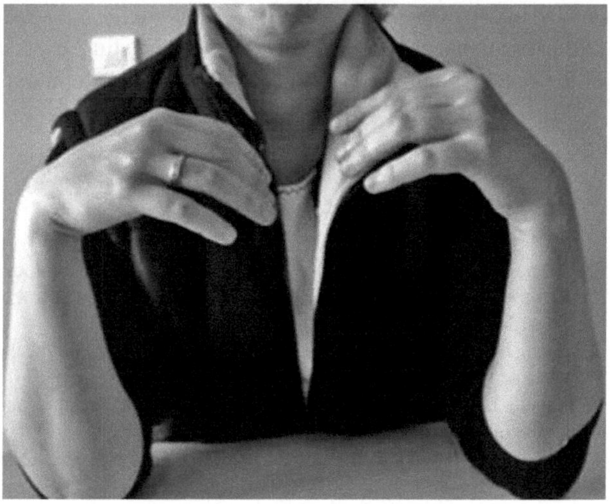

Fig. 11 Clinical result in palmar flexion

4 Results

The authors compared their results to the series of tenodesis to the flexor carpi radialis by Moran et al. [6], Garcia-Elias et al. [1], Talwalkar et al. [7], Chabas et al. [8] and the series of capsulodesis to the dorsal intercarpal ligament by Berger and Moran et al. [6] for the treatment of chronic scapholunate instability (Table 1).

5 Discussion

The benefit as far as strength and pain is the same as the other series. Post-operatory ranges of the wrist in flexion and in extension are less diminished with this technique. Thus, it can be considered as a therapeutic option to recover a stability of the scapholunate couple, since it is efficient and engenders little stiffening (Figs. 11 and 12). The exam

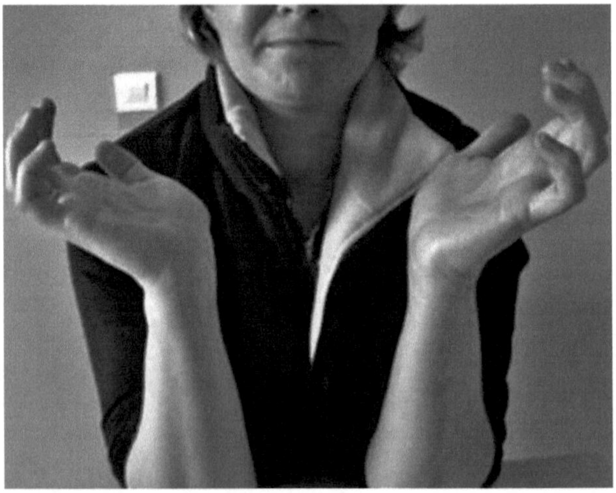

Fig. 12 Clinical result in dorsal flexion

of these patients in 10 years will be very interesting, especially as far as the maintenance of the scapholunate interval and the possible development of arthrosis are concerned.

References

1. Garcia-Elias M, Lluch A, Stanley JK (2006) Three-ligament tenodesis for the treatment of scapholunate dissociation: indications and surgical technique. J Hand Surg 31A: 125–134
2. Walsh JJ, Berger RA, Cooney WP (2002) Current status of scapholunate interosseous ligament injuries. J Am Acad Orthop Surg 10:32–42
3. Watson HK, Ballet FL (1984) The SLAC wrist: scapholunate advanced collapse pattern of degenerative arthritis. J Hand Surg 9A:358–365
4. Berger RA (2007) Palpable landmarks for dorsal wrist capsulotomy. J Hand Surg 32A: 1291–1295
5. Dreant N, Dautel G (2003) Development of an arthroscopic severity score for scapholunate instability. Chir Main 22(2):90–94
6. Moran SL, Ford KS, Wulf CA, Cooney WP (2006) Outcomes of dorsal capsulodesis and tenodesis for treatment of scapholunate instability. J Hand Surg 31A:1438–1446
7. Talwalkar SC, Edwards AT, Hayton MJ, Stilwell JH, Trail IA, Stanley JK (2006) Results of tri-ligament tenodesis: a modified brunelli procedure in the management of scapholunate instability. J Hand Surg Br 31(1):110–117
8. Chabas JF, Gay A, Valenti D, Guinard D, Legre R (2008) Results of the modified brunelli tenodesis for treatment of scapholunate instability: a retrospective study of 19 patients. J Hand Surg Am 33(9):1469–1477

Dorsal Scapholunate Capsulodesis: Viegas' Technique

E. Camus

1 Introduction

The existence of scapholunate instability signifies an association of intrinsic scapholunate ligament lesion and lesions of the extrinsic carpal stabilizing ligaments [1–8]. Many techniques for scapholunate stabilization have been described ranging from simple pinning [9] to wrist arthrodesis [10–12] including ligament repairs [13] and a variety of capsulodesis and tenodesis techniques [14].

After studying the dorsal carpal ligaments [1, 15], Viegas described a transverse dorsal capsulodesis technique [16] using the dorsal intercarpal ligament to reinforce the dorsal component of the interosseous scapholunate ligament.

2 Technique

Once the diagnosis of scapholunate instability is established – arthroscopically if need be – the indication of performing this technique depends on the duration of the lesion, its irreparability and the degree of laxity of the ligament. Anaesthesia is locoregional or general. The patient lies supine with the hand on an arm table. The hand is in pronation, with slight wrist flexion and positioned on a rolled crepe bandage. Under tourniquet, a longitudinal midline incision parallel to the finger extensors is used. Hemostasis is performed using bipolar diathermy and the extensor retinaculum is incised through the fourth extensor compartment. The radial border is dissected off Lister's tubercle exposing EPL followed by the radial wrist extensors. The EDC tendons are retracted ulnarly, while the radial extensors and EPL are

E. Camus
Hand Surgery Unit, SELARL Chirurgie de la Main, Polyclinique du Val de Sambre, 162, route de Mons, 59600 Maubeuge, France
e-mail: ejcamus@wanadoo.fr, emmanuel.camus@wanadoo.fr

E. Camus, L. Van Overstraeten (eds.), *Carpal Ligament Surgery*,
DOI 10.1007/978-2-8178-0379-1_22, © Springer-Verlag France 2013

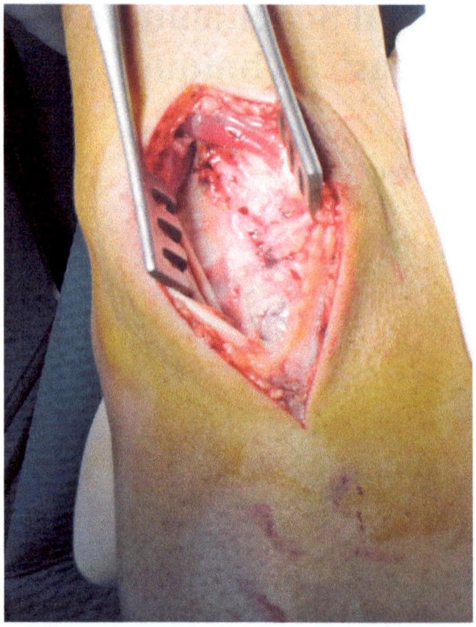

Fig. 1 Capsular exposure

retracted radially to expose the capsule (Fig. 1). The posterior interosseous nerve is identified at the dorsal border of the radius and resected about 1 cm proximally after coagulation. Fatty tissue covering the capsule may be resected to facilitate identification of the fibres. The dorsal intercarpal band of fibres of the dorsal intercarpal ligament (DICL) should then be identified palpating with fine closed forceps to mark the transverse thickening of fibres firmer than the rest of the capsule. Berger described specific landmarks to identify the bands of the dorsal ligament [17]. The capsule is incised at the proximal margin of this dorsal intercarpal ligament (Fig. 2a–b). The posterior aspects of the scaphoid and lunate are thus exposed and the scapholunate ligament lesion is identified. The dorsal pole of the scaphoid is usually subluxed dorsally and may be reduced by axial traction on the hand, pushing the proximal pole anteriorly – possibly using a K-wire as a 'joystick'. The lunate is likewise reduced by axial traction. If this is insufficient, wrist flexion will correct the lunate position which is maintained using a temporary radiolunate 1.6 mm K-wire. A scapholunate pinning is done with a 1.2 mm K-wire, completed using a scaphocapitate K-wire.

The dorsal intercarpal ligament is then prepared for reinsertion. After a chronic lesion, it is found to be retracted lying more distal to its anatomical position over the lunate and the dorsal groove of the scaphoid, and usually adherent to the carpus [16]. It can be dissected off using the scalpel, taking care not to section it (Fig. 3). The scaphoid groove and the dorsal horn of the lunate are freshened using a rasper (Fig. 4). The dorsal intercarpal ligament can now be transferred to the dorsal scapholunate interval. If the capsule is retracted and the DICL cannot be properly mobilized, it can be detached from the rest of the capsule by an incision parallel to the initial one (Fig. 5), along its distal border. Once it is at the scapholunate interval,

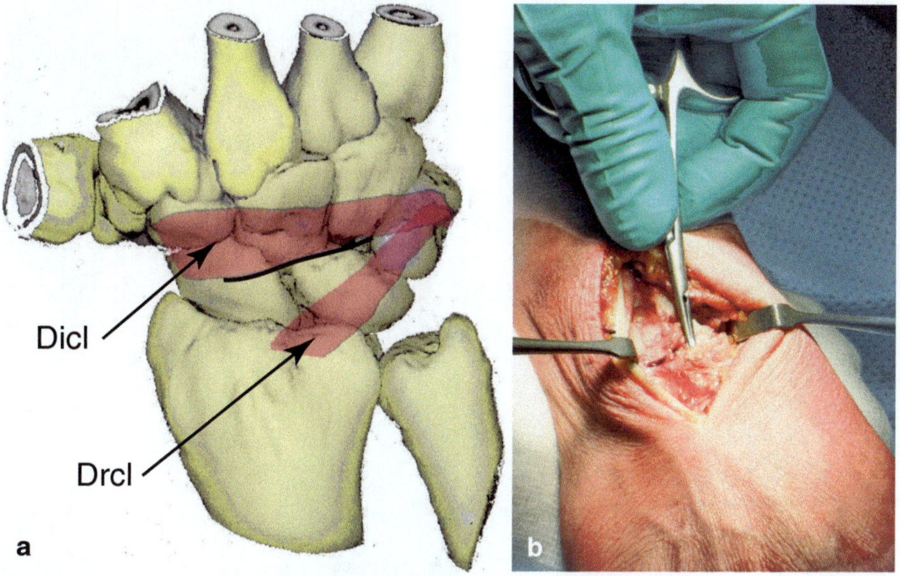

Fig. 2 (**a**) Dorsal capsular incision. *DRCL* dorsal radiocarpal ligament, *DICL* dorsal intercarpal ligament, — Capsular incision. (**b**) Dorsal capsular incision

Fig. 3 Detachment of dorsal intercarpal ligament (*DICL*). (*LICD*): Dorsal Inter Carpal Ligament. *Sca* scaphoïd, *Lu* lunatum

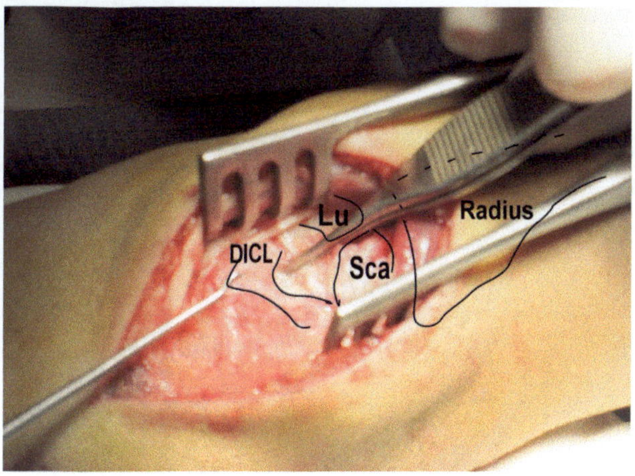

it is secured by two anchors, sometimes three or four, taking care to maintain transverse tension on the fibres of the DICL to maintain reduction and keep the scapholunate junction closed (Fig. 6).

The transverse capsular incisions are left open so as not to limit postoperative wrist flexion. Once the tendons are repositioned, the retinaculum is repaired by two x stitches with braided absorbable 2/0 suture. The K-wire is cut but kept long enough so that EPL does not pass over it and rupture. The skin is sutured using simple

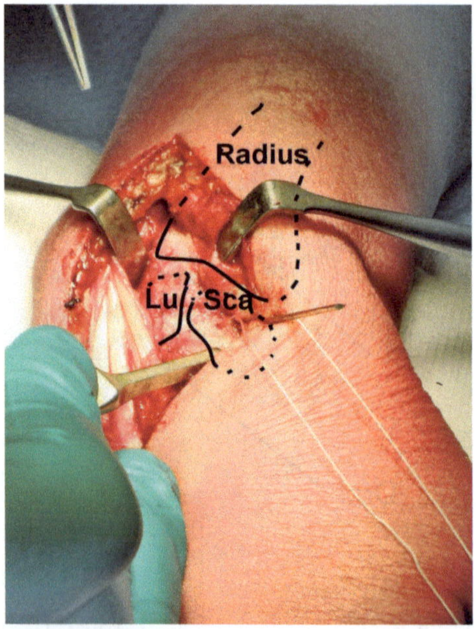

Fig. 4 Freshening of the scaphoid groove using a rasper. Scapholunate pinning and scaphoid anchor are in place. *Sca* scaphoïd, *Lu* lunatum

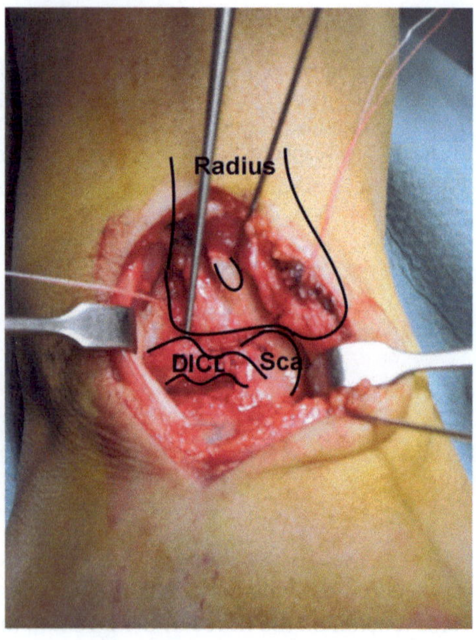

Fig. 5 Proximal transfer of DICL. *Sca* scaphoïd

stitches of nonabsorbable 4/0 monofilament over a drain. If the patient is compliant, a simple enforced removable splint is placed, facilitating dressings and allowing forearm swelling and remission. Fingers are allowed mobilization in space with no grip or loading to avoid any distraction at the scapholunate interval.

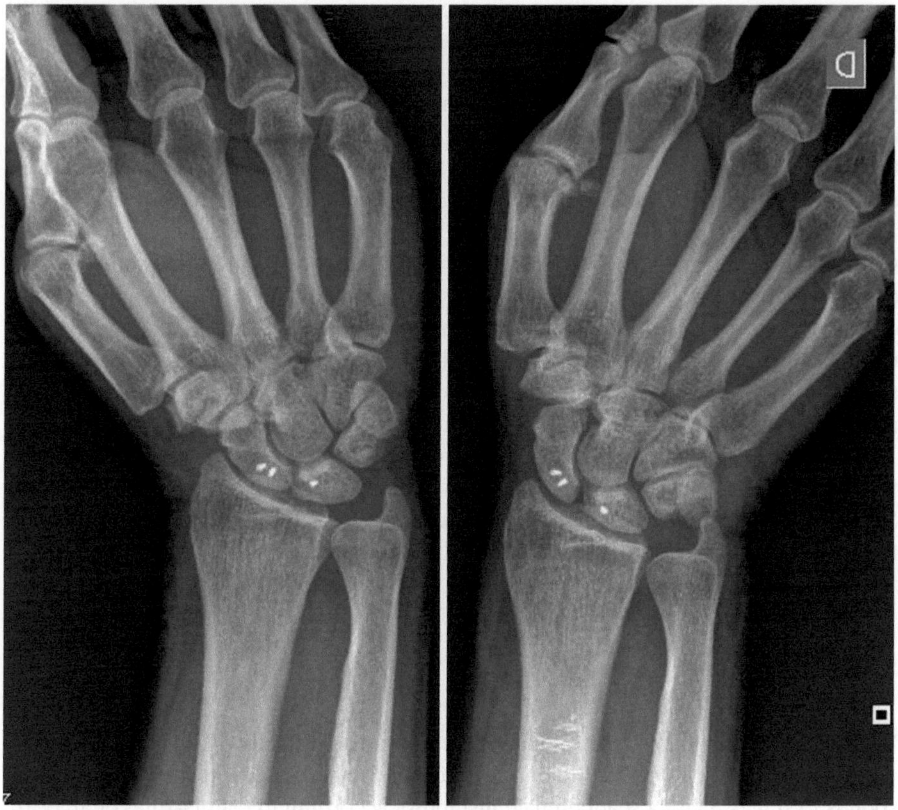

Fig. 6 Appearance on X-ray showing good scapho-lunate stability and motion

3 Preliminary Results of Our Series

We present results of our first 14 cases, with average follow-up of 21 months (18–31). There are 10 men of average age 31 years (19–42) and 4 women of average age 28 years (21–36). The average preoperative delay was 8 months (3–14). There were nine work-related accidents and five domestic accidents.

The procedure consisted of a capsulodesis with 2 anchors 8 times, 3 anchors 3 times, 4 anchors twice and 5 anchors once (suture breakage).

At follow-up wrist ROM was recorded. There was 49.8° flexion, 53.2° extension, 23° radial deviation and 40° ulnar deviation. The grip was 27.8 kgf; Pain using VAS (score 1–10) was 1.94 with preoperative pain score at 6.57. The PRWE global score moved from 58.2/150 preoperative to 25.4/150 postoperative. Ten patients had very good or good results, three satisfactory and one bad result.

There were four skin irritations cured by wire removal and one EPL irritation without rupture. Two cutaneous dysaesthesias disappeared at 4 and 9 months post-operative. One patient developed a stage 2 SLAC lesion at 30 months, not shown on X-ray but confirmed by scintigraphy and second look arthroscopy.

4 Discussion

Scapholunate instability is the most common carpal instability [16] due to concentrated loading on the carpus at this point [20]. By far, the commonest treatment is the Blatt capsulodesis [21, 22]. But results are disappointing. Capsulodesis does not suppress the pain nor the radiological misalignment and causes a clear decrease in wrist flexion [23, 24]. It seemed logical to design a capsulodesis more respectful of the physiological isometry of the wrist. Since it has been stated that the strongest component of the scapholunate ligament is the dorsal one [18, 19], we have considered a ligamentoplasty that is transverse and not axial. The Viegas' technique meets these requisites. The choice of the dorsal intercarpal ligament is also interesting since it is more resistant than the interosseous scapholunate ligament and thus more adapted to replacing it [15].

Clinical results do not give complete recovery; however, 10 out of 14 patients were satisfied or very satisfied with their outcome. Bad result corresponds to the SLAC lesion developed. These are only preliminary results; the sample size and follow-up time are not sufficient to draw definite conclusions.

5 Indications

We use this technique for cases of chronic scapholunate instability – dynamic or static – where the scaphoid is reducible and no arthritis is seen on arthroscopy. This corresponds to stages 3 and 4 scapholunate instability according to Garcia-Elias et al. [25].

References

1. Mitsuyasu H, Patterson RM, Shah MA, Buford WL, Iwamoto Y, Viegas SF (2004) The role of the dorsal intercarpal ligament in dynamic and static scapholunate instability. J Hand Surg 29A:279–288
2. Short WH, Werner FW, Fortino MD, Palmer AK, Mann KA (1995) A dynamic biomechanical study of scapholunate ligament sectioning. J Hand Surg 20A:986–999
3. Short WH, Werner FW, Green JK, Masaoka S (2002) Biomechanical evaluation of ligamentous stabilizers of the scaphoid and lunate: part 1. J Hand Surg 27A:991–1002
4. Short WH, Werner FW, Green JK, Masaoka S (2005) Biomechanical evaluation of ligamentous stabilizers of the scaphoid and lunate: part 2. J Hand Surg 30A:24–34
5. Short WH, Werner FW, Green JK, Sutton LG, Brutus JP (2007) Biomechanical evaluation of ligamentous stabilizers of the scaphoid and lunate: part 3. J Hand Surg 32A:297.e1–297.e18
6. Kuo CE, Wolfe SW (2008) Scapholunate instability: current concepts in diagnosis and management. J Hand Surg 33A:998–1013
7. Szabo RM, Slater RR, Palumbo CF, Gerlach T (2002) Dorsal intercarpal ligament capsulodesis for chronic, static scapholunate dissociation: clinical results. J Hand Surg 27A:978–984
8. Gajendran VK, Peterson B, Slater RR Jr, Szabo RM (2007) Long-term outcomes of dorsal intercarpal ligament capsulodesis for chronic scapholunate dissociation. J Hand Surg 32A: 1323–1333

9. Palmer AK, Dobyns JH, Linscheid RL (1978) Management of post-traumatic instability of the wrist secondary to ligament rupture. J Hand Surg Am 3:507–532
10. Watson HK, Ryu J, Akelman E (1986) Limited triscaphoid intercarpal arthrodesis for rotatory subluxation of the scaphoid. J Bone Joint Surg Am 68-A:345–349
11. Hom S, Ruby LK (1991) Attempted scapholunate arthrodesis for chronic scapholunate dissociation. J Hand Surg 16A:334–339
12. Pisano SM, Peimer CA, Wheeler DR, Sherwin F (1991) Scaphocapitate intercarpal arthrodesis. J Hand Surg 16A:328–333
13. Lavernia CJ, Cohen MS, Taleisnik J (1992) Treatment of scapholunate dissociation by ligamentous repair and capsulodesis. J Hand Surg 17A:354–359
14. Garcia-Elias M, Geissler WB (2005) Carpal instability. In: Green DP, Hotchkiss RN, Pederson WC, Wolfe S (eds) Green's operative hand surgery, vol 1, 5th edn. Elsevier/Churchill Livingstone, Philadelphia, pp 535–604
15. Viegas SF, Yamaguchi S, Boyd NL, Patterson RM (1999) The dorsal ligaments of the wrist: anatomy, mechanical properties and function. J Hand Surg 24A:456–468
16. Viegas SF, DaSilva M (2000) Surgical repair for scapholunate dissociation. Tech Hand Up Extrem Surg 4(3):148–153
17. Berger RA (2007) A method of defining palpable landmarks for the ligament-splitting dorsal wrist capsulotomy. J Hand Surg 32A:1291–1295
18. Berger RA (1996) The gross and histologic anatomy of the scapholunate interosseous ligament. J Hand Surg 21A:170–178
19. Berger RA, Imeada T, Berglund L, An KN (1999) Constraint and material properties of the subregions of the scapholunate interosseous ligament. J Hand Surg 24A:953–962
20. Camus EJ (2004) Biomécanique du scaphoïde. In: Lussiez B, Rizzo C, Lebreton E (eds) Le scaphoïde de la fracture à l'arthrose. Sauramps Médical, Montpellier, pp 45–54
21. Zarkadas PC, Gropper PT, White NJ, Perey BH (2004) A survey of the surgical management of acute and chronic scapholunate instability. J Hand Surg 29A:848–857
22. Blatt G (1987) Capsulodesis in reconstructive hand surgery. Dorsal capsulodesis for the unstable scaphoid and volar capsulodesis following excision of the distal ulna. Hand Clin 3(1): 81–102
23. Wyrick JD, Youse BD, Kiefhaber TR (1998) Scapholunate ligament repair and capsulodesis for the treatment of static scapholunate dissociation. J Hand Surg 23B:776–780
24. Deshmukh SC, Givissis P, Belloso D, Stanley JK, Trail IA (1999) Blatt's capsulodesis for chronic scapholunate dissociation. J Hand Surg 24B(2):215–220
25. Garcia-Elias M, Lluch AL, Stanley JK (2006) Three-ligament tenodesis for the treatment of scapholunate dissociation: indications and surgical technique. J Hand Surg 31A:125–134

The Capsulo-Fibrodesis: Horizontal Proximal Carpal Row Retightening Capsulodesis with Scapholunate 'Fibrodesis' – A New Surgical Option for Scapholunate Dissociation

O. Delattre, S. Joulie, J. Vogels, C. Alexieva, L. Stratan, and F. Duroux

Many techniques have been described for the treatment of pre-arthrosis scapholunate instabilities whether they consist in capsulodesis or tenodeses. All these techniques' aim is to correct the scaphoid rotatory subluxation, making it vertical again and closing the scapholunate gap. The multiplicity of the techniques is the consequence of their doubtful result on the repositioning of the scaphoid. Radiocarpal capsulodesis has the theoretical drawback to be efficient only when the wrist is placed in flexion and may limit wrist mobility in flexion. Scaphocapitate arthrodesis, which is still unknown to us, is efficient to straighten the scaphoid but at the expense of a significant stiffening of the wrist. The scaphocapitate arthrodesis probably less stiffens the wrist but the level of nonunion is close to 50 % due to the small size of the joint surfaces which are treated, but remains an interesting option to eliminate the scapholunate gap. Recent works insist on the importance of the dorsal intercarpal ligament (DIC) injuries associated with the scapholunate ligamentous injury [1]. Intercarpal capsulodesis which has recently been described by Berger [3] and Viegas [2] takes this notion into account. As we were inspired by the strong points of these two techniques and convinced, it really was a carpal ligamentous problem (intrinsic and extrinsic) and not a radiocarpal problem; we recently directed towards a new technique of dorsal intercarpal capsulodesis with retightening of the DIC by an overcoat suture (suture en paletot), associated with a scapholunate fibrodesis.

O. Delattre (✉) • S. Joulie • J. Vogels • C. Alexieva • L. Stratan • F. Duroux
Hand Surgery Unit,
CHU et SOS mains de Fort-de-France,
BP 63297200 Fort-de-France, Martinique
e-mail: olivier.delattre@chu-fortdefrance.fr; jerome.vogels@gmail.com

E. Camus, L. Van Overstraeten (eds.), *Carpal Ligament Surgery*,
DOI 10.1007/978-2-8178-0379-1_23, © Springer-Verlag France 2013

The big difference with the Viegas procedure is the longitudinal incision made over wrist capsule in the DIC, leaving a radial- and an ulnar-based flap, which permits this dishing and overcoat suture with an important retightening of the complete first carpal row. This capsulodesis is done after reduction of the scapholunate gap with a solid double osteosuture with one or more suture anchors placed in the proximal part of the scaphoïd and the lunate. These scapholunate osteosutures are tied after resecting the cartilage of the scapholunate joint. This is the second particularity of our procedure, the so-called scapholunate fibrodesis.

1 Scapholunate 'Fibrodesis'

It consists in a complete resection of the cartilage of the scaphoid articular facet of the lunate and the lunar articular facet of the scaphoid with several perforations down to the spongious bone. This accurate exposure of the articular surfaces is followed by a trans-articular osteosuture (thanks to anchors which are placed into the articular facets). The aim is to at close the scapholunate gap and to maintain, in time, this reduction as a fibrosis is created. This is not a bone fusion as the aim is not to block this joint, this would be antiphysiological, but to maintain the scapholunate gap closed thanks to fibrosis and thus to keep this joint space mobile. Hence, the name of fibrodesis seemed more appropriate to us. Thus, the idea is to close the scapholunate gap and to try and increase the chances to maintain the gap closed as long as possible with a fibrosis of all the articular facets and not only with the scapholunate ligament which remnants are sutured at the same time.

2 Horizontal First Carpal Row Retightening Capsulodesis

It is a horizontal retightening of the DIC ligament which will be overcoat sutured after a longitudinal incision at the base of the scapholunate interval at the beginning of the surgery during the radiocarpal capsulotomy which, in our technique, remains longitudinal (vertical). As fibrodesis is prepared, the ulnar traction exerced on the radial flap of the dorsal intercarpal ligament enabled a satisfactory reduction of the scapholunate gap and to correct the horizontality of the scaphoid. This ulnar traction on the radial flap of the DIC is perpetuated by an overcoat suture under tension in ulnar strip of this extrinsic ligament. The threads of the osteosuture of the fibrodesis are tightened and come to lay down by two U-shape points this dorsal intercarpal ligament which is retightened on the scapholunate space (Figs. 1 and 2).

Two technical details seem important to us:

1. The two DIC flaps are made at the beginning of the surgery and are high on purpose (between 8 and 10 mm long): it is important to remember that at the beginning of a surgery, it is not always easy to see the DIC whether it is a healthy or *a fortiori* a post-traumatic wrist. We locate the 'efficient' section of the radial strip as we

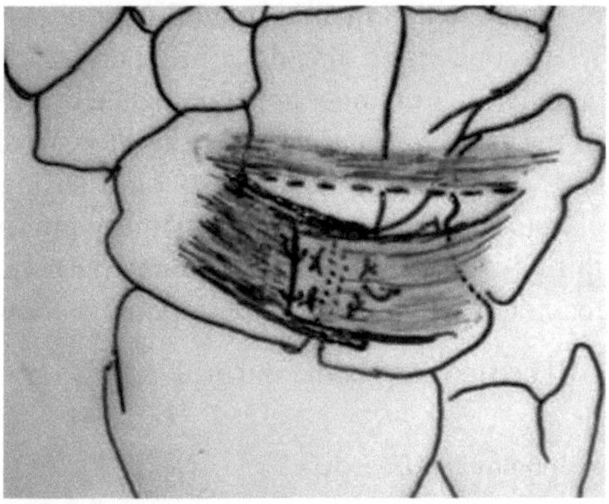

Fig. 1 Diagram demonstrating the horizontal retightening capsulodesis by dishing or suture 'en paletot' of the dorsal intercarpal ligament, with placement of the sutures

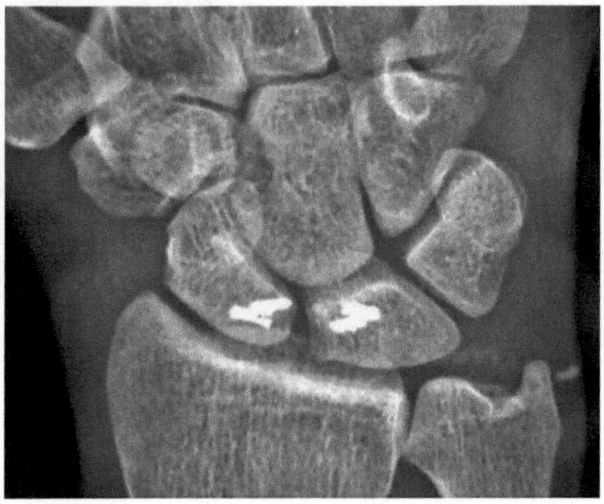

Fig. 2 Anteroposterior radiograph demonstrating the placement of the suture's anchors and the closing of the scapholunate gap at 2 years after surgery

isolate the strongest section which enables, by traction, to straighten the scaphoid. The ulnar flap takes the distal one-third of the radiocarpal ligament with the proximal part of the DIC, which thus reinforces it and enables a strong overcoat suture of the two flaps and an efficient retention to reposition the scaphoid.

2. To correct the dorsal bascule of the lunate, we end the surgery by a 'dorsal complementary capsulodesis' between the two carpal rows with a suture between the dorsal side of the lunate through the re-tensed dorsal intercarpal ligament and the distal capsule at the level of the capitate. Moreover, this surgery enables to close the articular capsule of the carpus while it is never made at the radiocarpal level. The wrist is immobilized in extension on a resin cast during 6 weeks.

3 Conclusion

This recent technique has to be ratified by a clinical study under way once more time has passed. It seems to be efficient on the long term to maintain the reduction of the scapholunate gap and the verticalization of the scaphoid. Better results are observed with dynamic instabilities and with a relatively poor loss of mobility of the wrist concerning the flexion. Acute or chronic injuries that have not developed degenerative changes are approached by this technique. The intraoperative efficiency of the retightening of the dorsal intercarpal ligament associated with this new concept of fibrodesis which rests on a strong osteosuture encouraged us to abandon classic scapholunate complementary pin fixation in certain cases with good reductibility of the scaphoïd. We show you here the three different steps of this surgical technique illustrated by intraoperative views.

The first step is the intrinsic time:

Scapholunate 'fibrodesis'

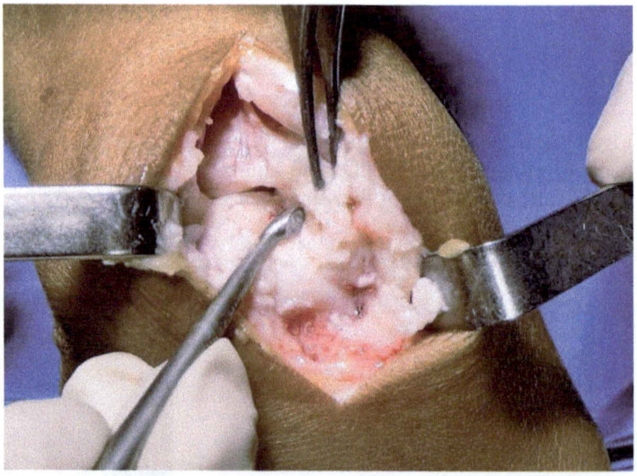

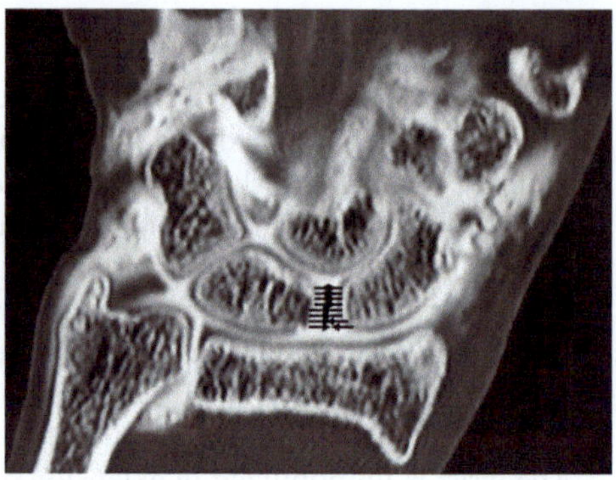

Complete resection of the cartilage of the scapholunate joint with several perforations down to the spongy bone

Second step is intrinsic time too:

Anchors in scaphoid and lunate with double osteosuture. We can see a good closing of the gap in this case

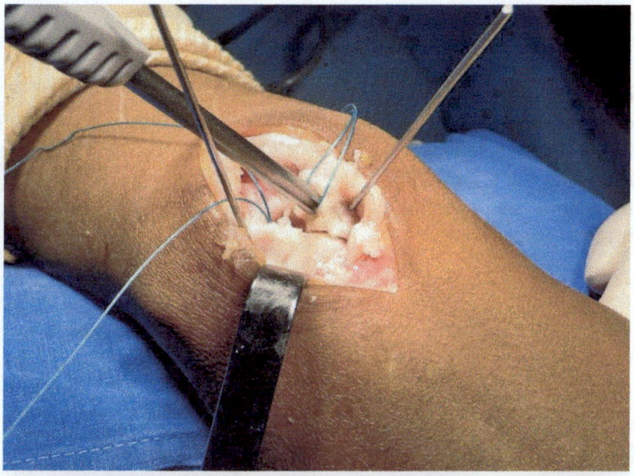

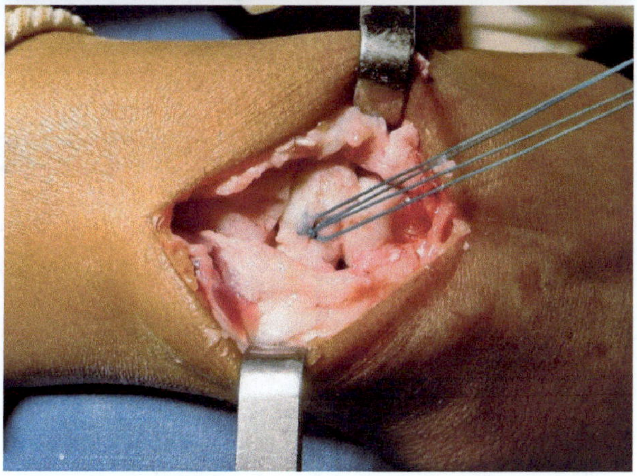

The third step is the extrinsic time: horizontal first carpal row retightening *capsulodesis*. For this capsulodesis, it is necessary to make a longitudinal capsulotomy at the beginning of the procedure

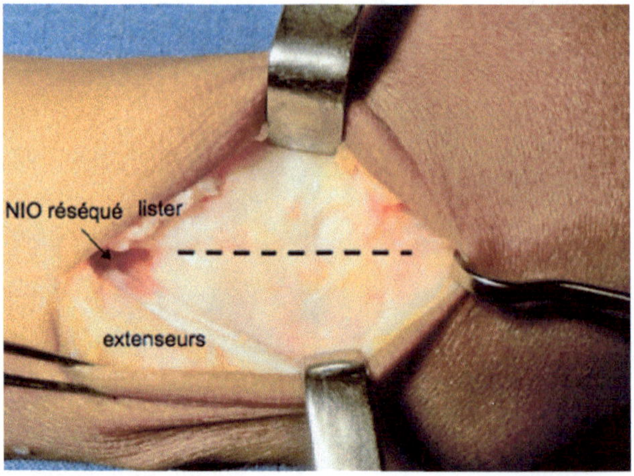

Drawing of the longitudinal capsulotomy just ulnar to Lister's tubercle after resecting the terminal branch of the posterior interosseous nerve

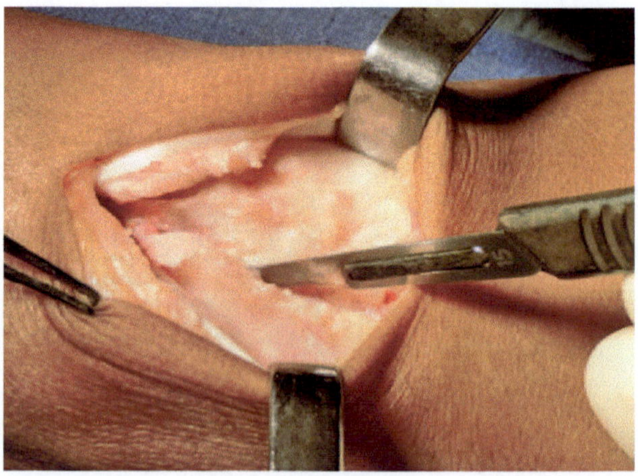

Longitudinal capsulotomy: section of the DIC

Dissection of the radial flap of the DIC

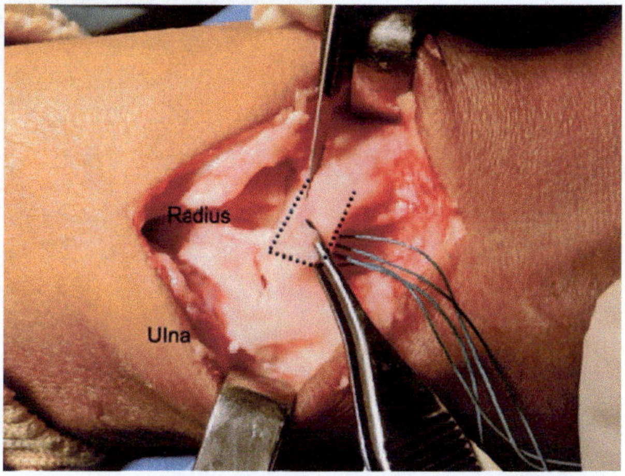

Dissection of the ulnar extrinsic flap (DIC + distal half of the DRC)

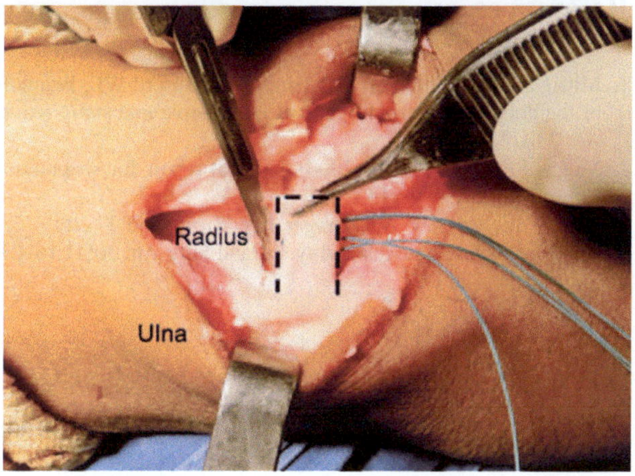

Suture "en paletot" (overcoat suture) of the two flaps with transversal retension by dishing two flaps of the DIC. With reinforcing and dorsal laying out by two U-shape points with the scapholunate anchor sutures

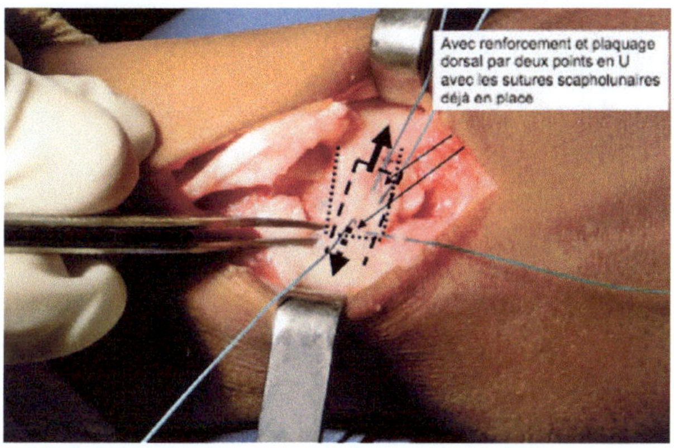

Final view

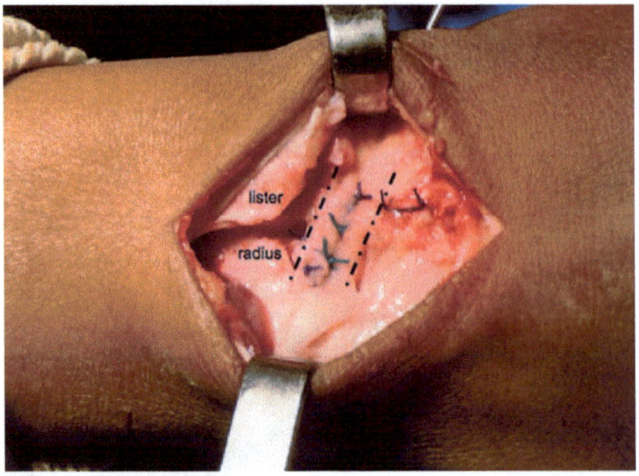

References

1. Mitsuyashu H, Patterson RM, Shah MA, Buford WL, Iwamoto Y, Viegass SF (2004) The role of the dorsal intercarpal ligament in dynamic and static scapholunate instability. J Hand Surg Am 29A(2):279–288
2. Viegas SF, Dasilva MF (2000) Surgical repair for scapholunate dissociation. Tech Hand Up Extrem Surg 4(3):14–153
3. Moran SL, Cooney WP, Berger RA, Strickland J (2005) Capsulodesis for the treatment of chronic scapholunate instability. J Hand Surg Am 30(1):16–23

The Brunelli's Tenodesis

F. Schuind and W. El Kazzi

1 Introduction

Of the many patterns of wrist osteoarthrosis, the SLAC wrist (scapholunate advanced collapse pattern) is one of the commonest. It was described in 1948 by Watson and Ballet [20] who studied the radiological progression of chondral degeneration in 210 patients. These authors described three stages of increasing severity, with the osteoarthrosis progressively affecting more joints. The term SLAC wrist is derived from what the authors thought to be the aetiology, namely, the rupture of the scapholunate (SL) ligament, leading to dorsal flexion of the lunate (the so-called DISI – dorsal intercalated segment deformity) and, more importantly, to pathological palmar flexion and dorsal subluxation of the scaphoid. These anomalies, initially dynamic, become over time fixed (Fig. 1). The malposition of the scaphoid leads to a decrease in the joint contacts between the scaphoid and the radius. The resulting excessive articular stresses cause the osteoarthrosis, first involving the radioscaphoid joint. The lunate dorsal flexion seems to have little consequences at the level of the radiolunate joint.

Experimentally, the isolated section of the SL membrane in a cadaveric wrist does not cause any kinematic alteration [3], except in some special radioscaphoid morphotypes [21]. Distal radius fractures are frequently complicated by intrinsic wrist ligament lesions, especially affecting the SL membrane, yet SLAC wrist is a rare occurrence after distal radius fractures. In fact, the SL ligament may have more a proprioceptive than a mechanical role [9]. As early as 1989, Jantea believed that the said SL dissociative instability resulted initially from insufficiency of the ligaments stabilizing the distal pole of the scaphoid at the scaphotrapeziotrapezoid

F. Schuind, M.D., Ph.D. (✉) • W. El Kazzi, M.D.
Department of Orthopaedics and Traumatology, Erasme University Hospital,
808, route de Lennik, B-1070 Brussels, Belgium
e-mail: frederic.schuind@erasme.ulb.ac.be; welkazzi@hotmail.com

E. Camus, L. Van Overstraeten (eds.), *Carpal Ligament Surgery*,
DOI 10.1007/978-2-8178-0379-1_24, © Springer-Verlag France 2013

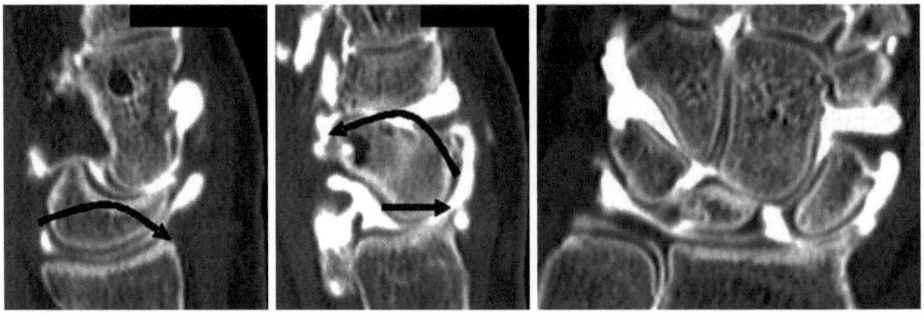

Fig. 1 SLAC wrist with dorsal flexion of the lunate (*left*), palmar flexion and dorsal subluxation of the proximal pole of the scaphoid (*centre*) and SL diastasis (*right*). Note the presence of radioscaphoid and lunocapitate chondral lesions

(STT) level, followed by distension and ultimately secondary rupture of the SL ligament (Jantea C., Mayo Clinic, Rochester, MN, USA, 1989, Personal communication). Brunelli considered the deep part of the flexor carpi radialis (FCR) sheath to be the principle stabilizer of the STT complex [2]. Garcia-Elias believed that the primary stabilizer of the scaphoid was the SL ligament, especially its dorsal component, the STT ligament complex and the scaphocapitate and radioscaphocapitate ligaments being secondary stabilizers [7]. Short reported that the secondary stabilizers were the scaphocapitate and scaphotrapezial ligaments [16, 17].

It is worthy of note that the term instability is incorrect; in fact, the new equilibrium reached in a fixed DISI deformity is quite stable and thus difficult to correct. We proposed in 1996 the term 'carpal dyskinetic syndrome' [14]. Garcia-Elias defined carpal instability as carpal kinetic dysfunction (load transmission) and/or dyskinematic (osseous alignment), but proposed keeping the term instability by right of use [7].

The results of repair of chronic SL lesions remain disappointing, probably owing to the difficulty of correcting scaphoid malposition by these reconstructions. We have abandoned our 1995 original technique of SL repair using a vascularized transfer of the interosseous membrane [13, 15], when in 1995 Brunelli described his technique of ligamentoplasty where a band of the FCR tendon, still attached to the second metacarpal, is tunnelled through the distal pole of the scaphoid and anchored to the dorsoulnar radius, thereby reducing the pathological scaphoid flexion, the dorsal subluxation of the proximal pole as well as the SL diastasis (Fig. 2). The lunate dorsiflexion tends to autocorrect spontaneously, following scaphoid reduction [2, 3].

2 Surgical Technique

The surgery is usually performed under regional anaesthesia. We like the approach through a dorsal radio-scapho-lunate incision parallel to the distal rim of the radius [6]. The dorsal sensory radial nerve branches are identified and spared. The third

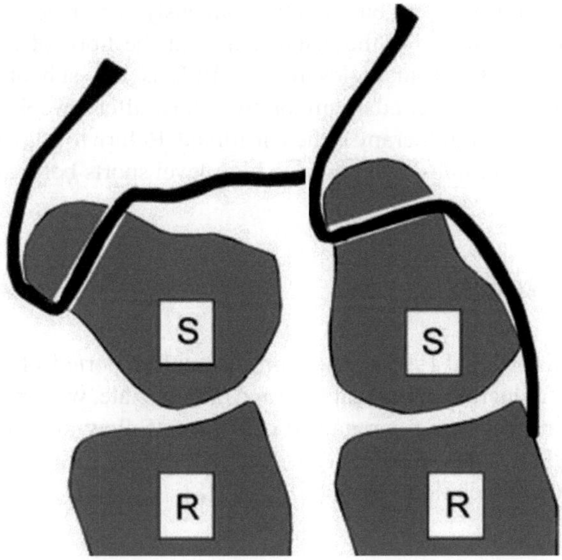

Fig. 2 The Brunelli's tenodesis using a band of the FCR tendon

compartment is incised and the extensor pollicis longus (EPL) tendon palmarly retracted. It is usually unnecessary to open the fourth compartment; it can be 'en bloc' dissected off the distal radius over several millimetres. The dissection proceeds on either side of the extensors carpi radialis, taking care not to damage distally the radial pedicle. The ligament lesions are thus exposed. There is usually an abnormal diastasis between the scaphoid and lunate, with extensive synovitis. There is often little left of the SL ligament, and any attempt at its direct suture is doomed to fail. There is evident dorsal subluxation of the proximal pole of the scaphoid, and the lunate, in DISI, is practically invisible under the capitate head which is situated very close to the radius glenoid. The SL synovitis is resected. Distally, the surgeon approaches the STT interval, which is not so easy to open due to the scaphoid malposition; the synovitis present at this level is as well resected. The reducibility of the scaphoid is now evaluated. A second 4-cm incision is then made along the FCR, centred over the scaphoid tubercle, easily palpable due to the malposition of that bone. The tendon sheath is opened, dividing some thenar muscle fibres. Through another transverse incision, 7 cm higher, a third (about one-half according to Brunelli [2]) of the FCR tendon is harvested, preserving its distal attachment to the trapezium, trapezoid and second metacarpal. At this level, the tendon sheath is not opened. The STT joint is approached, and a spatula is introduced in this joint, giving its orientation. A 2.8- or 3.2-mm tunnel is made through the distal pole of the scaphoid, parallel to this joint, and the tendon band is passed through it. By pulling on the ligamentoplasty, one can usually observe the 'automatic' reduction of the scaphoid and lunatum with disappearance of the SL diastasis. If this is not the case, the surgeon can use K-wires temporarily inserted in both bones as 'joysticks' to assist the reduction. The scaphoid is fixed in the reduced position using one scaphocapitate K-wire; in many cases, a second K-wire is used to transfix the SL joint. The wires are bent and buried subcutaneously. The tendon graft is fixed under tension using an anchor in the distal radius, at the floor of the third compartment. After meticulous capsular closure, the EPL is left subcutaneous. The wire(s) is(are) removed as a secondary minor procedure, after 6 weeks of immobilization in a plaster cast. Physiotherapy is then instituted. Return to heavy manual work is not allowed before 3 months, and return to high-level sports before 6 months.

3 Results

In his original 1995 publications, Brunelli reported 11 and then 13 cases of satisfactory reduction of the scaphoid and of the lunate, with restoration of the carpal height, the results being maintained over time (follow-up between 6 months and 2 years [2, 3]). Other publications reported results using modifications of the original Brunelli technique [4, 5, 8, 11, 12, 18].

4 Discussion

The natural evolution of the 'scapholunate dissociation instability' syndrome is delayed radiocarpal and midcarpal osteoarthrosis. It is especially the scaphoid subluxation which causes damage to the hyaline cartilage, at least in the first stages. The different types of SL ligamentoplasty described in the 1980s have been abandoned by most authors. Many patients operated during that era had to be reoperated by partial or total wrist arthrodesis. These failures discouraged attempting ligament reconstruction and favoured scaphoid reduction, followed by fixation of the reduced scaphoid by partial carpal arthrodesis, either STT or scaphocapitate fusion. However, these interventions caused substantial wrist stiffness. Watson proposed a technique for SLAC wrist reconstruction involving scaphoidectomy and 'four-corner' fusion of the capitate, lunate, hamate and triquetrum [20]. Other authors did not hesitate to proceed directly to first carpal row resection, especially when the lunocapitate joint was still normal. These different techniques were relatively aggressive, their complication rate was not negligible and their long-term results not well known. This is why the Brunelli technique, which durably corrects the scaphoid malposition, avoiding the evolution towards osteoarthrosis, is now favoured by many wrist surgeons. For us, it is the treatment of choice for treatment of SL dissociative instability without osteoarthrosis.

In order to avoid postoperative reduction of palmar wrist flexion, several authors have proposed to avoid to fix the tendon ligamentoplasty to the distal radius. In the technique of Van Den Abbeele, the graft was fixed to the dorsal radio-triquetral ligament [19]. Garcia-Elias and Stanley described the '3LT' technique (3-ligament tenodesis : STT complex, SL and luno-triquetral ligaments) where the trans-scaphoid tunnel is not any more parallel to the STT joint, but rather oblique, ending dorsally and proximally, adjacent to the SL joint – at the level of the strongest part of the SL ligament. The tendon band then follows a path transverse and dorsal to the previously reduced lunate, to which it is anchored. The tendon is finally passed around the dorsal radio-triquetral ligament (the ligament had been preserved throughout the Berger approach to the carpus [1]) and sutured to itself [8, 18]. This technique would have the advantage of reconstructing the most mechanically important portion of the SL ligament, of better reducing the gap between the two bones, as well as avoiding radial insertion and therefore wrist stiffness. It does not however allow the same reducing moment on the scaphoid. Howlett showed that the scaphoid tunnel must be distal to ensure the best SL correction [10]. We have ultimately returned to the original Brunelli procedure.

References

1. Berger RA (2007) A method of defining palpable landmarks for the ligament-splitting dorsal wrist capsulotomy. J Hand Surg Am 32:1291–1295
2. Brunelli GA, Brunelli GR (1995) Une nouvelle intervention pour la dissociation scapho-lunaire. Proposition d'une nouvelle technique chirurgicale pour l''instabilité carpienne avec dissociation scapho-lunaire (11 cas). Ann Chir Main 14:207–213
3. Brunelli GA, Brunelli GR (1995) A new technique to correct carpal instability with scaphoid rotary subluxation: a preliminary report. J Hand Surg Am 20(3 Pt 2):S82–S85
4. Chabas JF, Gay A, Valenti D, Guinard D, Legre R (2008) Results of the modified Brunelli tenodesis for treatment of scapholunate instability: a retrospective study of 19 patients. J Hand Surg Am 33:1469–1477
5. de Smet L, van Hoonacker P (2007) Treatment of chronic static scapholunate dissociation with the modified Brunelli technique: preliminary results. Acta Orthop Belg 73:188–191
6. dos Reis FB, Koeberle G, Leite NM, Katchburian MV (1993) Internal fixation of scaphoid injuries using the Herbert screw through a dorsal approach. J Hand Surg Am 18:792–797
7. Garcia-Elias M (1997) The treatment of wrist instability. J Bone Joint Surg Br 79:684–690
8. Garcia-Elias M, Lluch AL, Stanley JK (2006) Three-ligament tenodesis for the treatment of scapholunate dissociation: indications and surgical technique. J Hand Surg Am 31:125–134
9. Hagert E, Persson JK, Werner M, Ljung BO (2009) Evidence of wrist proprioceptive reflexes elicited after stimulation of the scapholunate interosseous ligament. J Hand Surg Am 34(4): 642–651
10. Howlett JP, Pfaeffle HJ, Waitayawinyu T, Trumble TE (2008) Distal tunnel placement improves scaphoid flexion with the Brunelli tenodesis procedure for scapholunate dissociation. J Hand Surg Am 33:1756–1764
11. Kuo CE, Wolfe SW (2008) Scapholunate instability: current concepts in diagnosis and management. J Hand Surg Am 33:998–1013
12. Links AC, Chin SH, Waitayawinyu T, Trumble TE (2008) Scapholunate interosseous ligament reconstruction: results with a modified Brunelli technique versus four-bone weave. J Hand Surg Am 33:850–856
13. Schuind F (1995) Scapholunate reconstruction using a vascularized flap of the interosseous membrane. J Orthop Surg Tech 9:21–26
14. Schuind F, Fumière E, Sintzoff S (1996) The value of standard and functional radiographs in diagnosing wrist instability. In: Büchler U (ed) Wrist instability. Martin Dunitz, London, pp 61–67
15. Schuind F, Alemzadeh S, Dhaene F, Feipel V (1997) New technique: reconstruction of the scapholunate ligament using a vascularized flap of the interosseous membrane. In: Saffar P, Amadio PC, Foucher G (eds) Current practice in hand surgery. Martin Dunitz, London, pp 299–305

16. Short WH, Werner FW, Green JK, Masaoka S (2005) Biomechanical evaluation of the ligamentous stabilizers of the scaphoid and lunate: part II. J Hand Surg Am 30:24–34
17. Short WH, Werner FW, Green JK, Sutton LG, Brutus JP (2007) Biomechanical evaluation of the ligamentous stabilizers of the scaphoid and lunate: part III. J Hand Surg Am 32:297–309
18. Talwalkar SC, Edwards AT, Hayton MJ, Stilwell JH, Trail IA, Stanley JK (2006) Results of tri-ligament tenodesis: a modified Brunelli procedure in the management of scapholunate instability. J Hand Surg Br 31:110–117
19. van den Abbeele KL, Loh YC, Stanley JK, Trail IA (1998) Early results of a modified Brunelli procedure for scapholunate instability. J Hand Surg Br 23:258–261
20. Watson HK, Ballet FL (1984) The SLAC wrist: scapholunate advanced collapse pattern of degenerative arthritis. J Hand Surg Am 9:358–365
21. Werner FW, Short WH, Green JK, Evans PJ, Walker JA (2007) Severity of scapholunate instability is related to joint anatomy and congruency. J Hand Surg Am 32:55–60

Chronic Lunotriquetral Ligament Injuries: Arthrodesis or Capsulodesis

L. De Smet, I. Janssens, and W. Van De Sande

1 Introduction

Several treatments for patients with isolated lunotriquetral (LT) tears have been described previously. The choice between an LT fusion (attempts to), repair and (complicated) ligament reconstruction, is not yet established [2, 3, 5–7, 9, 11].

LT arthrodesis gives variable outcomes and most ligament reconstructions are technically demanding, requiring extensive approaches. In 1996, Sennwald and collaborators [10] proposed a radially based flap of the extensor retinaculum to be inserted on the triquetrum and in so doing reconstructing a dorsal stabilizer of the LT joint (capsulodesis).

The purpose of this chapter is to compare Sennwald's technique with a similar group of patients previously treated at our department with an LT fusion.

2 Materials and Methods

2.1 Patients

We reviewed the patients treated for an isolated LT tear in our institution [12]. We considered the LT tear as the cause of the ulnar-sided wrist pain when the LT interval was tender, when the Reagan test was positive and when other causes of ulnar wrist pain were excluded. In all patients, the diagnosis was established or confirmed on arthroscopic findings.

L. De Smet (✉) • I. Janssens • W. Van De Sande
Department of Orthopedic Surgery, U.Z. Pellenberg,
Weligerveld, 1, B-3212 Lubbeek (Pellenberg), Belgium
e-mail: luc.desmet@uz.kuleuven.ac.be

E. Camus, L. Van Overstraeten (eds.), *Carpal Ligament Surgery*,
DOI 10.1007/978-2-8178-0379-1_25, © Springer-Verlag France 2013

Two groups were established. Group I underwent an LT arthrodesis. There were 17 patients: 8 men and 9 women with a mean age of 32.6 years (SD 10). The dominant side was involved in eight cases. The men follow-up was 5.6 years (SD 1.99). Group II consisted of 13 patients, treated with a capsulodesis according to Sennwald [10]. There were 5 men and 8 women with a mean age of 30 years (SD 11) with ten times the dominant wrist involved. The follow-up was 2 years (SD 1.5). The differences in age, gender and involved side were not significant ($p > 0.05$, t-test). This is not a randomized study. The LT fusion technique was largely abandoned in 2001 due to the high failure rate [12]. Sennwald's capsulodesis became our first choice of treatment since 1999.

A traumatic event was recalled in 15 patients. The dominant symptom was ulnar-sided wrist pain in 14 and radial wrist pain in 6. The radiographs were normal in 23; a static VISI (volar intercalated segment instability) was present in 7. In none of the radiographs, an interruption of Gilula's line was observed. Arthrograms were performed in 21 wrists with communication between the radiocarpal joint through the LT interval and the midcarpal joint in 17 cases. All patients underwent an arthroscopy. Instability of the LT joint was observed in all through the midcarpal portal. The patients were treated by different surgeons with different level of experience.

2.2 *Surgical Technique*

The wrist was approached through a ligament-sparing incision, and the LT was explored.

During surgery, a broad diastasis of the LT joint was obvious in all patients, indicating a complete rupture of the LT ligament.

In group I, the LT joint was exposed and the cartilage removed. Usually, an autologous cancellous bone graft was inserted in the gap, and the LT joint was fixed with K-wires (3×) or staples (2×) or a Herbert screw (12×). A forearm cast was applied for 6 weeks.

In group II, a radially based flap of the retinaculum extensorum, 1 cm broad, is prepared and passed deep to the fourth and fifth compartments and fixed with a bone anchor into the triquetrum. A forearm cast was applied for 6 weeks.

2.3 *Evaluation*

The patients were evaluated by two independent observers (I.J. and WVDS). They were asked for satisfaction (very, fair, poor), pain and function on a visual analogue score (VAS) and if they should have the same procedure again. Range of motion and gripping force were measured. Complications were noted. In group I, a control radiograph was taken and evaluated for fusion.

Table 1 Summary data

	Group I – LT fusion	Group II – ligament reconstruction	*p* value
N	17	13	
M/F	8/9	5/8	
Age	32.6 years (10)	30 years (11)	
Follow-up (years)	5.6 years (1.99)	2 years (1.5)	
Satisfaction	8/9	8/5	0.43
Pain (VAS)	5.8 (1.84)	4.3 (2.69)	0.078
Function (VAS)	3.2 (3.83)	6.8 (1.84)	0.007*
Grip (in kg)	27.7 (12.37)	32.0 (16.29)	0.15
Extension	37 (21.3)	61 (18.5)	0.33
Flexion	40 (25.3)	55 (19.9)	0.44
Reoperation (Y/N)	11/6	3/11	0.02*

( ) standard deviation, *significant

3 Results

In group I, two patients were very satisfied, six were satisfied, nine were not, and ten should have the procedure again. They scored 5.8 on the pain score (0=no pain, 10=intolerable pain) and 3.2 (0=no impairment, 10=severe impairment) on the functional score. The grip strength was 28 kg; the key pinch was 7.3 kg. The extension was 37°, flexion was 40°, and forearm rotation was 141°. Complications were numerous: one had a reflex sympathetic dystrophy, five had a paresthesia in the dorsoulnar side of the hand, two had a pisohamatum impingement, and eight developed a pseudarthrosis of the LT fusion.

In group II, three were very satisfied, five were satisfied, five were not, and eight should have the same procedure again. The mean score on the pain score was 4.3 (SD 2.69). On the function score, it was 6.8 (SD 1.84). The grip strength was 32 kg; the key pinch was 7.3 kg. The extension was 61°, the flexion was 55°, and forearm rotation was 177°. Complications were less frequent 3 (23%) and consisted in paresthesia in the territorium of the dorsal branch of the ulnar nerve, one case with tendon adhesions and one painful scar. Significancy ($p<0.05$) was reached for function (*t*-test) and reoperation ratio (Chi Square) (Table 1).

In group I, a reoperation was required in 11 patients (29 procedures including removal of hardware), and in group II, it was necessary in 3 patients (three procedures) (Chi Square, $p<0.05$).

4 Discussion

Based on the observation that patients with congenital lunotriquetral coalition are usually without symptoms, LT arthrodesis has been the standard treatment option for LT ligament ruptures. The outcome however is not uniformly favorable, and complications are numerous. The rate of nonunion varies between 0 and 57 % [4, 9]. High complication rates are mostly due to technical errors: nonunion, neurapraxia of the dorsal branch of the ulnar nerve and midcarpal joint discongruency. Patient satisfaction was only 57.1 % in the series of Shin et al. The rate of complications, others than nonunion, varies between 22 and 46 % [5]. The outcome is very variable, and the evaluation of results in the published series is not very detailed. Sennwald et al. called the LT arthrodesis a "controversial" procedure [9]. On the contrary, Guidera et al. [4] in a recent survey had very favorable results in 24 patients.

Reported results on LT ligament reconstructions in literature are less numerous. The available techniques are complicated, but in a comparative series of Shin et al. [5], the outcome for the patients with a reconstruction was better with less complications [11]. The procedure described by Sennwald et al. [10] is technically less demanding and reconstructs the dorsal intercarpal ligaments by a strip of the retinaculum. In the sequential section experiments of Ritt et al. [8], a VISI deformity can be obtained when both the LT and the dorsal extrinsic ligaments are divided; LT ligament section only had only partial effect on the overall carpal configuration: a full blown VISI is only seen after sectioning the extrinsic ligament. The Sennwald procedure is very similar to Blatt's capsulodesis in scapholunate dissociations [1].

Based on our survey, reconstruction of the LT is our first choice since it preserves better motion, has similar subjective outcomes compared to the LT arthrodesis and has, in a training hospital, a lower complication rate.

References

1. Blatt G (1987) Capsulodesis in reconstructive hand surgery: dorsal capsulodesis for the unstable scaphoid and volar capsulodesis following excision of the distal ulna. Hand Clin 3:81–102
2. Guidera P, Dwyer T, Orlando G, Zeppieri J, Yasuda M (2002) Lunotriquetral arthrodesis using cancellous bone grafts. J Hand Surg 26A:422–427
3. Kirchenbaum D, Coyle M, Leddy JP (1993) Chronic lunotriquetral instability: diagnosis and treatment. J Hand Surg 18A:1107–1112
4. McAuliffe J, Dell P, Jaffe R (1993) Complications of intercarpal arthrodesis. J Hand Surg 18A:1121–1127
5. Nelson D, Manske P, Pruitt D, Martin R (1993) Lunotriquetral arthrodesis. J Hand Surg 18A: 1113–1120
6. Pin P, Young V, Gilula L, Weeks P (1989) Management of chronic lunotriquetral ligament tears. J Hand Surg 14A:77–83
7. Reajan D, Linscheid R, Dobyns J (1984) Lunotriquetral sprains. J Hand Surg 9A:502–514
8. Ritt M, Linscheid R, Cooney W, Berger R, An K (1998) The lunotriquetral joint: kinematic effects of sequential ligament section, ligament repair and arthrodesis. J Hand Surg 23A:432–445
9. Sennwald G, Fischer M, Mondi P (1995) Lunotriquetral arthrodesis: a controversial arthrodesis. Hand Surg 20B:755–760
10. Sennwald G, Fischer M, Zdravkovic V (1996) The value of arthroscopy in the evaluation of carpal instability. Bull Hosp Joint Dis 54:186–189
11. Shin A, Weinstein L, Berger R, Bishop A (2000) Treatment of isolated injuries of the lunotriquetral ligament. J Hand Surg 83B:1023–1028
12. Vandesande W, De Smet L, Van Ransbeeck H (2002) Lunotriquetral arthrodesis, a procedure with a high failure rate. Acta Orthop Belg 67:361–367

Scapholunate Ligament Reconstruction Using a Bone-Ligament-Bone Autograft

J. Goubau, P. Van Hoonacker, B. Berghs, and D. Kerckhove

Injuries of the scapholunate ligament are often underestimated. In the acute phase, radiographs are often misleading. Initially, patients have quite sharp pains which tend to decrease over a couple of weeks with rest, immobilization and painkillers.

Moreover, many general practitioners underestimate the long-term consequences of these 'sprains'. Some stages of scapholunate dissociation result in important long-term functional handicaps.

The traumatic mechanism is generally a high-velocity trauma: the most known one is the hyperextension of the wrist with a variable degree of ulnar deviation and/or radio-metacarpal pronation of the carpus. For instance, falls from an important height, motorbike accidents or rotatory injuries using power tools are part of the possible mechanism.

The injury of the scapholunate ligament has several stages which depend on the severity of the injury. In 1980, Mayfield described the different stages of perilunate injury. The first stage is scapholunate dissociation. Scapholunate dissociation has variable degrees of severity and repercussion on the kinematics of the carpus.

The experimental isolated scapholunate injury causes less dissociative instability in vitro than the same injury in vivo. These differences are easily explained by the

J. Goubau (✉)
Hand and Upper Limb Unit, Department of Orthopaedics and Trauma,
AZ St Jan AV Brugge – Oostende,
Campus Bruges, Ruddershove 10, Bruges 8000, Belgium

Department of Orthopaedics and Traumatology, University Hospital Brussels,
Laarbeeklaan 101, Brussels, Belgium
e-mail: jean.goubau@azsintjan.be, jean@goubau.eu

P. Van Hoonacker • B. Berghs • D. Kerckhove
Hand and Upper Limb Unit, Department of Orthopaedics and Trauma,
AZ St Jan AV Brugge – Oostende,
Campus Bruges, Ruddershove 10, Bruges 8000, Belgium

E. Camus, L. Van Overstraeten (eds.), *Carpal Ligament Surgery*,
DOI 10.1007/978-2-8178-0379-1_26, © Springer-Verlag France 2013

concomitant injuries at the level of the capsula and the ligaments which link the scaphoid, the trapezoid, the trapezium and the capitate. Since most of these injuries are not always detected, even rarely diagnosed in emergency, a classification which takes into account the delay before the patient is seen in a specialized consultation for the first time is useful. Injuries are divided into three groups: an acute, a subacute and a chronic group.

In the acute group, the injury is less than a week from the original trauma: it allows a reinsertion suture of the ligament. The subacute group is composed of injuries which have been seen between one and six weeks posttraumatically where the potential of ligamentous recovery as far as scarring is concerned is reduced. Finally, the group of chronic injuries, more precisely at least 6 weeks after the trauma and when the recovery-healing using a simple reinsertion becomes difficult, is even impossible. The only case for which the management of the chronic injuries is possible is when the injury has an osseous avulsion at the level of the lunate. It sometimes enables, in chronic cases, a surgical osteosynthesis reinsertion of the fragment with an 8 weeks' temporary immobilization and an antebrachial plaster cast. Outcome is nevertheless unpredictable.

As far as the repair of the scapholunate ligament using a bone-tissue-bone transplant is concerned, we rather indicate it at stages III and IV of Garcia-Elias, Lluch and Stanley classification [6] which correspond to a complete and unrepairable rupture of the scapholunate ligament with or without a reducible rotatory subluxation of the scaphoid.

This classification mostly depends on the quality of the scapholunate ligament, the potential of recovery of the scapholunate ligament and the quality of the radiocarpal and midcarpal cartilage.

The history of bone-tissue-bone autografts started in 1995 when Svoboda [8] suggested a biomechanical testing of the dorsal metatarsal ligaments of the fourth and fifth metatarsals, the dorsal metatarsal ligament and the calcaneo-cuboidal ligaments. The first short-term result was published in 1997 by [1] Weiss who proposed a series of 19 patients with a follow-up of 3.6 years with a bone-retinaculum-bone autograft to reconstruct the scapholunate ligament.

Since then, several articles have been published on the subject: Harvey [3, 4] and Cuénod [7] both established an in vitro biomechanical analysis of the different carpo-metacarpal ligaments and compared them to the scapholunate ligament.

In 2007, the article published by the same Harvey et al. [5] confirmed the lack of long-term study but underlined the very interesting early results.

The surgical technique is rather simple and requires a dorsal longitudinal approach with a radiocarpal and midcarpal ligamentotomy which respects the orientation of the ligamentous fibres, such as described by Berger and Bishop [2]. The reduction of the scapholunate dissociation and the correction of the rotary instability of the scaphoid are made by pinning of the semilunate and the scaphoid with a joystick. This allows an easy reduction of the intercalated instability. Then, we put the arthrorhisis K-wires bridging the scapholunate joint with two 1.2-mm K-wires, followed by a single pinning of the scaphocapitate joint. Pins can be left

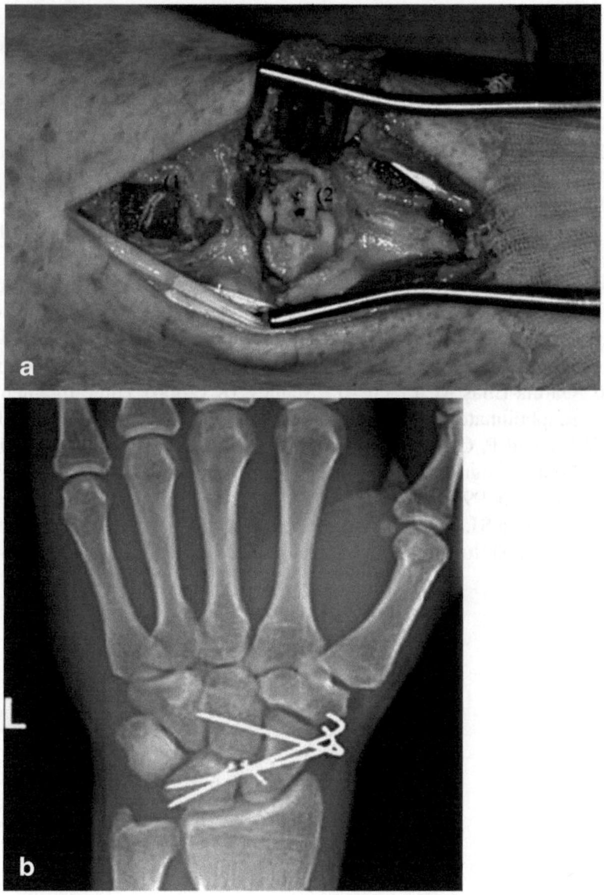

Fig. 1 (**a**) Removal of the CMC III bone-ligament-bone graft (*1*) and fixation at the anatomic location of the dorsal scapholunate ligament (*2*). (**b**) Reducing correction of the instability by K-wire pinning of the scaphoid, lunate and capitate

percutaneously, but preferably buried subcutaneously (Fig. 1b). Then we locate the carpo-metacarpal joint and ligament of the third ray, which corresponds to the ligament which has the most common characteristics and biomechanics compared to the scapholunate ligament. The ligament is harvested together with a piece of bone – a square with and edge of maximum 3 mm – on the capitate and on the base of the third metacarpal (Fig. 1a 1). At the level of the scaphoid and lunate, bone is resected sufficiently – no conflict is allowed between the graft and the joint of the radial epiphysis after placement – on the exact location where the bony attachments of the donor ligaments will be fitted. This is screwed by 1.3-mm screws or slightly bigger (Fig. 1a 2). Postoperatively a forearm cast is fitted. After 8 weeks, the cast and pins are removed.

As far as our personal experience is concerned, it matches the reports of Weiss: although a result can be very satisfactory at midterm, total recovery can be very long (12–18 months) to get.

References

1. Weiss APC, Providence RI (1998) Scapholunate ligament reconstruction using a bone-retinaculum-bone autograft. J Hand Surg 23A:205–515
2. Berger RA, Bishop AT (1997) A fiber-splitting capsulotomy technique for dorsal exposure of the wrist. Tech Hand Up Extrem Surg 1(1):2–10
3. Harvey EJ, Hanel D, Knight Beng JB, Tencer AF, Seattle WA (1999) Autograft replacements for the scapholunate ligament: a biomechanical comparison of hand-based autografts. J Hand Surg 24A:963–967
4. Harvey EJ, Sen M, Martineau P (2006) A vascularized technique for bone-tissue-bone repair in scapholunate dissociation. Tech Hand Up Extrem Surg 10(3):166–172
5. Harvey EJ, Berger RA, Lee Osterman A, Fernandez DL, Weiss AP (2007) Bone-tissue-bone repairs for scapholunate dissociation. J Hand Surg 32A:256–264
6. Garcia-Elias M, Lluch AL, Stanley JK (2006) Three-ligament tenodesis for the treatment of scapholunate dissociation: indications and surgical technique. J Hand Surg 31 A:125–134
7. Cuénod P, Charrière E, Papaloïzos MY (2002) A mechanical comparison of bone-ligament-bone autografts from the wrist replacement of the scapholunate ligament. J Hand Surg 27A:985–990
8. Svoboda SJ, Eglseder WA Jr, Belkoff SM (1995) Autografts from the foot for reconstruction of the scapholunate Interosseous ligament. J Hand Surg 20A:980–985

Reduction and Association of the Scaphoid and Lunate (RASL)

J. Goubau, P. Van Hoonacker, B. Berghs, and D. Kerckhove

In 1984, Faithfull and Timothy Herbert described the use of the Herbert screw for small joint fusion of the hand in the *Journal of Hand Surgery* [4]. It was their way to illustrate the quality of a wonderful headless compression screw, which would mark the end of the century in interfragmentary screwing of small bones. It was the first time that internal splinting of the small bones was described and more specifically scapholunate synostosis – syndesmosis – with a headless compression screw.

In 1991, Timothy Herbert described in the *World Journal of Surgery* his new technique of scapho-lunate repair using a Herbert screw (Fig. 1) [6].

RASL stands for reduction and association of the scaphoid and lunate, and the goal is to recreate an association between the two bones (scaphoid and lunate) with a bony or fibrous link. Biomechanics are not restored but are more physiological than the alternative procedures (Blatt dorsal capsulodesis, scapho-trapezoideo-trapezial arthrodesis, Brunelli standard or modified).

The indications are subacute ligamentary repair (stage III and IV as described by Garcia-Elias et al. [5]). This means reducible, dissociative instability with good cartilage quality. Contraindications for this operation are pre-existing arthrosis whether radio-carpal or between scaphoid, trapezoid and trapezium. Radio-styloid arthritis is not a contraindication.

J. Goubau (✉)
Hand and Upper Limb Unit, Department of Orthopaedics and Trauma,
AZ St Jan AV Brugge – Oostende,
Campus Bruges, Ruddershove 10, Bruges 8000, Belgium

Department of Orthopaedics and Traumatology, University Hospital Brussels,
Laarbeeklaan 101, Brussels, Belgium
e-mail: jean.goubau@azsintjan.be, jean@goubau.eu

P. VanHoonacker • B. Berghs • D. Kerckhove
Hand and Upper Limb Unit, Department of Orthopaedics and Trauma,
AZ St Jan AV Brugge – Oostende,
Campus Bruges, Ruddershove 10, Bruges 8000, Belgium

E. Camus, L. Van Overstraeten (eds.), *Carpal Ligament Surgery*,
DOI 10.1007/978-2-8178-0379-1_27, © Springer-Verlag France 2013

Fig. 1 Immediate Postop view showing the Herbertscrew in place (X-Ray Courtesy of Dr Jean Michel Cognet, Reims, France); note the styloidectomy of the Radius

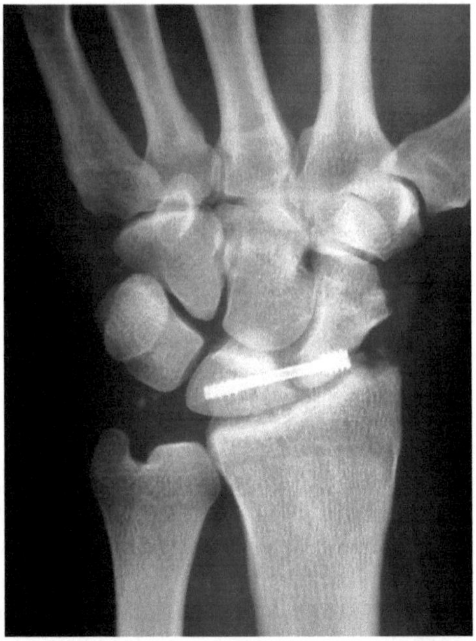

The technique described by Faithfull et al. is based on a dual incision dorsal and radial in a longitudinal way. The dorsal incision is for the actual surgical procedure; the radial approach is used to perform the styloidectomy and insert the headless compression screw (Herbert, HCS, etc.).

The dorsal approach is a 3–4 extensor compartment incision with a U-shaped distally based flap of the capsule. Other approaches described by Berger and Bishop are also possible [2]. Inspection of the scapholunate gap and quality of the cartilage is performed, and placement of two 1.5-mm K-wires in the distal radial portion of the lunate and the distal ulnar portion of the scaphoid is performed to act as joysticks. Care is taken to place the K-wire in a maximal divergent angle in order to correct the instability by clamping both K-wires together with a Kocher [7]. With a knife, we perform the sharp removal of the ligament remnants, and we remove with a bur and rongeur the cartilage until cancellous bone is exposed.

With the radial approach, the styloid is removed through the first extensor compartment, which is reclined in a volar way. After resection of the styloid, exposure of the scaphoid is realised. The removal of the styloid diminishes the impingement of the scaphoid, eases the insertion of the bone screw and can also enhance the results by removal of degenerated articular surface of the styloid of the radius.

Afterwards, a reduction of the scaphoid and lunate is performed with the joysticks by clamping them with a Kocher; a K-wire is placed between scaphoid and lunate from radial to ulnar, slightly distal to the mid-waste of the scaphoid taking care not to penetrate the midcarpal joint space. The cannulated bone screw (Herbert) is inserted from radial to ulnar under image intensifier.

After placing the screw, joysticks are removed and the mobility is tested in flexion and extension. Next, closure of the capsular is performed to avoid capsulodesis.

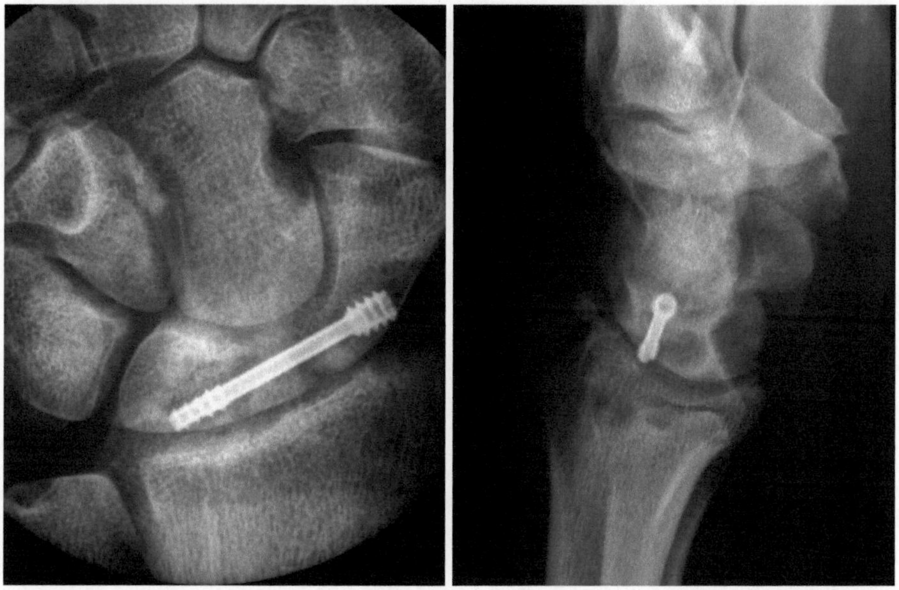

Fig. 2 Same patient as in figure 1, 3 months after the RASL procedure: note the lysis around the screw (*left*) and perforation of the screw in the radiocarpal joint (*right*) (Courtesy of Dr Jean Michel Cognet, Reims, France)

Postoperatively, a short arm spica cast is applied for 4–6 weeks and rehabilitation is started.

The long-term results of this procedure are not well documented in the literature. Two articles report good results: Zubairy et al. [8] report in 2003 a 70 % overall satisfactory result; Alnot, with a slightly different procedure, reports a 90 % satisfactory [1].

Overall, the RASL procedure is not very popular; publications are rare but the early reported results were satisfactory. The aim is not a consolidation but a tight fibrous fusion, as you would expect in a hypertrophic pseudarthrosis. Recent publications by Cognet et al. report an overall bad result (Fig. 2) and recommend abandoning this technique [3]. It should be reminded as a historic option for treatment of a chronic non-arthritic radio-scapho-lunate dissociation.

References

1. Alnot JY, De Cheveigne C, Bleton R (1992) Instabilité scapho-lunaire chronique post-traumatique traitée par arthrodèse scapho-lunaire. Chir Main 11(2):107–118
2. Berger RA, Bishop AT (1997) A fiber-splitting capsulotomy technique for dorsal exposure of the wrist. Tech Hand Up Extrem Surg 1(1):2–10
3. Cognet JM, Levadoux M, Martinache X (2011) The use of screws in the treatment of scapholunate instability. J Hand Surg Eur Vol 31(8):690–693
4. Faithfull DK, Herbert TJ (1984) Small joint fusions of the hand using the Herbert screw. J Hand Surg Br 9B:167–168

5. Garcia-Elias M, Lluch AL, Stanley JK (2006) Three ligament tenodesis for the treatment of scapholunate dissociation. J Hand Surg Am 31A:125–134
6. Herbert TJ (1991) Acute rotatory dislocation of the scaphoid: a new repair using Herbert screw fixation across the sapho-lunate joint. World J Surg 15:463–469
7. Rosenwasser MP et al (1997) The RASL procedure: reduction and association of the scaphoid and lunate using the Herbert screw. Tech Hand Up Extrem Surg 1(4):263–272
8. Zubairy A, Jones WA (2003) Scapholunate fusion in chronic symptomatic scapholunate instability. J Hand Surg 28(4):311–314

Results of the Modified Brunelli Technique for Chronic Static Scapholunate Instability

L. De Smet, P. Van Hoonacker, and S. Goeminne

1 Introduction

Scapholunate instability is the most common pattern of carpal instability. Despite their frequency, these lesions are often missed or poorly treated, and this may lead to an important amount of wrist dysfunction and degeneration [1]. Treatment of chronic scapholunate instability remains controversial. There is no consensus between different stabilization procedures such as capsulodesis, tenodesis, and intercarpal fusions [1].

In 1995, Brunelli and Brunelli [2] introduced a new technique in the treatment of chronic scapholunate dissociation, using a flexor carpi radialis (FCR) tendon slip to reduce the rotatory subluxation of the scaphoid and to reduce the scapholunate distance. Van Den Abbeele et al. [3] developed a three-ligament tenodesis based on Brunelli's technique, reconstructing the scapholunate interosseous ligament, the scaphotrapeziotrapezoidal ligament and the dorsal radiotriquetral ligament. This study evaluates the outcome of the treatment of chronic, static scapholunate instability with a three-ligament tenodesis at our institution.

L. De Smet (✉) • S. Goeminne
Hand Surgery Unit, Department of Orthopedic Surgery, U.Z. Pellenberg, Weligerveld, 1, B-3212, Lubbeek (Pellenberg), Belgium
e-mail: luc.desmet@uz.kuleuven.ac.be; s.goeminne@uz.kuleuven.ac.be

P. Van Hoonacker
Hand and Upper Limb Unit, Department of Orthopaedics and Trauma, AZ St Jan AV Brugge – Oostende, Campus Bruges, Ruddershove 10, 8000 Bruges, Belgium

E. Camus, L. Van Overstraeten (eds.), *Carpal Ligament Surgery*,
DOI 10.1007/978-2-8178-0379-1_28, © Springer-Verlag France 2013

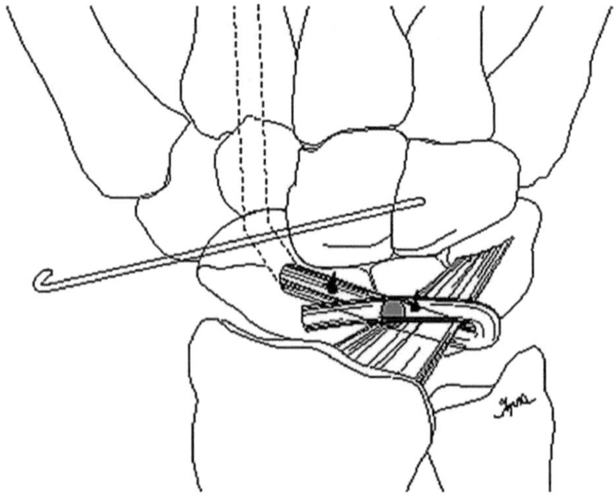

Fig. 1 Schematic represenatation of the technique used

2 Material and Methods

At UZ Leuven, 46 patients with chronic static scapholunate instability underwent a modified Brunelli procedure between 1998 and 2010. Twelve patients were excluded for this review because they needed a salvage procedure (wrist arthrodesis or proximal row carpectomy), and two patients were excluded because of a fall on the operated hand. Of the remaining 32 patients, 21 were willing to come to the hospital for clinical and radiological evaluation. In this group of 21 patients, mean age at the time of surgery was 39 years (range 26–47) and male to female ratio was 16:5. Mean follow-up was 33.5 months (range 8–69). In ten patients diagnosis was made on plain radiographs, three patients needed an MRI scan, and in eight patients, diagnosis was made arthroscopically. Nineteen patients sustained a fall on the outstretched hand more than 1 year before the diagnosis was made.

Postoperative pain, grip strength (Jamar dynamometer), and range of motion (hand held goniometer) were clinically evaluated. A quick DASH score was calculated. Standard radiographs were taken to measure scapholunate distance and angle and to evaluate carpal collapse using the Nattrass coefficient (carpal height divided by length of the capitates).

The modified Brunelli technique as described by Van Den Abbeele et al. [3] and Garcia-Elias et al. [4] was used.

A dorsal approach to the wrist joint described by Berger was made. First the scapholunate interval was evaluated, and then the scaphoid was released distally and reduced. A tunnel was made in the distal pole of the scaphoid from dorsal to volar. A suture anchor was placed in the lunate. A transverse palmar incision was made along the flexor carpi radialis (FCR), proximal to the scaphoid, and the cutaneous nerve branch of the radial nerve is protected. A second transverse palmar incision was made more proximally, over the musculotendinous junction of the

FCR, and the radial half of the tendon was retrieved to form a distally based FCR tendon strip. The tendon strip was then passed through the tunnel in the scaphoid, from volar to dorsal. The end of the tendon strip was passed under the dorsal radiocarpal ligament slip and attached to the lunate with the suture anchor placed earlier (Fig. 1). The tendon slip does not pass the radiocarpal joint. One or two K-wires were placed: one from scaphoid to capitate and (occasionally) one from scaphoid to lunate. Wrist capsule and skin were carefully sutured. A short arm and thumb cast is applied for 6 weeks. After 6 weeks of immobilization, K-wires were extracted and mobilization was initiated (Fig. 1).

3 Results

Mean satisfaction was 7.5/10 (range 2–10), mean pain visual analog score was 2.7/10, and mean quick DASH score was 15.5 (range 5–33) with a maximum possible DASH of 55. All patients would have the same surgery again and only two patients had not returned to work because of the wrist. Range of motion was significantly reduced compared to the contralateral side as illustrated in Table 1 but was in all case within the functional range. Grip strength was also significantly reduced (Table 1). Results of the radiographical measurements are shown in Table 2. No significant differences are seen here.

Table 1 ROM and grip strength of the operated hand compared to the contralateral side

	Mean (range)		
	Operated hand	Normal hand	*p*-value
Flexion	50 (20–75)	74 (40–90)	<0.001
Extension	51 (28–90)	71 (45–100)	<0.001
Ulnar deviation	33 (30–50)	42 (25–50)	<0.001
Radial deviation	19 (10–30)	29 (20–50)	<0.001
Grip strength	39 (21–61)	47 (26–71)	<0.001

Table 2 Preoperative radiological measurements compared to postoperative values

	Mean (range)		
	Preoperative	Postoperative	*p*-value
SL angle	66.5 (32.9–94.4)	61.9 (30–97.2)	0.03
SL interval	3.3 (1.5–7.9)	2.9 (1.5–5.4)	0.15
Nattrass coefficient	1.394 (1.27–1.51)	1.385 (1.22–1.55)	0.41

4 Discussion

Isolated rupture of the scapholunate ligament leads to dynamic scapholunate instability. If the scaphotrapeziotrapezoidal ligament and the dorsal radiotriquetral ligament are also damaged, a static scapholunate instability occurs [3].

In 1995, Brunelli and Brunelli [2] designed a new technique using a FCR tendon slip to reduce the scaphoid, correct the scapholunate dissociation and restore carpal height. They report on 13 cases with a short follow-up period of maximum 2 years. There is a limitation in wrist flexion of 30–60 % compared to the contralateral wrist and a limitation in grip strength of mean 35 % less than the contralateral hand. All 13 patients could return to work, 11 had no pain left and all 13 patients were satisfied.

Van Den Abbeele et al. [3] slightly modified Brunelli's technique by tunneling the FCR tendon slip under the dorsal radiolunotriquetral ligament and attaching it upon itself or directly to the lunate. Consequently the radiocarpal joint is not longer crossed in order to avoid loss of radiocarpal flexion. As this tendon reconstruction actions as the scapholunate, lunotriquetral and scaphotrapeziotrapezoid ligament, it is called a three-ligament tenodesis. Twenty-two patients with a mean follow-up period of 9 months were included in this study. Fifteen of them had predynamic instability, 4 dynamic instability and 3 had static scapholunate instability. Postoperative radiographic evaluation showed no changes in the average scapholunate angle compared to the preoperative X-rays. Postoperative ROM was compared to preoperative ROM resulting in a loss of wrist flexion of 18 % and a loss of extension of 20 %. Mean grip strength was 58 % of the contralateral hand. Fourteen patients had returned to work at the time of follow-up and 17 told they would have the operation again. Two patients needed a neuroma excision and two patients developed a reflex sympathetic dystrophy.

Talwalkar et al. [5] clinically reviewed 55 patients: 32 of them had static instability, 23 had dynamic instability. An additional 62 patients answered a questionnaire. Thirty-one percent loss of flexion, 20 % loss of extension and 12 % loss of radio-ulnar deviation was noted when compared to the contralateral wrist. Mean grip strength was reduced by 30 % of the contralateral side. A difference between the static and dynamic group was not found. Mean pain VAS was 3.7, 79 % of the patients were satisfied and 88 % would have the same procedure again after a mean follow-up period of 4 years. Two patients needed scaphocapitate fusion, two needed wrist fusion, two needed an ulnar shortening. Four patients needed a neuroma excision and one patient developed a reflex sympathetic dystrophy.

They conclude three-ligament tenodesis has a role in the treatment of scapholunate dissociation in patients with a reducible scaphoid and without degenerative changes.

In 2006, Garcia-Elias et al. [4] reported their results of the three-ligament tenodesis. They reviewed 38 patients with an average age of 31 years: 21 had a dynamic instability and 17 had a static instability. After a mean period of 46 months, 28 patients were completely pain free at rest, and 29 patients had returned to their normal activity level. Measurement of ROM resulted in a flexion of 74 % of the contralateral side, an extension of 77 %, an ulnar deviation of 92 % and a radial deviation

Table 3 Reported outcome data in the recent literature

Study	Patient number	Mean follow-up (months)	ROM		Grasp strength	Mean age	Male/female	No pain (%)	Mean pain VAS	Satisfied (%)
			Flexion	Extension						
Brunelli's original report	13	15	30–60 % CL		65 % CL			85		100
Van Den Abbeele	22	9	82 % Pre Op	80 % Pre Op	58 % CL	30	1/1		3/10	77
Talwalkar	117	47	69 % CL	80 % CL	70 % CL	38	50/67	62	3.7/10	79
Garcia-Elias	38	46	74 % CL	77 % CL	65 % CL	31	24/14	74		
UZ Leuven	21	33.5	68 % CL	72 % CL	83 % CL	39	16/5	77	2.7/10	85

of 78 %. Average grip strength was 65 % of the contralateral side. Two patients developed a DISI deformity and nine patients developed degenerative changes. Secondary surgical treatment was not necessary.

When comparing our results (excluding those patients who needed a salvage procedure) to those given in literature (Table 3), we can conclude similar results although our study only includes patients with static scapholunate instability, whereas other studies include patients with predynamic, dynamic, and static instability.

5 Conclusion

The results of our study are similar to those published in literature so far. We also report encouraging results on satisfaction, pain relief, ROM, and grasp strength. There are however two difference between our study and previously published works. Firstly, we report a large need for salvage procedures in our patient population. Additional research is needed to search for an explanation for this difference. Secondly, our study only includes patients with a chronic, static scapholunate instability, whereas other studies include patients with predynamic, dynamic, and static instability. Finally, we can conclude a modified Brunelli's tenodesis has its place in treating chronic, static scapholunate instability.

References

1. Walsh JJ, Berger RA, Cooney WP (2002) Current status of scapholunate interosseous ligament injuries. J Am Acad Orthop Surg 10:32–42
2. Brunelli GA, Brunelli GR (1995) A new technique to correct carpal instability with scaphoid rotatory subluxation: a preliminary report. J Hand Surg Am 20:S82–S85
3. Van Den Abbeele KL, Loh YC, Stanley JK, Trail IA (1998) Early results of a modified Brunelli procedure for scapholunate instability. J Hand Surg Br 23:258–261
4. Garcia-Elias M, Lluch AL, Stanley JK (2006) Three-ligament tenodesis for the treatmend of scapholunate dissociation: indications and surgical technique. J Hand Surg Am 31A:125–134
5. Talwalkar SC, Edwards ATJ, Hayton MJ, Stilwell JH, Trail IA, Stanley JK (2006) Results of tri-ligament tenodesis: a modified Brunelli procedure in the management of scapholunate instability. J Hand Surg Br 31B:110–117

Scaphocapitate Arthrodesis

F. Delétang

1 Introduction

Chronic scapholunate instability is a serious ligamentous wrist injury.

Whether of traumatic or degenerative origin, these lesions cause a functional disability of the wrist with limitation of mobility, loss of force and pain with force and grip.

The progression of this instability to arthritis is due to deficiency of the constraints of the scapholunate ligaments causing rotatory and posterior dislocation of the scaphoid [1]. The timeline of the arthritic progression of this instability has been well defined. The resulting articular congruence between the scaphoid fossa on the radius and the proximal pole of the scaphoid leads to radioscaphoid arthritis.

The ligament constraints for scapholunate stability are well known – these are the distal scaphotrapezoidal ligament complex [2] or the scapholunate attachments of the dorsal intercarpal ligament [3, 4]. However, it is difficult to determine the importance of each of these lesions in the genesis of instability and especially the predominance in culpability of one ligamentous structure over another.

In chronic scapholunate instability, ligament lesions are not reparable. The different surgical techniques available are destined to restore radioscaphoid congruence, decrease functional signs, alleviate pain and allow return to work or recreational activity. They also presume to avoid recurrence of instability and protect the carpus from the progression to arthritis. Soft tissue as well as bony procedures such as fusion have been proposed.

The aim of scaphocapitate arthrodesis is to permanently restore this radioscaphoid congruence to protect from carpal arthritis while improving wrist function.

F. Delétang
SOS Hand Emergencies Orléans Val de Loire, Polyclinique des Longues Allées,
25 rue Mondésir, Saint-Jean-de-Braye 45800, France
e-mail: dr.fabiendeletang@me.com

E. Camus, L. Van Overstraeten (eds.), *Carpal Ligament Surgery*,
DOI 10.1007/978-2-8178-0379-1_29, © Springer-Verlag France 2013

2 Surgical Technique

Scaphocapitate arthrodesis is performed under locoregional anaesthesia with an upper arm tourniquet after exsanguination of the upper limb to maintain a bloodless field. A posterior approach is used, the extensor retinaculum which is incised between the third and fourth compartments. The EPL and finger extensors are retracted. Partial wrist denervation is systematically performed by resection of the posterior interosseous nerve. An H-shaped or Berger capsulotomy with a triangular flap on an ulnar hinge is used to access the joint [5] (Fig. 1).

The radiocarpal and midcarpal intervals are examined to exclude a cartilage lesion with subchondral osseous lesion, which – if present – is a contraindication to this arthrodesis. The scapholunate ligament remnants are excised to allow optimal reduction of the scaphoid. Scaphocapitate interval surfaces are freshened down to cancellous bone. Rotatory subluxation of the scaphoid is reduced with a 10/10-mm Kirschner wire introduced into the proximal pole of the scaphoid and used as a 'joystick' (Figs. 2, 3 and 5). A temporary scaphocapitate arthrodesis using a 12/10-mm Kirschner wire maintains this reduction. Good scaphocapitate congruence is verified: the radioscaphoid angle should be about 45° on lateral view on intraoperative fluoroscopy.

A cancellous bone graft is harvested from the radius at the tubercle of Lister after radial corticotomy through the same approach. The graft is used to improve congruence at the arthrodesis interface. The fixation is secured using 2–4 standard or shape memory scaphocapitate staples (Fig. 4). Intraoperative wrist mobilization is done to exclude dorsal conflict with the hardware. A radial styloidectomy may be performed if a styloscaphoid conflict is detected. The capsule and retinaculum are reconstructed. Skin is closed in two planes with a suction drain. The preoperative forearm wrist splint is replaced by a fibreglass splint until radiological consolidation as judged by the surgeon is achieved. This is around 10 weeks. Rehabilitation is then begun.

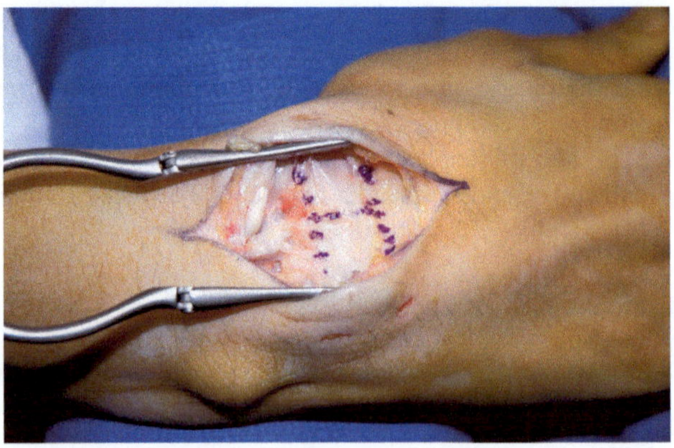

Fig. 1 Dorsal approach 3–4, capsulotomy design

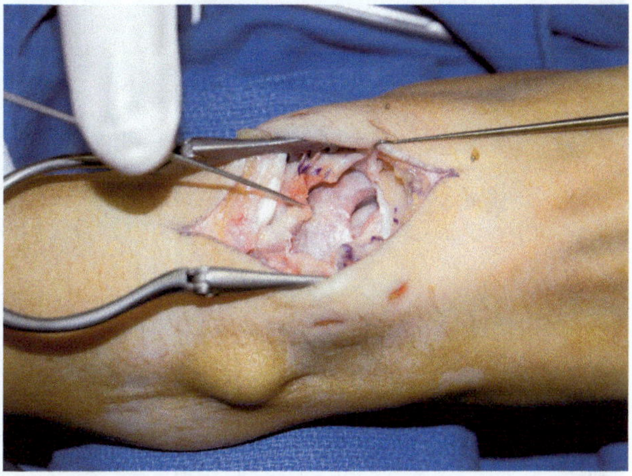

Fig. 2 Joystick K-wire in the pole of the scaphoid is used for reduction of rotatory subluxation

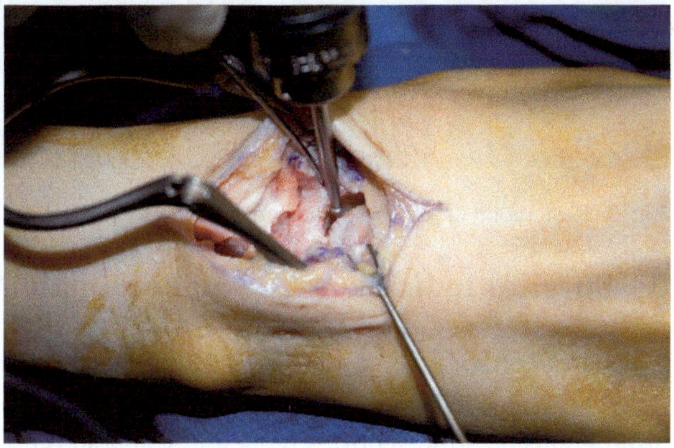

Fig. 3 Scaphocapitate freshening

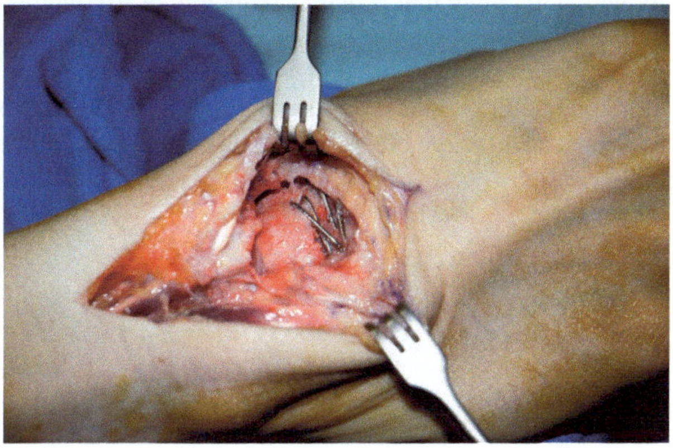

Fig. 4 Scaphocapitate arthrodesis using bipodal staples

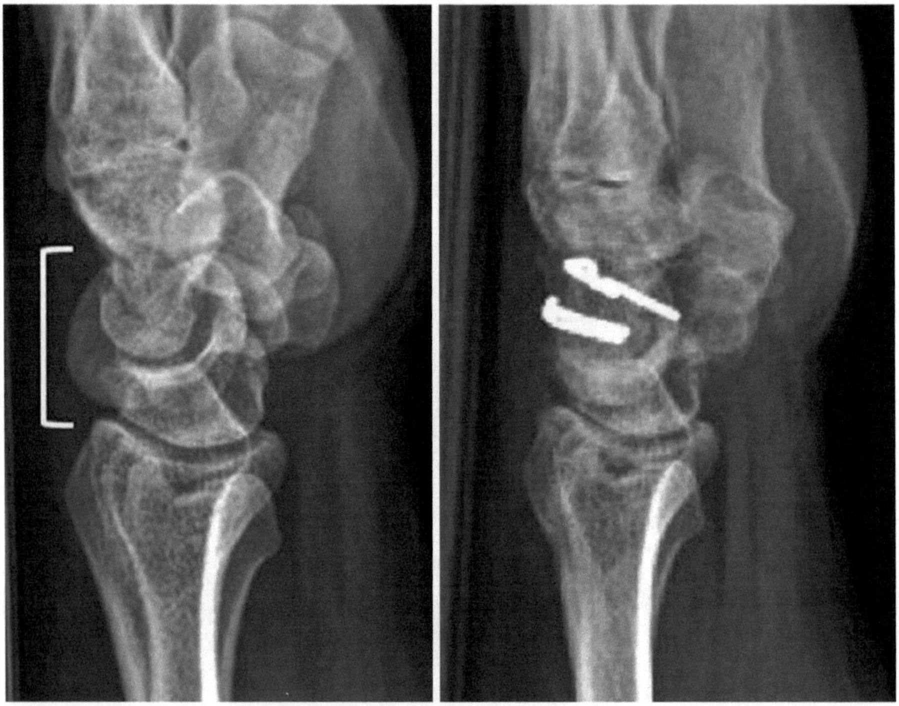

Fig. 5 Restoration of radioscaphoid congruence by scaphoid reduction

3 Surgical Indications of Scaphocapitate Arthrodesis

In chronic scapholunate instability, a complete description of ligament lesions, cartilage lesions and scaphoid reducibility should be precise and documented by CT arthrogram and arthroscopy. A reducible scaphoid is essential for the success of soft issue stabilization techniques [6] (Fig. 5).

Scaphocapitate arthrodesis is indicated in late, fixed chronic scapholunate instability with a scaphoid that is hardly reducible or irreducible. This corresponds to stage 5 in the algorithm of Garcia-Elias et al. [6]. It is also indicated if surgical approaches at the dorsum of the wrist preclude soft tissue procedures. It can also be used after failure of stabilization or failed primary ligament repair. Radioscaphoid arthritis and more advanced arthritis are contraindications to scaphocapitate arthrodesis.

4 Clinical Series

4.1 Material

Our study is retrospective monocentric including 58 scaphocapitate arthrodesis procedures for chronic scapholunate instability performed in our unit between 1999 and

2007. Thirty-one arthrodeses in 30 patients (24 men and 6 women) were reviewed by an independent examiner. Mean age at operation was 43 years (20–65). Mean follow-up was 5 years (8 months–8 years). The dominant hand was affected in 70 % of cases. Distribution of injury mechanisms was as follows: indirect wrist trauma 74 % (23/31) with associated high-energy lesions in 16 % (3 articular distal radius fractures, 1 perilunate dislocation, 1 distal radius fracture with perilunate dislocation), without trauma in 26 % (7/31) and with one case after trapezectomy for basal thumb arthritis. The series included 57 % work accidents. All patients presented with symptomatic chronic scapholunate instability, with 35 % after failed primary ligament surgery – either by attempt at reinsertion or after bone-ligament-bone procedures. The arthrodesis was performed at an average of 25 months after the first surgery (8–72). All patients had clinical and radiological evidence of scapholunate instability. Diagnostic arthroscopy was performed in 23 wrists to exclude a possibility for ligament reinsertion and any contraindication to scaphocapitate arthrodesis as in radiocarpal or midcarpal arthritis. Scapholunate instability was of grade 3 in 61 % and grade 2 in 39 % according to the classification of Dréant and Dautel [7]. The delay between the onset of symptoms and the surgery was on average 15.8 months (1–48). The mean time-off work duration was on average 5.2 months (0–36).

4.2 Method

Follow-up included clinical examination, radiologic and functional assessment.

Bilateral wrist examination was used to compare mobility of the operated wrist to the contralateral one, grip strength and pinch grip using the Jamar dynamometer. Preoperative and follow-up X-rays were used to compare carpal height and index of lateral deviation in the frontal view [8] before and after. Radioscaphoid, radiolunate and scapholunate angles were also compared. The duration of consolidation, the degree of nonunion, radiocarpal or midcarpal arthritis and styloscaphoid conflict were assessed. Complications to the procedure were documented.

Functional assessment was done using DASH and PRWE scores [9].

The PRWE evaluates overall wrist disability more precisely, comparing it to healthy wrist. The patient reports on pain at rest or on activity and the ability of performing specific activities involving the wrist. Values are reported as disability percentages. The time-off work was noted, as well as return to same position versus vocational reclassification.

4.3 Results

Scaphocapitate arthrodesis diminishes wrist mobility (Table 1). Flexion was at 41° (−37 % of contralateral) and extension 39° (−29 %). Radial inclination was limited to 11° (−52 %), and ulnar inclination is at 32° (−18 %). Flexion-extension range was at 80°, and radioulnar inclination was 43°.

Table 1 Scaphocapitate arthrodesis series

	Delay (months)	n-SLI	Follow-up (months)	Age	% TOW	F°	E°	RI°	UI°	Jamar (kg/force)	Nonunion %
Pisano et al. [11]	16	11–4	23.4	32	–	32	42	10	24	29	12
Chantelot et al. [12]	16	13–13	26	40	38	28	48	13.8	25.8	14	23
Saffar [19]	18	33–33	26	39.4	40	37.2	51.3	10.3	29.2	–	15
Delétang et al. [27]	16	31–31	60	43	57	41	39	11	32	32.5	13(8)

Mean grip strength Jamar was 35.5 kg (−19 %), and the pinch grip was minimally affected at 6 kg (−10 %).

DASH score was 27 %. PRWE score showed global disability of 25 % compared to the healthy side. Pain at rest was absent in 50 % of fused wrists and scored 1.5/10 for the other patients. It increased with increased loading or repetitive movements, reaching a maximum of 4/10. Ninety-four percent of patients were satisfied with the procedure and would choose to have it done again. Return to work was 71 % with 22 % professional reclassification. The mean time-off work postoperative was 5.8 months.

Radiologic analysis showed duration of consolidation to be 10.1 weeks postoperative [6–13]. The carpal height and index of deviation on front view were conserved at follow-up – they were normal preoperatively. Radioscaphoid angle went from 60° preoperative to 55° postoperative; the radiolunate angle showed little change, −6° to −9°. The mathematical resultant – the scapholunate angle – showed a small shift from 66° to 63° postoperative.

In 84 % of cases, there was no radioscaphoid arthritis. A radial styloscaphoid conflict was found in 22 % of wrists with little clinical impact. A complementary styloidectomy (same setting) had been performed in 32 % of operated cases to avoid styloscaphoid conflict.

Radiocarpal or midcarpal arthritis was found in 16 % of operated wrists; these had all presented with distal radius fractures +/− perilunate dislocation. Two wrists required an additional palliative procedure: four-corner arthrodesis in one and total wrist arthrodesis in the other due to symptomatic progression of arthritis.

The fixation was performed using bipodal staples with no shape memory in 86 % of cases. A radial cancellous bone graft was used in 81 % of fusions.

Nonunion was found in 13 % of cases – 8 % for the 58 scaphocapitate arthrodesis performed in the unit.

We had CRPS type I in 5 % cases and no infections.

Several criteria may influence results analysis: arthrodesis in a patient over 40, preoperative time-off work of more than 12 months, the 'work accident' concept and a previous scapholunate ligament repair. There were no statistically significant differences for clinical, functional and radiological results in relation to these criteria. However, patients with work accidents did tend to have worse functional results and longer time-off work (8.3 months on average).

5 Discussion

5.1 Functional Results

The technical description of scaphocapitate arthrodesis dates back to 1950 [10, 13], yet clinical series using this technique are sparse in the literature (Table 1 and Fig. 6).

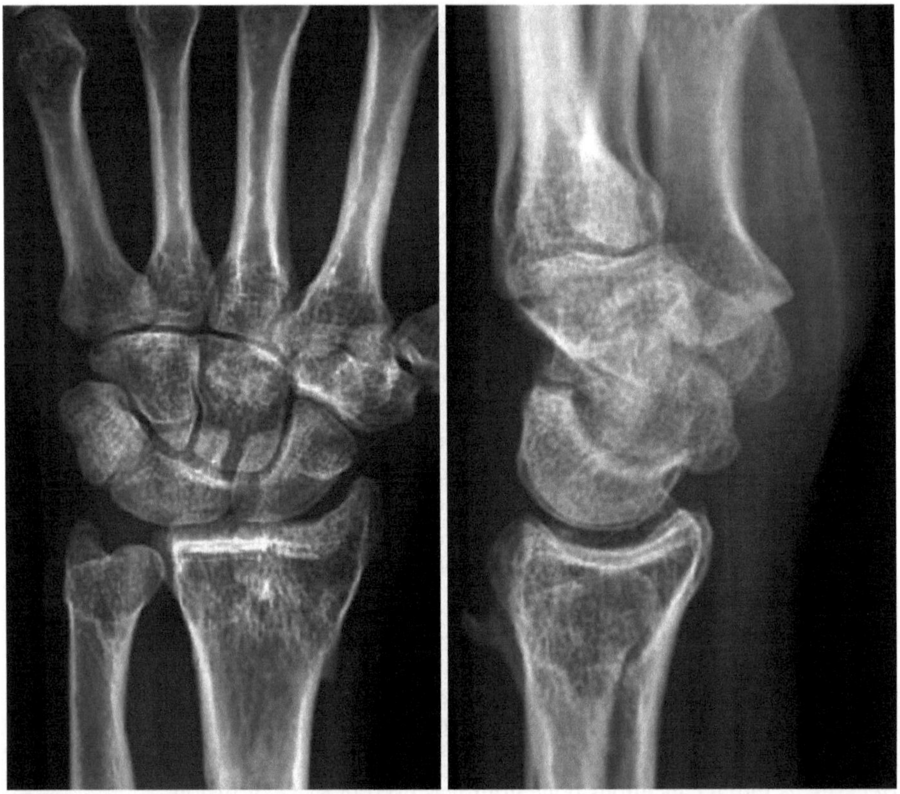

Fig. 6 Late chronic scapholunate instability

Arthrodesis diminishes wrist mobility in all series. Experimentally, this limitation comes from blocking the scaphocapitate joint during wrist movements [14]. In flexion and radial inclination, the scaphoid has no more flexion pronation around the capitate which limits the mobility of the scaphocapitate unit. Extension and ulnar inclination are less affected since the default mobility of the scaphocapitate unit is smaller during these movements. However, clinical mobility is smaller than experimental mobility probably due to capsuloligamentary scarring and scarring from previous operations.

These movements allow most daily activities and work. Most of our patients returned to work with 78 % at the same job post despite the high rate of work accidents (57 %).

Force restoration and pain relief also contribute. This pain relief varies in the literature, and a pain-free state for all patients is not achieved. At rest, 50 % of our patients are pain-free, and 50 % have bouts of seasonal pain that decreases with time (13–46 %) [11, 12, 15]. Pain increases with forceful activities and daily activities but is overall moderate (23–41 %) [11, 12, 15]. The PRWE is a good test which allows breakdown of pain to correlate to different activities. Experimentally, on a wrist in neutral position, scaphocapitate arthrodesis transfers load from the radiolunate to the radioscaphoid joint [16–18]. Forced movements of the scaphoid in radial inclination against the radial surface add to this load transfer. The load increase to cartilage on the proximal pole of the scaphoid may account for the residual pain.

5.2 *The Osteosynthesis of the Scaphocapitate Arthrodesis*

Nonunion is a dreaded complication with dire impact on functional results and prognosis. The rate of nonunion varies between 12 and 23 % in the literature [11, 12, 15, 19].

It falls to 8 % for arthrodesis performed in our unit. The mode of osteosynthesis is still debated. Compression is not a guarantee for consolidation. As in any arthrodesis, the quality of freshening of the articular surfaces is crucial. A graft usually taken from the radius is indispensable, and exaggerated compression should not artificially decrease the prepared scaphocapitate space. Compression screws frequently require an additional approach with risk to the radial nerve. We used two or three bipodal staples; this seems to be a good compromise compared to compression screws. Strict immobilization of the wrist in a below-elbow splint is routine in all cases until evidence of consolidation.

5.3 *Scaphocapitate Congruence and Protection Against Carpal Arthritis*

The scaphocapitate congruence and the radioscaphoid angle are the two most important control criteria intraoperatively. The reduction of scaphoid subluxation using a joystick K-wire as well as the temporary scaphocapitate arthrodesis are key steps in this technique. Experimentally, a radioscaphoid angle between 30° and 57° allows the achievement of 60 % mobility of a healthy wrist compatible with most habitual daily activities [20]. The radioscaphoid angle should be verified by intraoperative fluoroscopy and ideally set at 45°. The aim of this arthrodesis is the restoration of physiological radioscaphoid congruence. The stability of this congruence protects the wrist from major scaphocapitate arthritis in the long run.

Scaphocapitate arthrodesis does not reduce the DISI deformity of the lunate since the constraining ligaments of the scapholunate complex are damaged. The postoperative scapholunate angle is thus less important than for soft tissue techniques since only the radioscaphoid angle is deliberately modified.

A radiologic styloscaphoid conflict exists in 22 % of cases with little clinical impact.

The benefit of routine radial styloidectomy in scaphocapitate arthrodesis in terms of pain relief and mobility has not been shown in the literature or in this study, as for STT arthrodesis. We have performed complementary styloidectomy in only 7 % of cases (Fig. 7).

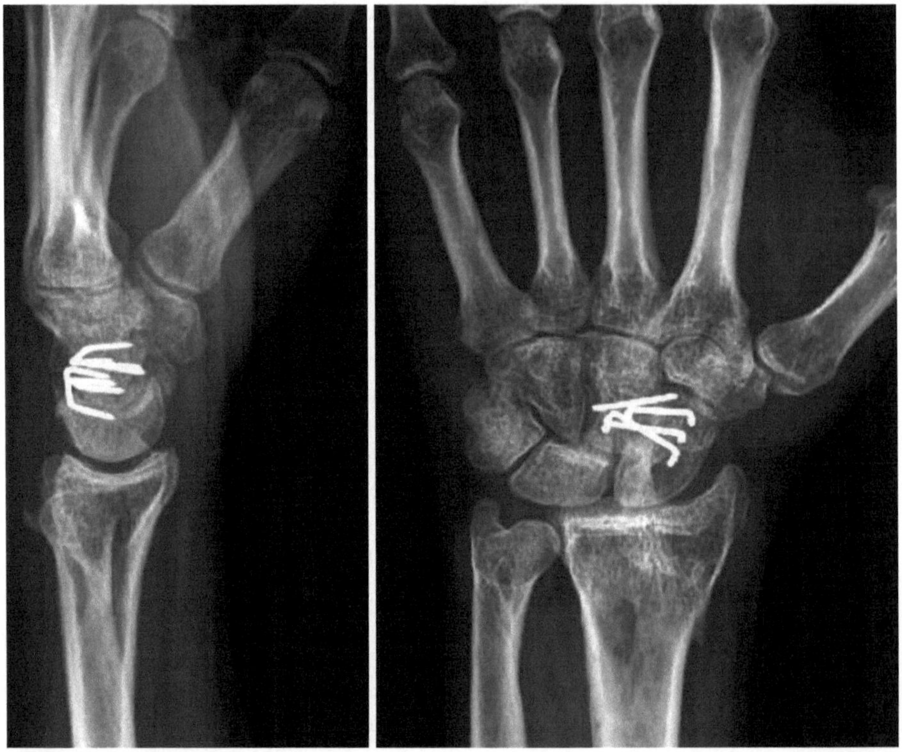

Fig. 7 Scaphocapitate arthrodesis

From this study and from the literature, we can conclude that scaphocapitate arthrodesis protects against carpal arthritis with at least 5 years of follow-up. The few identified failures can be explained by severe cartilage lesions upon initial injury.

5.4 Other Techniques for Treatment of Chronic Scapholunate Instability

Other partial arthrodesis techniques are used for the treatment of chronic scapholunate instability.

STT arthrodesis is used by many authors and follows the same logic of stabilization of the horizontal 'rocking chair' tilt of the scaphoid. Watson et al. [21], who promoted this technique, published excellent results with better mobility, less pain and frequent return to the same work post. These results are generally superior to those with scaphocapitate arthrodesis or soft tissue procedures.

A meta-analysis on 258 cases by Siegel and Ruby [22] showed different results than Watson. In comparison to our study, range of motion was identical; strength was similar with a similar nonunion rate. However, the complication rate (excluding nonunion) was 43 %, which included hardware-related infections, radioscaphoid arthritis, CRPS type I or persistent irritation of the radial nerve. In our study, the complication rate was 5.4 %. STT fusion is technically more difficult. It is more difficult to set the angle of the scaphoid on its base; the experimentally defined radioscaphoid angle needed to obtain acceptable wrist range of motion is more acute, between 30° and 47° [20]. In the light of these results, we no longer perform STT fusion in scapholunate instability.

Scaphocapitate arthrodesis and other techniques aiming at mechanically competent fibrous nonunion [23] have been described. Experimentally, this fusion causes minimal limitation of wrist mobility. However logical, it does not compensate for all lesions of the scaphoid ligament constraints, especially the distal scaphoid ligament complex. A high rate of nonunion of 35–72 % [24] is reported with this fusion, and the results are less predictable even if good clinical results have been observed, with better subjective than objective assessment values [25].

Scaphocapitolunate arthrodesis has also been described [26] aiming at a better radial load distribution on the scapholunate complex to avoid overloading of the radioscaphoid interval leading to degenerative arthritis. Experimental as well as clinical mobility is smaller than in scaphocapitate fusion. Results in terms of pain and return to work are inferior to those of scaphocapitate fusion. At 5-year follow-up, the radioscaphoid compartment does not show degenerative arthritis in scaphocapitate fusion. In the light of these results, scaphocapitolunate arthrodesis is not included in our armamentarium for treatment of scapholunate instability.

Soft tissue procedures follow the same logic of improving function and scaphoid stabilization. They aim to reduce mobility limitation by not blocking the midcarpal joint. Capsulodesis and ligamentoplasties require a reducible scaphoid – a key prerequisite that must be properly assessed. These techniques are probably indicated at an earlier stage of scapholunate instability than scaphocapitate arthrodesis. These techniques and their indications will be discussed elsewhere in this work.

6 Conclusion

Scaphocapitate arthrodesis promotes better wrist function with less pain in daily activities at the expense of mobility. It allows many patients to return to work. It protects against carpal degenerative arthritis for at least 5 years' follow-up while restoring radioscaphoid congruence. It is the treatment of choice in chronic late fixed scapholunate instability, with a barely reducible scaphoid.

It is also the treatment of choice in failed ligament repairs or other failed soft tissue procedures.

References

1. Watson HK, Ballet FL (1984) The SLAC wrist: scapholunate advanced collapse pattern of degenerative arthritis. J Hand Surg Am 9(3):358–365
2. Boabighi A, Kuhlmann JN, Kenesi C (1993) The distal ligamentous complex of the scaphoid and the scapho-lunate ligament. An anatomic, histological and biomechanical study. J Hand Surg Br 18(1):65–69
3. Mitsuyasu H, Patterson RM, Shah MA, Buford WL, Iwamoto Y, Viegas SF (2004) The role of the dorsal intercarpal ligament in dynamic and static scapholunate instability. J Hand Surg Am 29(2):279–288
4. Viegas SF, Yamaguchi S, Boyd NL, Patterson RM (1999) The dorsal ligaments of the wrist: anatomy, mechanical properties, and function. J Hand Surg Am 24(3):456–468
5. Berger RA, Bishop AT, Bettinger PC (1995) New dorsal capsulotomy for the surgical exposure of the wrist. Ann Plast Surg 35(1):54–59
6. Garcia-Elias M, Lluch AL, Stanley JK (2006) Three-ligament tenodesis for the treatment of scapholunate dissociation: indications and surgical technique. J Hand Surg 31A:125–134
7. Dréant N, Dautel G (2003) Development of a arthroscopic severity score for scapholunate instability. Chir Main 22(2):90–94
8. Youm Y, McMurthy RY, Flatt AE, Gillespie TE (1978) Kinematics of the wrist. I. An experimental study of radial-ulnar deviation and flexion-extension. J Bone Joint Surg Am 60(4):423–431
9. Voche P, Dubert T, Laffargue C, Gosp-Server A (2003) Patient-rated wrist questionnaire: preliminary report on a proposed French version of a North American questionnaire designed to assess wrist pain and function. Rev Chir Orthop Reparatrice Appar Mot 89(5):443–448
10. Sutro CV (1946) Treatment of nonunion of the carpal navicular bone. Surgery 20:536–540
11. Pisano SM, Peimer CA, Wheeler DR, Sherwin F (1991) Scaphocapitate intercarpal arthrodesis. J Hand Surg Am 16(2):328–333
12. Chantelot C, Becquet E, Leconte F, Lahoude-Chantelot S, Prodomme G, Fontaine C (2005) Scaphocapitate arthrodesis for chronic scapholunate instability: a retrospective study of 13 cases. Chir Main 24(2):79–83
13. Helfet AJ (1952) A new operation for ununited fracture of the scaphoid. J Bone Joint Surg 34:329
14. Garcia-Elias M, Cooney WP, An KN, Linscheid RL, Chao EY (1989) Wrist kinematics after limited intercarpal arthrodesis. J Hand Surg Am 14(5):791–799
15. Young Szalay MD, Peimer CA (2002) Scaphocapitate arthrodesis. Tech Hand Up Extrem Surg 6(2):56–60
16. Horii E, Garcia-Elias M, Bishop AT, Cooney WP, Linscheid RL, Chao EY (1990) Effect on force transmission across the carpus in procedures used to treat Kienbock's disease. J Hand Surg Am 15(3):393–400
17. Short WH, Werner FW, Fortino MD, Palmer AK (1992) Distribution of pressures and forces on the wrist after simulated intercarpal fusion and Kienbock's disease. J Hand Surg Am 17(3):443–449
18. Viegas SF, Patterson RM, Peterson PD et al (1990) Evaluation of the biomechanical efficacy of limited intercarpal fusions for the treatment of scapho-lunate dissociation. J Hand Surg Am 15(1):120–128
19. Saffar P (2007) Arthrodèse scapho-capitale. In: Cours européen de pathologie chirurgicale du membre supérieur et de la main. Sauramps Médical, Montpellier, pp 199–204
20. Minamikawa Y, Peimer CA, Yamaguchi T, Medige J, Sherwin FS (1992) Ideal scaphoid angle for intercarpal arthrodesis. J Hand Surg Am 17(2):370–375
21. Watson HK, Wollstein R, Joseph E, Manzo R, Weinzweig J, Ashmead D 4th (2003) Scaphotrapeziotrapezoid arthrodesis: a follow-up study. J Hand Surg Am 28(3):397–404
22. Siegel JM, Ruby LK (1996) A critical look at intercarpal arthrodesis: review of the literature. J Hand Surg Am 21(4):717–723

23. Rosenwasser MP, Miyasajsa KC, Strauch RJ (1997) The RASL procedure: reduction and association of the scaphoid and lunate using the Herbert screw. Tech Hand Up Extrem Surg 1(4):263–272
24. Chick G, Daunois O, Alnot JY (2007) L'arthrodèse scapho-lunaire dans la dissociation scapho-lunaire. In: Cours européen de pathologie chirurgicale du membre supérieur et de la main. Sauramps Médical, Montpellier, pp 205–213
25. Zubairy AI, Jones WA (2003) Scapholunate fusion in chronic symptomatic scapholunate instability. J Hand Surg Br 28(4):311–314
26. Rotman MB, Manske PR, Pruitt DL, Szerzinski J (1993) Scaphocapitolunate arthrodesis. J Hand Surg Am 18(1):26–33
27. Deletang F, Segret J, Dap F, Dautel G (2011) Chronic scapholunate instability treated by scaphocapitate fusion: a midterm outcome perspective. Orthop Traumatolo Surg Res 97(2):164–171.

Medicolegal Aspects of Traumatic Wrist Ligament Injuries

L. Van Overstraeten

1 Memo of Theoretical Repair of Corporal Damage

1.1 In Common Law

In common law, in case of damage due to a third party (Article 1382 of the French 'Code Civil'), it is required to repair 'all the damage, and nothing but the damage' [1].

This is why an existing previous state excludes damage [10]. It then seems obvious that an adaptive carpal arthritis SLAC III seen on X-ray immediately after a trauma will not be accepted as damage due to a road traffic accident (RTA). However, in a wrist fracture treated by closed reduction fixation 15 years preceding trauma, the evolution of adaptive instability cannot be excluded. It is even less acceptable that a previously asymptomatic patient who sustains a recent wrist sprain caused by a third party is deprived of complete treatment and, after arthroscopic diagnosis of an old instability, is told that the lesion will be treated conservatively 'until return to the previous state of affairs' (Chap. 8) [9].

Corporal damage in civil code corresponds to the following criteria of Simonin [5]:

1. Type of the trauma
2. Type of lesion
3. Correspondence of site
4. Anatomopathologic sequence
5. Condition of time
6. Previous pathology
7. Exclusion of previous cause

Time coincidence is frequently used to exclude a lesion [6, 7, 8].

L. Van Overstraeten
Hand and Foot Surgery Unit SPRL,
Rue Pierre Caille N° 9, Tournai B-7500, Belgium
e-mail: l.v.o@skynet.be

E. Camus, L. Van Overstraeten (eds.), *Carpal Ligament Surgery*,
DOI 10.1007/978-2-8178-0379-1_30, © Springer-Verlag France 2013

A compression fracture of L1 seen on thoracic views 6 weeks after a car accident will not be accepted by the company. In the same way, an intracarpal ligamentary injury which is diagnosed after arthroscan or arthroscopy 6 months following a fall on the hand has little chance of being accepted as chargeable damage [7, 8].

This is why immediate management and complete workup are necessary even for a seemingly minor hand injury.

And this becomes all the more important because, with accidents in common law, proof of the lesion is the responsibility of the victim.

Even if these are not the prerogatives of the treating surgeon, in common law, not only the physical disability is addressed but also the economical disability (the financial repercussions of loss of physical capacity as regards training and experience on the general work market), the inability to perform household chores and moral and cosmetic damage, pain and help of a third party.

It is also worth noting that in common law, we can declare certain reservations about the future. These reservations allow the reopening of the file in case of development of tardive complications. These reservations must be very carefully expressed. In case of interosseous ligament lesions which are known to remain silent very long and have a long evolution history, the wording of these reservations is essential [7, 8].

In common law, the cost is undertaken by medicolegal insurance.

1.2 In Work Accidents (Law)

Contrary to common law, here, the previous condition can be covered by insurance companies. However, the accident must correspond to the definition 'a sudden incident suffered by a contractual employee during or on the way to work'.

Scaphoid nonunion advanced collapse with definite carpal arthritis that is subjected to bony contusions in a work accident and remains disabling after orthopaedic treatment can be covered by work's insurance company for a vascularized Matti-Russe graft. Similarly, an old silent instability that becomes disabling by a minor trauma will be covered for a capsulodesis by company.

Even if the silent previous pathology is not clear, the worker gets the benefit of the doubt.

By law, only loss of economic capacity following loss of function is compensated. In Belgium, unlike physical disability, this economic disability is not quantified. An estimate by the medical expert is resorted to.

A review of deterioration can be done 3 years following the consolidation of the original injury; the worker should be informed of an eventual possible clinical and radiological instability that must be evaluated and followed up. Whatever the duration of evolution, a SLAC will be covered if it is indisputably attributable to a work accident. Vibrating machine work accidents will be discussed later.

Note that the employee undertakes his or her own defence costs and may be assisted by his syndicate.

2 Natural History of Ligament Lesions

2.1 *Stable Lesions*

Stable lesions rarely present problems. After arthroscopic identification of the stable character of a sprain (articular and extrinsic stability), temporary disability and orthopaedic treatment are modulated by pain. Usually, time-off work does not exceed 4 weeks. Consolidation is the state obtained 6 months following the final X-ray, usually without permanent disability (IP: 0 %).

2.2 *Unstable Lesions*

Unstable lesions can be more problematic. In the emergency setting, the treatment is always accepted. K-wire fixation of a recent lesion within 6 months should have a favourable outcome. Ledoux reports good results with the fixation of the lunotriquetral complex but reports a progressive horizontalization with scapholunate complex which is more loaded and mobile [2].

Complications aside, the disability period for manual worker rarely exceeds 5 months (6 weeks of workup, 6–8 weeks with K-wire fixation in place, 4–6 weeks of physiotherapy). Consolidation is usually achieved within a year, with permanent disability of ±5 % related to stiffness, residual pain and loss of force with usually identical economical consequences.

Not all authors agree with these results. In 1998, Lucas and Stehman reported a series of 17 cases including 15 cases of arthroscopically unstable ligament lesions. The results of surgical fixation techniques are mediocre. The average permanent disability and time-off work (TOW) are 3 times greater for patients treated conservatively following arthroscopy [3].

Older instability cases are more problematic. Arthroscopy, which is the diagnostic tool essential for instability assessment, is not accepted by the insurance body, as any subsequent stabilization procedure (suture, capsulodesis, ligamentoplasty) [4]. This makes the situation difficult; clinical symptoms may disappear within 4–6 months (even with increased radiological instability), but the physical and economic disabilities are still evaluated using essentially clinical criteria. The clinician or doctor of appeal must give subtle arguments to make the insurance doctor acknowledge the importance of treatment. He must demonstrate that treatment (stabilize and arrest the adaptative decompensation) and the financial interest of the insurance body (to limit the residual disability and especially the probability that the reserve is not effective) are related. A court decision is frequently necessary.

3 View of the Medical Advisor

The insurance-advising doctor who evaluates and defends an insurance case has the tendency to minimize the adverse sequelae in his evaluation and even sometimes underestimate the damage.

In common law, he would not voluntarily accept a reservation on an unstable ligament lesion. The appeal doctor defending the patient or the clinician must present irrevocable evidence to support the acceptance of these reservations.

In work accidents, the insurance advisor will always try to refute a preexisting state or to precipitate the return to it.

4 Expectations of the Patient and Duty of the Appeal Doctor or Therapist: The Traps

4.1 Accountability and Criteria of Simonin

In common law, 'condition of time' (i.e. the shortest time possible between trauma and diagnosis) and rapid management are essential.

4.1.1 New Lesion in Work Accident

This is the case of a 37-year-old prisoner escort who suffered a fall at work on 21/10/2011.

He presented with pain, functional impairment and abnormal standard X-rays; CT arthrogram showed a passage of contrast through scapholunate, lunotriquetral intervals and a TFCC lesion.

CT arthrography at 4 weeks showed no hemarthrosis, normal synovial fluid turbidity, mild hematic synovitis, stage 3 chondritis with exposed proximal pole of scaphoid, Dautel 3 instability denoting apparently very old perilunate lesions and instability (SLAC II).

No pinning was done, waiting for return to previous state.

In case of no improvement, first carpal row excision was offered and proposed to insurance.

5 Reopening of the Patient Case in Case of Decompensation (Even After 20 Years)

It must be possible to question the patient on causes of an old instability:

What insured and declared sport does he perform?

Accident in common law: Did a reservation exist?

Declared work accident? Could it have been aggravated?

6 Work Accident and Work-Related Diseases: Vibrating Tools

In anterior scapholunate instability in a young manual worker, a history of regular use of vibrating tools should orient the clinician or the appeal doctor to address in Belgium the 'basis of work-related disease' or in France 'la Commission Technique d'Orientation et de Reclassement Professionnel 'COTOREP' and file a request for management.

This is readily accepted.

References

1. Feron P. (1999) Vade-mecum of medicolegal evaluation: l'invalidité, l'incapacité, le handicap et le dommage corporel en droit belge Edition "De Boek Universite" Bruxelles 241–2
2. Ledoux P (1998) Treatment of ligamentary injuries of wrist. In: Lucas P, Stehman M (eds) Séquelles traumatiques coude et poignet, vol 4, Actualité du Dommage corporel collection médico-legale. Edition Juridoc, Bruxelles, pp 201–208
3. Lucas P, Stehman M (1998) Séquelles traumatiques coude et poignet, vol 4, Actualité du Dommage corporel collection médico-legale. Edition Juridoc, Bruxelles
4. Potaznik A (1998) Arthroscopy of the wrist. In: Lucas P, Stehman M (eds) Séquelles traumatiques coude et poignet, vol 4, Actualité du Dommage corporel collection medico-legale. Edition Juridoc, Bruxelles, pp 143–148
5. Simonin C (1947) Médecine légale judiciaire. Maloine, Paris
6. Lurquin P (1989) L'expertise médicale amiable, judiciaire et pénale. Bruylant, Bruxelles
7. Lurquin P (1985) Traité de l'expertise en toutes matières, tome I. Bruylant, Bruxelles
8. Lurquin P (1985) Traité de l'expertise en toutes matières, tome II. Bruylant, Bruxelles
9. Dreant N, Dautel G (2003) Development of an arthroscopic severity score for scapholunate instability. Chir Main 22(2):90–94
10. Van Overstraeten L, Camus EJ (2012) Arthroscopic criteria for dating wrist sprains. Chir Main 31:171–175

Socioeconomic Aspects of Traumatic Wrist Ligament Injuries

L. Van Overstraeten

1 Introduction

Scapholunate ligament injuries are a main cause of instability causing great wrist dysfunction, time off work and cessation or modification of activity [1].

2 Material and Methods

It is difficult to obtain precise information about wrist ligament injury patients.

Attempts at information retrieval from insurance companies have been unsuccessful – data is guarded as secrets of state.

The department of statistics at the Belgian National Institute of Disease and Invalidity INAMI does not have precise diagnostic information about wrist pathology. The data consists largely of costs of different services (Chap. 30). We can find the cost of fractures with and without wrist reduction and the cost of fixation, but no information is available on the cost of wrist sprains. This is the same for stabilization of unstable intracarpal lesions.

We were able to collect precise data from the Belgian Database of Work Accidents – FAT [2–5].

L. Van Overstraeten
Hand and Foot Surgery Unit SPRL,
Rue Pierre Caille N° 9, Tournai, B-7500, Belgium
e-mail: l.v.o@skynet.be

E. Camus, L. Van Overstraeten (eds.), *Carpal Ligament Surgery*,
DOI 10.1007/978-2-8178-0379-1_31, © Springer-Verlag France 2013

3 Incidence of Wrist Injuries

Wrist injuries are quite frequent and represent an important proportion of work accidents. Analysis of data obtained from FAT showed that wrist injuries represent 6.5 % of the 164,951 accidents in 2006 and 5.1 % of the 163,928 accidents in 2007. They occupy sixth place after finger injuries (21 %), knee and leg (9 %), eyes (8 %), hands (7 %) and feet (6.5 %) [4].

Wrist fractures represent more than 25 % of bone and joint injuries of the wrist (27.3 % in 2006 and 25.2 % in 2007) and more than 11 % of all wrist lesions (13.2 % in 2006 and 11.5 % in 2007); ligament lesions (labeled 'dislocations' and sprains) represent about three-fourth of all bone and joint wrist work-accident lesions (72.8 % in 2006 and 74.8 % in 2007). They represent more than one-third of all wrist work-accident lesions grouped together (35.17 % in 2006 and 34.1 % in 2007) (Table 1).

4 Wrist Trauma and Disability

About a fourth of wrist work trauma does not cause time off work and activity cessation, irrespective of the nature of the lesion.

The proportion is greater for sprains (34.73%) than for fractures (20.32 %).

5 Proportion and Total Time of Temporary Disability

The total time of temporary disability TTD following a work accident involving the wrist is greater in sprains (55.3 % of TTD for ligament lesions and 32.5 % for fractures – 2006 and 2007 together). One out of two fractures will lead to permanent disability (47.1 %), whereas this is true for less than 10 % of ligament lesions (9.94 %) (Table 2).

TTD is greater for fractures or ligament lesions than other wrist lesions. Among patients with wrist fractures and sprains, 71.41 % return to work within a month from the injury, while 89.19 % patients with other wrist lesions return to work within the month.

TTD seems shorter for sprains than for fractures. 81.5 % of wrist sprain patients return to work within a month from the injury, while only 33.9% fracture patients do so. Similarly, 16 % sprain patients return to work within 6 months, while 50 % fracture patients do so.

The proportion of 'long duration TTD' (>6 months) is significantly greater for fractures and sprains than for other lesions. 3.76% patients with bone and joint wrist lesion (fracture or ligament lesion) will have TTD greater than 6 months. This proportion falls to 1.58 % for patients with other wrist lesions.

Table 1 Distribution of wrist lesions in accidents at the workplace according to the year of occurrence – 2006 and 2007

	Nature of the lesion								
Year	Closed fractures	Open fractures	Unspecified fractures	Dislocations	Sprains	Dislocations and nonspecific sprains	Total fractures, dislocations, and sprains	Other injuries	General total
2006	293	11	1,142	102	2,340	1,420	5,308	5,672	10,980
2007	262	6	687	115	1,814	910	3,794	4,536	8,330
Total	555	17	1,829	217	4,154	2,330	9,102	10,208	19,310

Table 2 Distribution of wrist lesions in accidents at the work place according to the outcome of the accident – 2006 and 2007

	Nature of the lesion								
Outcome	Closed fractures	Open fractures	Unspecified fractures	Dislocations	Sprains	Nonspecific dislocations and sprains	Total fractures, dislocations, and sprains	Other injuries	General total
No outcome	126	2	360	71	1,416	840	2,815	4,416	7,231
Temporary disability	176	1	604	126	2,339	1,243	4,489	5,214	9,703
Permanent disability	253	14	865	20	399	247	1,798	576	2,374
Mortality	0	0	0	0	0	0	0	2	2
Total	555	17	1,829	217	4,154	2,330	9,102	10,208	19,310

The percentage of long duration TTD accidents (6 months to 1 year) is significantly greater for wrist fractures (4.8 %) than for ligament lesions (1.0 %) and other wrist lesions (0.62 %).

The percentage of work accidents with very long TTD (>1 year) is tiny for fractures (0.37 %) and ligament lesions (<0.10 %) (Table 3).

6 Rate of Permanent Disability PD

The majority of work-related wrist sprains recover without economic disability (*PD*=0 %) This is not the case for wrist fractures. Thus, 90.4 % of sprains recover without PD, and 52.9 % fractures do so.

Around 5% of sprains will have a residuel permanent disability of 1 to 5 % and 15% of wrist fracture will have the same economic disability. While 25 % of wrist fracture work-accident patients will have a residual permanent disability of 10 %, less than 4 % of sprains will have the same economic disability (Table 4).

7 Socioeconomic Profile of the Trauma Patient

7.1 Sex Incidence

According to the FAT statistics for the years 2006–2007, it is clear there is male sex predominance (71.10 %) for all wrist lesions grouped together.

There is a marked prevalence of fractures (73.6 %) in men over sprains (67.1 %). Inversely, women have more sprains (32.9 %) than fractures (26.4 %) (Table 5).

8 Incidence According to Age of the Patient and Nature of the Lesion

The majority of work-related wrist trauma patients – all lesions included – are in their 30s and 40s (65.7 %). The younger age group 15–24 represents 23.23 % and manual workers over 50 are 11.05 %. In the 25–49 age group, the prevalence of fractures (62.43 %) is almost the same as ligament lesions (66.8 %).

In the 15–24 age group, about 1/4th of lesions are wrist sprains (23.34 %).

In the ‘over 50’ age group, fractures are almost as frequent (43.52 %) as carpal ligament lesions (56.48 %), while in the 25–39 age group, 25 % are fractures while 75 % are sprains. In the young age group, fractures represent only 20.16 %, while sprains 79.84 % (Table 6).

Table 3 Distribution of wrist lesions in accidents at the workplace according to the duration of temporary disability – 2006 and 2007

Duration of temporary disability	Nature of the lesion								
	Closed fractures	Open fractures	Unspecified fractures	Dislocations	Sprains	Nonspecific dislocations and sprains	Total fractures, dislocations, and sprains	Other injuries	General total
0 days	172	4	536	73	1,470	880	3,135	4,494	7,629
1–3 days	1	0	16	14	396	165	592	1,213	1,805
4–30 days	59	1	248	86	1,537	842	2,773	3,396	6,169
1–6 months	294	11	905	36	630	384	2,260	944	3,204
6 months–1 year	17	1	98	2	55	25	198	63	261
More than 1 year	1	0	8	0	4	0	13	9	22
Unknown	11	0	18	6	62	34	131	89	220
Total	555	17	1,829	217	4,154	2,330	9,102	10,208	19,310

Table 4 Distribution of wrist lesions in accidents at the workplace according to the expected rate of permanent disability – 2006 and 2007

	Nature of the lesion								
Expected percentage of permanent disability (%)	Closed fractures	Open fractures	Unspecified fractures	Dislocations	Sprains	Nonspecific dislocations and sprains	Total fractures, dislocations, and sprains	Other injuries	General total
0	302	3	964	197	3,755	2,083	7,304	9,632	16,936
<5	84	4	361	9	212	134	804	332	1,136
5–10	143	8	391	11	165	96	814	180	994
10–16	19	2	86	0	20	15	142	45	187
16–20	2	0	6	0	1	1	10	4	14
20–36	5	0	14	0	0	1	20	13	33
36–66	0	0	6	0	1	0	7	2	9
66–100	0	0	1	0	0	0	1	0	1
Total	555	17	1,829	217	4,154	2,330	9,102	10,208	19,310

Table 5 Distribution of wrist lesions in accidents at the workplace according to sex of the patient – 2006 and 2007

Sex	Nature of the lesion								
	Closed fractures	Open fractures	Non specified fractures	Dislocations	Sprains	Nonspecified sprains	Total fractures dislocations, and sprains	Other lesions	General total
Woman	173	4	457	80	1,407	712	2,833	2,741	5,574
Man	382	13	1,372	137	2,745	1,617	6,266	7,464	13,730
Unknown	0	0	0	0	2	1	3	3	6
Total	555	17	1,829	217	4,154	2,330	9,102	10,208	19,310

Table 6 Distribution of wrist lesions in accidents at the workplace according to age – 2006 and 2007

	Nature of the lesion								
Age group	Closed fractures	Open fractures	Nonspecified fractures	Dislocations	Sprains	Nonspecified sprains	Total fractures dislocations, and sprains	Other lesions	General total
15–24	84	1	310	47	1,015	502	1,959	2,527	4,486
24–49	335	12	1,152	151	2,732	1,594	5,976	6,711	12,687
Over 50	136	4	367	19	406	233	1,165	970	2,135
Unknown	0	0	0	0	1	1	2	0	2
Total	555	17	1,829	217	4,154	2,330	9,102	10,208	19,310

9 Incidence of Sprains and Type of Work

Expectedly, the incidence of wrist injury is higher with manual work than intellectual work. This is confirmed by the 2006–2007 FAT data [4]. In 2006–2007, 83.56 % of work-accident wrist injuries occurred in manual workers. 73.20 % of bone and joint wrist lesions were ligament injuries. During this period, one-third of manual workers wrist lesions were ligamentous (34.30 % cases).

Intellectual workers presented with ligament injuries in 75.67 % of cases.

The typical socioeconomic profile of a work-related wrist injury is a 25–49-year-old manual worker. This cohort includes 594 accidents in 2006 and 437 in 2007 (Table 7).

10 Evolution of Unstable Lesions

Upon data analysis, one can only be surprised by the low prevalence of economic permanent disability associated with ligament lesions. As mentioned above, 90.4 % sprains recover with no permanent disability, 5 % have a residual economic disability of 1–5 %, and less than 4 % consolidate with a permanent disability of 5–10 % (Table 4).

In current practice, over 25 % of recent wrist sprains examined in a clinic are unstable lesions (Dautel 1–3 [6]). Even without specific treatment, the majority of these lesions tend to become painless, and sometimes they can stay so for a very long time. Without treatment, evolution towards arthritis is classic [1]. So where do these lesions then figure in the FAT database if 81.5 % of wrist sprains are back to work within 1 month (Table 3), and 90.4 % of sprains recover without permanent disability (Table 4)? It seems that these lesions do not appear at all in the data or are grouped with those that 'recover' within 1 month.

Thorough research failed to reveal the management of progressive lesions.

It seems that the FAT data collection ends with return to work. This can explain the lack of correlation between reality and the FAT results of long-term evolution of wrist ligament lesions.

It is up to the practitioner to trace the lesion back to a work accident.

In case of worsening outcome of a declared work accident, it is up to the advisor doctor to reopen the patient file.

Table 7 Distribution of wrist lesions in accidents at the workplace according to the type of work – 2006 and 2007

	Nature of the lesion								
Type of work	Closed fractures	Open fractures	Nonspecified fractures	Dislocations	Sprains	Nonspecified sprains	Total fractures dislocations, and sprains	Other lesions	General total
Intellectual	78	3	294	33	764	369	1,541	1,633	3,174
Manual	477	14	1,535	184	3,390	1,961	7,561	8,575	16,136
Total	555	17	1,829	217	4,154	2,330	9,102	10,208	19,310

Acknowledgment I thank Mrs. Benedicte Van Cutsem from the databank statistics of Work Accidents for her help.

References

1. Kuo CE, Wolfe SW (2008) Scapholunate instability: current concepts in diagnosis and management. J Hand Surg Am 33(6):998–1013
2. Thème 7 (2007) Secteur privé : caractéristiques des lésions causées par les accidents de travail en 2007 sur les lieux du travail, Fonds des accidents de travail – Fonds voor Arbeisongevallen: www.faofat.fgov.be
3. Thème 19 (2007) Secteur privé : caractéristiques des lésions causées par les accidents de travail en 2007 sur le chemin du travail, Fonds des accidents de travail – Fonds voor Arbeisongevallen: www.faofat.fgov.be
4. Thème 7 (2006) Secteur privé : caractéristiques des lésions causées par les accidents de travail en 2007 sur les lieux du travail, Fonds des accidents de travail – Fonds voor Arbeisongevallen: www.faofat.fgov.be
5. Thème 19 (2006) Secteur privé : caractéristiques des lésions causées par les accidents de travail en 2007 sur le chemin du travail, Fonds des accidents de travail – Fonds voor Arbeisongevallen: www.faofat.fgov.be
6. Dreant N, Dautel G (2003) Development of a arthroscopic severity score for scapho-lunate instsability. Chir Main 22(2):90–94

MIX
Papier aus verantwortungsvollen Quellen
Paper from responsible sources
FSC® C105338

If you have any concerns about our products,
you can contact us on
ProductSafety@springernature.com

In case Publisher is established outside the EU,
the EU authorized representative is:
Springer Nature Customer Service Center GmbH
Europaplatz 3, 69115 Heidelberg, Germany

Printed by Libri Plureos GmbH
in Hamburg, Germany